NATIVE HEALERS

NATIVE HEALERS
Foundations in Western Herbal Medicine

Anita Ralph and Mary Tassell

AEON

First published in 2020 by
Aeon Books
PO Box 76401
London W5 9RG

British Library Cataloguing in Publication Data

A C.I.P. for this book is available from the British Library

ISBN-13: 978-1-91280-711-6

Typeset by Medlar Publishing Solutions Pvt Ltd, India
Printed in Great Britain

www.aeonbooks.co.uk

CONTENTS

PREFACE

The salmon is able to jump upstream, not by fighting against the current, but by utilizing its knowledge of the reverse current which flows beneath the surface current.

—P. Carr-Gomm and S. Carr-Gomm[1]

We see the practice of Western herbal medicine as an example of the confluence of a multitude of streams of knowledge, ancient and modern, flowing into a harmonious pool of wisdom. All traditions of healing have their truths, their strengths and their weaknesses. As with so many things in life cooperation and integration yield the best results. We seek to combine the best that scientific research and development has to offer with the wisdom of ancient traditions and the powerful healing and tonic benefits of whole plants with whom we have co-evolved, to move towards a system of healing that is flexible, supportive, powerful and kind.

Native healers, the title of this book, refers to healing plants that exist in ecological niches across the planet. The term 'native healers' also resonates with the archaic tradition of herbalism and the wisdom passed down by our ancestors. 'Native healers' could also refer to you—by connecting with plant medicines and using what grows locally to you to help and heal yourself and your loved ones you are a native healer—thriving in nature!

Practising forms of medicine which are not considered to be biomedicine in the conventional sense can, on the surface, seem to be a daunting proposition for many of us. Herbal medicine is not part of mainstream-funded medicine here in the UK, and this can be used to imply that state-funded healthcare is the only bone-fide medicine. Unlike many other countries this artificial polarity sometimes leads to misunderstanding about herbal medicine. It can feel as if we are operating in opposition to current medical thinking. Under the surface, however, lie rich streams of knowledge and wisdom to carry us forward.

One of the central aims of this book is to provide a source of knowledge which forms the basis of the counter-current mentioned above; a source of complementary knowledge that in fact offers a fundamentally useful system of medicine to complement conventional biomedicine. Of central importance is the opportunity to offer help to those that have not been helped by conventional biomedicine. Equipped with this knowledge we can then progress with ease along the paths of our individual rivers, navigating potential obstacles and opposing energies with more assurance and finesse, to finally reach the transformative pool of healing wisdom that awaits us all.

This book reaches out to herbalists, health care professionals and all those interested in healing, and bridges the gap between thinking of plant medicines as simply 'natural' drugs, and across into the rich landscape of herbalists' ideas: ideas about the human body and how we function, and how plants might contribute positively to that dynamism.

We are from the Earth, and so are the plants that heal us.

Anita Ralph and Mary Tassell, 2019

Reference

1. Carr-Gomm, P. and S. Carr-Gomm, *Druid Animal Oracle*. 2007: Connections Book Publishing.

ACKNOWLEDGEMENTS

We would love to very enthusiastically thank the following people for all their help and support with the production of this book: Heartwood— an organization that is truly in the right place, at the right time for providing fertile ground for the establishment of the Foundation Course in Western Herbal Medicine, that is also the foundation for this book -It's founders, its tutors and its students, all are inspirational. Especially to Paul and Frances Hambly and Nic Rowley, for their invitation for us to be involved at all we owe a debt of gratitude. To Aeon, our bright and brilliant publishers, for their unerring guidance and enthusiasm. To Tony Smith for his help with diagrams, annotation of images, and the design of our cover. To Annette Hughes for providing beautiful plant drawings, and Bee McGovern for her botanical accuracy and photograph of chamomile. To Stephen Buhner for kind permission to use his poem, and to Henriette Kress for her incredible resource of old herbals and her help in sourcing botanical illustrations. To Ian Lawrence and John Tassell for being themselves—truly vital for so many reasons. Love and blessings to you all.

INTRODUCTION

Context: Introducing herbal medicine

Herbal medicine must have been there right at the very beginning of human history. Our ancestors were deeply embedded in the landscape in a way that is difficult to imagine for us modern humans. *Innately, we must have used herbal medicine.* Consider the complex meanings and significance to the earliest people, of animals, birds, trees and plants, when these things provided *everything*—all shelter, food, clothing and tools; it is less problematic then to see how knowledge of plant medicine will have begun very early indeed.

Animals are known to use plants as medicine.[1] Many recorded examples exist, and substantiation for Neanderthal medicinal plant use has recently been demonstrated by archaeologists.[2] Humans will have witnessed and copied the behaviours of other-than-human-beings, as we know we copied them in hunting and other skills. Consider also, the fact that *we are animals*, and therefore this instinct to track down and identify healing substances from the natural world is innate to us. We are a product of our environment, and that environment (until very recent times) has always been the natural world.

Definition—*Native*: Belonging inherently, and thriving innately, in nature.

In the world of information technology it denotes software, data, etc., that is specifically designed for the system on which it is run.

Native healers—those local plants with a capacity to heal reliably—will have been learned by our emergent species. At some point, *human* native healers, specialised in keeping and sharing knowledge of healing plants, will have begun a lineage that can still be found in all remaining native peoples, and even in technological societies today, all over our beautiful Earth.

Herbal medicine has been utilised in every inhabited continent on the planet, and has been adapted and updated as civilisations have progressed, and as our understanding of human physiology, and understanding of our relationship to the environment, has increased. Many sophisticated herbal medicine systems with ancient origins still exist and are utilised alongside any conventional biomedicine that may now be practised. Ayurveda, Traditional Chinese Medicine, Tibetan, Unani Tibb and many others have functioning educational institutions and practitioners in our modern world. The World Health Organization (WHO) recognises herbal medicine as the major form of healthcare for over 60% of the world's population.[3]

The focus of this book is partly an exploration of the fundamental usefulness of plants for healing to all people whatever their training or skills. Plants have been utilised as healing food and medicine by families and in homes across the world, and they can still play an important role today. We introduce recipes and strategies for using herbal medicine as kitchen pharmacy and home first aid throughout this book.

The focus of this book is also partly upon the professional practice of herbal medicine by the medical herbalists of the European tradition and, in particular, those of the UK in the 21st century. In Europe the term for medical herbalist is more usually phytotherapist, and phytotherapy refers to the subject of modern herbal medicine more broadly. Modern Western herbal medicine/phytotherapy has multiple and global origins, but is also intimately linked with the development of modern conventional biomedical science.

Definition—*Phytotherapy*: Phyto comes to us from the Greek, and means 'derived from or pertaining to plants'. Therapy also comes to us from Ancient Greece and means 'curing or healing'.

Medical herbalists do not use plants as direct alternatives to synthetic drugs however. The fundamental principles of Western herbal medicine lie in the recognition of the unity of the body-mind, and in the core principles of the restoration of dynamic function and enhancing the resilience of our physiology. By acknowledging complexity and interconnectedness, and by directing herbal medicine strategies at these root causes, the herbalist aims to help others re-build that resilience and help restore health and wellbeing.[3] We explore these concepts in more detail in this book.

Note: The word health is used here in its original meaning: health derived from the Old English *haelth*, meaning 'whole'.

Modern Western medical herbalists seek to combine up-to-date scientific advances in the study of physiology and medicine with everything that is known about medicinal plants in order to apply plant therapy to aid the dynamic ecosystem of the body to actively restore and balance function and resilience. In fact, Western medical herbalists exist as a result of a unique historical context whereby Europe became a melting pot of ideas derived from revived manuscripts of the ancient Egyptian, Greek and Roman worlds, from localised folk medicine and mediaeval monastic practice, through to the American botanical movement and its significant influence on herbalists in Britain. The effect of the plant medicines arriving in the UK and Europe from the First Nations peoples of the Americas, and the ideas of that time, led to a divergence from conventional medical practice that continues to this day. This divergence is still undergoing change with our ever-greater understanding of Eastern traditional medical systems, combined with an evolving acknowledgement of the importance of psychological health. New concepts of complexity in biology and modern discoveries in physiology are also informing the modern herbalist's practice today.

As scientific knowledge has increased, and as biomedical research has focussed on the search for new single-chemical drugs isolated from natural substances, ancient ideas about illness and the plants originally used to treat illness, have been largely discarded by modern medicine. The 20th century saw the steady, and all but complete, removal of once official plant medicines from the British pharmacopoeia by 1980. Subjects concerned with the nature and effects of these phytomedicines died out as well, without having been tended to and updated, and because this was before the age of the internet, formerly officially accepted knowledge about phytotherapy remains largely inaccessible to modern biomedical practitioners.

Much of Western herbal medicine is therefore based on empirical knowledge, and most modern herbalists acknowledge that historical ideas about health and disease can either seem out-dated or incompatible with conventional biomedicine. It is important to remember, however, that traditional concepts and ideas of health and disease were based on pre-modern descriptions of what was experienced, and reflected the extent of accepted knowledge of the time. Phenomenologically, these ideas are describing something useful. The use of plants was observed and recorded by people in much closer contact with the natural world than we can perhaps imagine today ...

It was empirical observation that led to plants being developed into drugs used in pain relief and surgical anaesthesia, such as belladonna (*Atropa belladonna* L.) for atropine eye drops used in eye surgery; opiates—alkaloids found in opium poppy (*Papaver somniferum* L.); and curare (*Chondrodendron tomentosum* Ruiz & Pav.)—which acts by blocking the action of the neurotransmitter acetylcholine at neuromuscular junctions allowing surgery to take place more easily whilst a patient is anaesthetised. The recent history of conventional biomedicine is full of doctors (and others) testing substances on themselves. Chemicals, plants and hormones were all examined in this way, and this form of experimentation helped our eventual understanding of their nature and mechanisms, as well as occasionally producing the odd medical charlatan who could temporarily cash-in on this.

Some traditional 'folk' remedies were adopted by conventional medicine and became synthesised into drugs. The discovery that the foxglove plant (*Digitalis purpurea* L.) could have benefits for patients with heart problems was attributed to William Withering, who had a patient who had been helped by a local traditional healer in

Staffordshire, England. He studied one of the herbs in her recipe (a species of *Digitalis*), identified cardiac alkaloids and developed these into what later became digoxin, a drug still used today.[4] Dr Withering of course was lucky enough to be wealthy and educated: the female traditional healer (we don't know her name), not being granted either wealth nor a right to education due to gender, was developing her empirical knowledge nevertheless.[5]

It is our hope that, like that native healer from whom Dr Withering found inspiration, this book will enable you to develop your own empirical knowledge of plant medicines, and bring those healing benefits into the lives of yourselves and those dear to you.

References

1. Engel, C., *How Animals Keep Themselves Well And How We Can Learn From Them*. 2003: Phoenix Press.
2. Hardy K. et al., *Neanderthal medics? Evidence for food, cooking and medicinal plants entrapped in dental calculus*. Naturwissenschaften—The Science of Nature, 2012.
3. Mills, S., *Out Of The Earth: The Essential Book of Herbal Medicine*. 1991: Penguin Books.
4. Griggs, B., *Green Pharmacy: The Story of Western Herbal Medicine*. 1997: Vermillion.
5. Brooke, E., *Women Healers Through History*. 1993: The Women's Press.

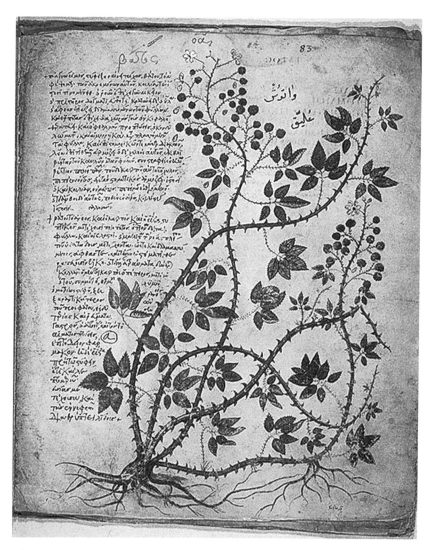

Blackberry (*Rubus fructicosa* L.) Illustration from the Vienna Dioscurides, early 6th Century.

CHAPTER ONE

Drawing from the deep pool: the history, scope and core principles of herbal medicine in the West

History and origins

As stated in the introduction, the origins of herbal medicine worldwide have an unknown lineage into archaic time and in other-than-human-beings. It is with the development of writing that ideas about health and disease, and the plants used as medicines, began to be recorded from oral traditions. Western herbal medicine, as practised by modern herbalists and members of the National Institute of Medical Herbalists today, has an eclectic and global heritage. Starting with information from oral cultures such as Ancient Greece, Ancient Egypt and beyond; concepts, theories and practical medicine of ancient times eventually became written texts.[1] The Roman Empire enabled the spread of these texts, and the collection of new ideas. Romanised physicians such as Dioscorides wrote their own works on medicine and the practical application of medicinal plants and of surgery. Pedianus Dioscorides (c. 40–90 CE) was originally from Greece, and his most famous work *De Materia Medica* was a precursor to modern pharmacopoeias (a technical book identifying and describing the preparation and use of medicines).

The ancient Greeks and Romans hailed the source of inspiration and knowledge of healing as coming from the Ancient Greek god Asclepius. It is thought by some scholars that Asclepius, also known as Thoth or Hermes Trismegistus could be based on the Ancient Egyptian architect Imhotep, although there is no evidence that he was a physician. Hieroglyphic carvings from Imhotep's stepped pyramid at Saqqara however state that Merit-Ptah was the 'chief physician', and so she would have existed about 2700 BCE, making her possibly the earliest recorded female physician.[2]

The Arabic scholars of the 9th–11th centuries then revived many of these texts, providing us with copies of works by Hippocrates and Galen, for example. Many of these Arab physicians, including people such as Avicenna, added to this information, practised medicine and surgery, and formed medical schools and hospitals that were very advanced for their time. Their work translating and adding to ancient texts meant that the knowledge and written work was picked up by the monastic traditions, copied and practised by monks and nuns (such as Hildegard of Bingen), and it also found its way to the original and first universities of Europe (and to medical practitioners of that time such as Trotula).

Works copied into Latin by monasteries and also new works from the early universities have allowed very ancient texts (such as Hippocrates

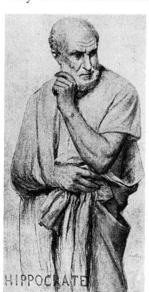

HIPPOCRATE

and Dioscorides) to survive today in the form of 'herbals', eventually being written in the English language (a key purpose of Nicholas Culpeper). Each culture left its mark on the work, so that many copies of the same book exist—in different languages and with slight variations.

Let's look at some of the key people from the history of Western herbal medicine.

Hippocrates c. 460–377 BCE was the son of a Greek physician, who, at that time were part of the rhizotomi or root gatherers. Rhizotomi were also known as Asclepiadiae after Aesclepius the Greek god of medicine (see above). Hippocrates is probably the most famous of all the Ancient Greek physicians and is known to this day as the father of medicine. The Hippocratic oath was named after him.

A number of different texts on medicine were originally ascribed to Hippocrates, but are now believed to have been written and edited by at least two different authors over approximately two centuries.

Texts include:

> *Ancient medicine*: This text emphasises the importance of balance within the body, and how essential it is to health. This is a forerunner to the modern-day concept of homeostasis in the body.
>
> *Airs, waters, places*: In this text physiological systems are aligned with definitions of body, soul and cosmos. This text also showed an in-depth understanding of the importance of the impact of environmental factors on health.
>
> *The nature of man*: This text expands on the theme of humoral medicine and how important it is to balance the humours within the individual for optimal health.

There are at least 50 other texts in this body of work. Hippocrates emphasised treating the physical body alongside emotional and mental states: an early record of holistic thinking perhaps.

> *It is far more important to know what person has the disease than what disease the person has.*
>
> —Hippocrates

Definition—*Holistic*: The term holistic was actually coined by General J. C. Smuts in 1926, and refers to the practice of looking at whole systems rather than breaking things down into their individual component parts (a mechanistic viewpoint). *Holon* is from Greek meaning 'whole'— *holos* (masculine) *holi* (feminine).

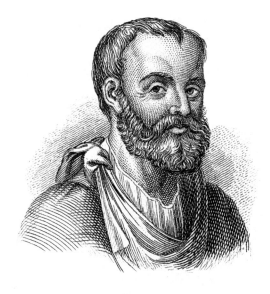

Galen.

Galen of Pergamon, 130–201 CE was born in the vibrant, intellectual Roman centre of Pergamon. His father had a dream given to him by the god Asclepius himself that Galen should study medicine. His 10-year training took him on to Smyrna and then Alexandria where he learned theories of medicine from ancient writings including those of Hippocrates, and more practical medicine such as surgery. His first job was as chief physician to the Roman gladiators, and this gave him much-needed experience in human anatomy. He went on to become personal physician to the Roman emperor Marcus Aurelius (ruled 161–180 CE). Galen published a huge corpus of works on language, logic, philosophy and many medical works on subjects such as diet, pharmacology, anatomy and physiology and surgery.

Galen was particularly influenced by the theory of the four humours, and he elevated this theory by attributing it to Hippocrates himself. He was also a practical observer and experimenter, and is considered to be the originator of the experimental method in medicine. This extended into pharmacology where he also suggested a method to observe the properties of herbal 'drugs'. He became so well known for this that he was often sent medicines from far around the Roman Empire to test. Some of his physiological observations were new for his time and were accurate (such as proving that urine is formed by the kidney not the bladder).

Galen also believed in individualised medicine, and that any medical training should be accompanied by the study of philosophy. The quotation, 'The best doctor is also a philosopher' is attributed to Galen. He was much admired and 400 years later his ideas were taken up by other great 'philosopher doctors' of the Arabic world such as Maimonides (1135–1204 CE). The 'medical logic' of Galen was subsequently absorbed by the new universities of Europe. These were founded as theoretical institutions based on Greek, and Arabic medical works translated into Latin, the dominant language of that time.

Galen's influence was such that after he died his works and theories became heavily modified, re-invented and re-interpreted and led to a sort of Galen-ism, that remained the predominant form of medicine practised in Europe right up to the 1600s.

It took 1500 years, until the Renaissance, for Galen's theories to be successfully challenged. First to do this was the Flemish anatomist Andreas Vesalius (1514–1564) who realised Galen's anatomy (based on animal dissection) was not always correct (in the ancient world, dissection of humans was forbidden). Then, William Harvey (1578–1657), credited with the discovery of the circulation of the blood, challenged and condemned Galen's inaccurate theory of blood, although it should be remembered that Harvey himself thought his own discovery *proved* humoural theory, and even he did not fully complete our understanding of the circulation.

Galenism, the dogmatic, rigid and sometimes just plain incorrect application of Galenic ideas, did much to discredit Galen into our modern time. He was however a polymath, a keen observer and empiricist, a thinking physician and surgeon, who believed in listening deeply to the patient as an individual.

Official plant medicines once found in the British Pharmacopoeia alongside chemical medicines up until the 1970s and 1980s, were known as 'Galenicals'. This has perhaps not helped the acceptance of modern phytotherapy among conventional doctors who may remember herbs being referred to in this way, and who think of Galen(ism) as holding back the progress of 'modern' medicine.

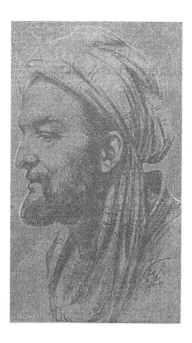

Probably the most famous of the Arabic scholars was Avicenna (Abū 'Alī al-Ḥusayn ibn 'Abd Allāh ibn Sīnā), (980–1037 CE) another polymath, physician and philosopher. Avicenna was born in what is now present-day Uzbekistan and lived during what has been called the Islamic Golden Age. At this time the West was going through what we now refer to as the Dark Ages (a mediaeval period of history), and medical knowledge from the Middle-East was significantly advanced by comparison. Muslim scholars had access to many sources of knowledge including that of Ancient Greco-Roman, Byzantine, Indian, Egyptian and Persian civilisations. It was the late middle ages before this wealth of knowledge became available to the West.

As another polymath, Avicenna is known to have written over 450 works including 40 on medicine. Possibly his most famous work on medicine is The *Canon of Medicine* which became one of the standard texts in medical universities in the mediaeval West.

> *There are no incurable diseases—only the lack of will. There are no worthless herbs—only the lack of knowledge.*
>
> —Avicenna

9th-century Arabic electuary for a cough caused by catarrh.
Equal parts of:

- Flax seed (Linseed) ground into a powder
- Sweet raisin (free from seed) pounded into a paste
- Pine nuts ground into paste
- Liquorice root ground into a powder
- Mix with honey (bereft of broth)

It is taken in the morning and at bedtime, it helps, God willing.

Adapted from *The Medical Formulary of Aqrabadhin of Al-Kindi (c. 800–870 CE) Arabian physician and philosopher.*

Works by Greek, Roman and Arabic physicians and others were preserved by the practice of monastic manuscript copying and translation.

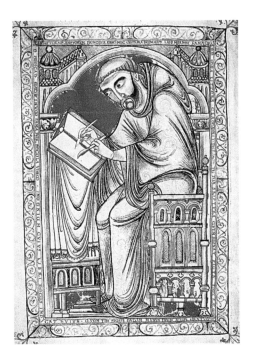

Many ancient texts survive because of this painstaking practice, and fuel the popular association between monks and herb gardens. Uniquely in Britain, records were kept on Anglo-Saxon medicine and so we can see the influence of Latin texts on traditional Leechbooks from around the 9th century CE (leech was the term for a doctor in those times) such as the Leechbook of Bald.[3,4] Bald was a monk, and set about recording and copying contemporary medicine into a written document that survives to this day. Monastic life also allowed for the development of new ideas within health and medicine, an example being the Abbess Hildegarde of Bingen whose writings on health and, uniquely, womens health, contributed to this corpus of knowledge.

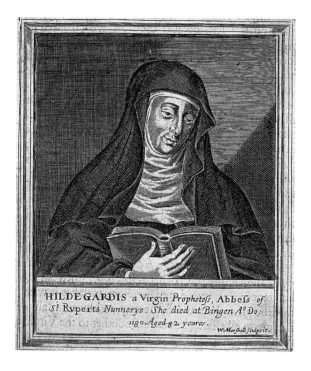

HILDEGARDIS a Virgin Prophetess, Abbess of St Ruperts Nunnerye. She died at Bingen A° Do: 1180 Aged 82 yeares.

W. Marshall sculpsit.

Hildegarde of Bingen, (1098–1179) abbess of Eibingen Abby, near Bingen, Germany. In addition to being one of the most important musical composers of the period, Hildegarde wrote extensively about health and medicine.

Her books on many subjects including *Physica* written during the period 1150 to 1158 and *Cause et Curae* were originally combined in *Liber subtilitatum diversarum naturarum creaturarum* (the *Book of the Subtleties of the Diverse Nature of Creatures*).

According to Hildegard of Bingen, disease is not a process, but an absence of process, a failing in the course of nature. Thus, from a holistic perspective, the presence of disease suggests a shortfall that can be improved upon. Her works describe over 2000 herb recipes, as well as ways of eating, and Hildegarde also had advice on wellness and living, that is regarded as a forerunner to the strong tradition of herbal medicine and naturopathy in Germany, and Northern Europe. These can be translated as:

- *Viriditas*—The drawing of energy from nature's 'greenness' and life force.
- Healthy and balanced nutrition found from the healing power of food.
- Regeneration of strained nerves with healthy sleep and dream regulation.
- Finding the harmonious balance between work and leisure.
- Removal of waste products and purification with regular fasting and sweat baths.
- Optimism of mind and strength of psychological defences.

Monastic preservation of medical texts provided an intellectual starting point for the study of medicine or *physic* in the first universities. In Padua, Salerno, Bologna, Oxford and throughout Europe, medicine was taught and pharmacy was demonstrated in the physic garden—some of these physic gardens remain open to visitors today.

Another contributor from this time was the medical practitioner and scholar Trotula—we do not know her full name. There are three books largely attributed to her that also contain new ideas for the time about health, and about women's health and wellbeing.[5]

The Christian requirement for charity throughout the Middle Ages was expressed in the formation of hospitality for pilgrims, and thus the formation of 'spittals' or 'hospitals', which cared for and treated those in need.

Medico-archaeology such as that at Soutra Aisle close to the Scottish border, reveals the use of medicinal plants on a large scale (as well as other medical interventions of the time such as blood-letting). Archaeological evidence found at Soutra Aisle, such as well-preserved seeds of *Valeriana officinalis* L. and *Hypericum perforatum* L. (still formed into a bolus), has been linked to contemporary 12th-century recipes in manuscripts from around the time of the hospital such as 'The armpit package of St Columba' a possible remedy for swollen lymph glands made from these plants.[6]

As the printing press took over from handwritten manuscripts, herbals began to be printed and circulated. An extraordinary number of herbals are still available to us today and many of them repeat and elaborate on information from existing or even long lost manuscripts. The popularity of herbals has ensured the survival of many for our continued enjoyment and learning. Familiar names include: John Gerard, Nicholas Culpeper, William Turner and John Parkinson.[7]

Two types of herbal knowledge existed; Latin texts for those wealthy enough to be educated, and secondly, a folk tradition, often in the form of practical medicine infused with some exotic remedies from Latin texts right alongside native and local plants. In the UK, some resources survive, often in the form of recipes, of the people's everyday herbalism. For example recipes from Wales and the physicians of Myddfai,[8] and 20th-century information collected from the country folk of England[9,10] and Scotland.[11]

One significantly negative outcome from this period of history in Europe was the witch-hunt genocide (gendercide). In Europe during the Middle Ages, many women (and some men) were persecuted supposedly for being witches. It has been regularly suggested that many of these so-called witches who were put to death, were in fact herbalists or simply people offering other people healing or midwifery services. The link between herbalists and witchcraft is still resonant today—albeit jokingly.[2] A brief read of the *Malleus Maleficarum* (*Hammer of the Witches*) by Heinrich Kramer in 1487—the work that sparked the notorious witch trials of Europe and early settlers of America, reveals a far more sinister misogyny at work.

Matilda Joslyn Gage, suffragette, has said that

> *The persecution of witches had nothing to do with fighting evil or resisting the devil—it was simply entrenched misogyny, the goal of which was to repress the intellect of women. A witch was not wicked, did not ride a broomstick naked in the dark nor consort with demons. She was instead likely to be a woman of superior intellect.*
>
> —Matilda Joslyn Gage

As a thought experiment Matilda suggested that for 'witches' we should instead read 'women', for their histories run hand in hand.

The witch trials had undoubtedly a suppressive effect on a living tradition of plant medicine throughout Northern Europe, and continues to lend an unfortunate negative association with herbal medicine and women healers.

Wealthy and literate women of the 16th–19th centuries continued to keep and record recipes for food, medicine and medicinal foods, for use within the home. Meanwhile paid professionals went on to create and protect the title of doctor, leading to the formation of medical societies.

The steady development of chemistry as a profession enabled the evolution of a whole new area of drug development, which orthodox medicine fully embraced. However, plant-based medicines were still recommended as part of the pharmacopoeia well into the 20th century. The British Pharmacopoeia of 1932 lists ointment of capsicum, gum of tragacanth, tincture of ginger, tincture of valerian, common tincture of rhubarb, and tinctures of myrrh, gentian, quassia and lobelia, to name just a few. The British Pharmaceutical Codex of 1954 included tincture of lemon, squill, rose fruit, rosemary oil, and peppermint in its list of recommended substances for medicines. The British National Formulary (BNF) of 2016 still includes peppermint oil as one of its recommendations, among a list of medicines that are otherwise overwhelmingly mono-chemical in nature.

During the 19th century, the success of the American Botanical Movement led to the formation of the National Association of Medical Herbalists (NAMH) in the UK in 1864, eventually becoming the National Institute of Medical Herbalists (NIMH).

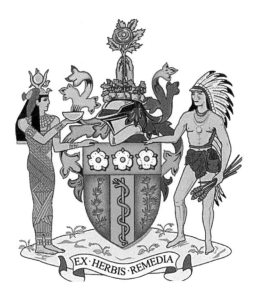

Coat of Arms, National Institute of Medical Herbalists.

There is acknowledgement (as can be seen from the former coat of arms of the NIMH pictured here), that the corpus of knowledge from the ancient and new worlds has informed what we today call modern herbal medicine, and phytotherapy. It also represents the strong connection to and yet difference from, conventional medical origins.

The influence from America cannot be underestimated. The pioneers from the old world had to live and survive in the unfamiliar newly settled lands of America. The survival of these early settlers can be seen as a direct result of First Nations peoples' knowledge of medicine and medicinal plants. Many European settlers were helped by them, then they copied and formalised herbal medicine techniques from those native peoples of Canada, and of North and South America. This new influence upon European herbal medicine set in motion a clear distinction between conventional and herbal medicine, and a revival in the use of plant medicines in contrast to the growing popularity of chemical medicines among most professional doctors.

In the 18th and 19th centuries, use of bleeding, mercury, opiates, arsenic, emetics and purgatives by regular doctors in America and Britain often resulted in the death of the patient. This influenced the creation of a strong alternative medicine system, which borrowed heavily from First Nations' sweat baths, herbal practice, and also from New England folk remedies.

Samuel Thomson (1769–1843), a New Hampshire farmer, formalised his system of medicine that was similarly 'heroic' but much less toxic and extreme than the current conventional options, and relied on medicinal plants. The principle that 'heat is life and cold is death' was behind a simple system of steaming and purging remedies, and the use of many herbs familiar to Western herbalists today such as chilli, ginger, prickly ash bark, yarrow, lobelia, bayberry, skullcap and boneset can be traced back to Thompsonian medicine.[12]

Thompson's original theory was later supplanted and developed into Physiomedicalism by Alva Curtis (1797–1881). This sectarian medical school, at its height in the 1880s in the USA, drew from energetic theories similar to Traditional Chinese Medicine and promoted a study of the patients' constitution and relevance of organ systems in the practice of herbal medicine.

The most resilient of the medical-botanical schools to emerge in the 19th century were the *eclectic physicians* founded in 1820 by Wooster Beach (1794–1868).[13]

The eclectic physicians introduced many American botanicals to the herbal pharmacopoeia of the UK, including echinacea (*Echinacea angustifolia* DC and *E. purpurea* (L.) Moench), wild indigo (*Baptisia tinctoria* (L.) R.Br.), black cohosh (*Actaea racemosa* L. formerly known as *Cimicifuga*) and golden seal (*Hydrastis canadensis* L.). Huge numbers of patients were treated and data about herbal interventions recorded.

John Milton Scudder MD (1829–1894) enhanced and continued the eclectic medical system. Its key features were the use of specific indications in herbal medicine practice. The patient was seen as an individual, and their unique symptoms were investigated using pulse, tongue and differential and physical diagnostics. Herbal medicines, conventional medicine, homoeopathy and hydrotherapy could be employed to help the patient.[14]

The history of Western herbal medicine in the UK in the 20th century is full of twists and turns. In 1941, against a backdrop of pharmaceutical 'wonder drugs' being continually discovered, the wartime government rushed the Pharmacy and Medicines Act onto the statute books. Overnight, members of the National Association of Medical Herbalists found that they could no longer supply herbal remedies directly to their patients. In effect it became illegal to practice as a consulting medical herbalist in the UK. Public reaction to this was generally hostile. NAMH members continued to practice and there were no prosecutions.

The 5th July 1948 is generally recognised as the birth of the National Health Service (NHS) in the UK. Its primary aim was to make healthcare available to everyone, not just to those who could afford it. Access to free healthcare, the fast-developing world of pharmaceutical companies and the accompanying enthusiasm engendered by the concept of 'magic bullet' medicine, and the 1941 Pharmacy and Medicines Act, all conspired to suppress the practice of Western herbal medicine in the UK.

This situation continued until 1964 when (in the wake of the thalidomide tragedy) the newly formed British Herbal Medicines Association (formed by Frederick Fletcher Hyde and Frank Powers) was ultimately successful in overthrowing the 1941 Pharmacy and Medicines Act.

Albert Orbell FNIMH, medical herbalist and president of the NIMH in its centenary year, played a pivotal role in founding the *Hospital for Natural Healing* (HNH) in Stratford, E14, in 1934, and was the Chairman of the Hospital Board for most of its 40-plus years existence. A charitable enterprise, the HNH was a most ambitious project, providing professional herbal health care to the people of London's deprived East End, regardless of their ability to pay.

The HNH also played a key role in the survival of the herbal profession in the UK during the difficult post-war years, when NIMH membership dropped to double figures. In an agreement with NIMH, the HNH provided professional training for herbal students from the 1950s until its closure in 1975. When it closed, the sale of the premises provided a substantial tranche of funds for the NIMH's Education Fund, a charity enabling the purchase of a building in Tunbridge Wells that established the School of Herbal Medicine run by Hein Zeylstra for the next 25 years or so.

Modern practitioners of herbal medicine, and members of the National Institute of Medical Herbalists, recognise the important discoveries and advancement of our understanding of the practical application of herbs due to the various American botanical movements, and their native First Nations' teachers. Established in 1864, the National Association of Medical Herbalists (now the NIMH), still aims to use herbal medicines (in association with areas such as advice on diet and lifestyle changes) to heal and relieve suffering. The NIMH has continued to educate and provide professional membership ever since its inception. This was formalised into University-based BSc and MSc qualifications in the late 1990s, and continues as equivalent professional training to the present day.

> We shall continue to treat each person as a unique entity and prescribe according to our judgement as to his needs.
> —Fred Fletcher Hyde, Presidential address to the NIMH

The UK legislative provisions for herbal medicine are to be found in the Medicines Act 1968, and they were successfully prevented from being removed in 1993, and again in 2011, by, among others, the courageous and indomitable medical herbalist and past-president of the NIMH, Michael McIntyre. Although he was not successful in gaining statutory regulation for herbalists in 2017, this was at least partly because herbal medicine poses so little threat to public safety. The European Herbal and Traditional Practitioners Association founded at the request of the UK government maintains a record of political events regarding herbal practitioners via their website.

The National Institute of Medical Herbalists maintains a register and professional standards for modern medical herbalists and liaises with government bodies and departments on matters pertaining to professional herbal treatment. Although herbal medicine in the UK is legislated for, it is currently outside of National Health Service funding and is therefore sometimes misunderstood in terms of its scientific rigour and professional standards. In some ways, the state-funded NHS has created a situation where any form of healing that is not conventional biomedicine is in some way pseudo-scientific or ineffective. Different countries worldwide have their own rules on herbal medicine provision, and in many countries other forms of healing are valued and integrated, including herbal medicine and naturopathy.

Some historical sources and people who have influenced the practice of Western herbal medicine are listed below for your information:

Greco-Roman

Dioscorides 50–80 CE, Pliny the Elder c. 23–79 CE, Galen of Pergamon c. 130–200 CE, Pseudo-Asclepeius 5th century CE.

Arabic

Abn Sina (Avicenna) c. 980–1037 CE, Serapo the Younger (Ibn Wafid) 13th century.

Anglo-Saxon/late Middle Ages

The Old English Herbarium c. 1000, Macer 9th–12th century, The Salernitian Herbal 12th century, Hildegarde of Bingen 1098–1179, Physicians of Myddfai 14th–18th century.

Renaissance/early modern

Leonhart Fuchs 1501–1566, Pietro Andrea Mattioli 1501–1577, William Turner 1509–1568, Rembert Dodoens 1516–1585, Jaques D'Alechamps 1513–1588, Jean Bauhin 1541–1613, John Gerard c. 1545–1612, John Parkinson 1566–1650, Nicholas Culpeper 1616–1654.

18th-century sources

William Salmon 1710, John Quincy d. 1722, Joseph Miller d. 1748, John Hill 1714–1775, William Cullen 1710–1790.

19th-century American and British sources

Albert Isiah Coffin 1790–1866, William Fox, William Cook 1832–1899, Finley Ellingwood 1852–1920.

20th-century texts

Richard Cranfield Wren, Richard Hool, Maud Grieve 1858–after 1941, Wilhelm Pelikan 1893–1981, Rudolf Weiss 1895–1991, The National Botanic Pharmacopoeia 1921, Albert Priest and Lilian Priest, British Herbal Pharmacopoeia 1983, Thomas Bartram 1913–2009.

21st-century texts

Julian Barker, Kerry Bone, Dr Mary Bove, Peter Bradley, Andrew Chevallier, Alison Denham, Graeme Tobyn, Midge Whitelegg, David Hoffman, Elizabeth Williamson, Christopher Menzies-Trull, Simon Mills, Aviva Romm, Ruth Tricky and Matthew Wood.

Key concepts of Western herbal medicine

Medical herbalists study conventional medical science, but they also study and practice using key principles and concepts distinct from conventional medical thinking today. Herbalists study a functional and ecological approach to health and disease that informs their use of herbal medicines, and the advice that they give. These key principles and concepts are implemented alongside conventional medical diagnosis to analyse the individual's health, and in the application of herbal therapy. This deeper analysis of the patient and their symptoms,

Definition—Medicine:

- The science or practice of the diagnosis, treatment and prevention of disease (in technical use often taken to exclude surgery).
- A drug or other (non-surgical) preparation for the treatment or prevention of disease.
- A spell, charm or fetish believed to have healing, protective or other power.

—Oxford English Dictionary

beyond the conventional diagnosis, ensures that herbal treatment remains person-centred.[15] The plant medicines applied in this way have the capacity to act within us to restore specific tissues of the body and also therefore the function of our own bodies.

Throughout this book, we shall revisit these core principles and concepts and develop the themes of this ecological view of health and of the plants themselves.

Core foundational principles of herbal practice

- That wellness and illness are made up of a mosaic of factors, and time is needed to discover and respond to these in an individualised way.
- Symptoms and not just the diagnosis are seen as important.
- The consultation is conducted in a fundamentally positive setting.
- Lifestyle, diet and psychological wellbeing are recognised as significant in disease causation and treatment outcome. The herbalist is therefore acting as a health guide not just as a prescriber of plants as medicine.
- Humans have an innate vitality or resilience that can be negatively or positively impacted.
- Herbalists assess the individual using pattern recognition[16] and a persistent theme within all traditions of herbal medicine is the assessment of a person's unique 'constitution'.
- Our physiological functions act as an interconnected whole, and so the practice of herbalism is more like that of the science of ecology— the study of complex interconnected systems.[17]
- Some areas of human function are so fundamental as to be pillars of wellbeing. These 'health drivers' are good digestive function, restorative sleep, regular relaxation, and the promotion of circulation and tissue health. Improvement in these areas will positively impact other essential physiological functions such as the hormonal system, the immune system or the skin, and will act on the trophic state of tissues and organs.
- Restoring resilience or 'bounce-back' can be a result of correcting the pillars of health with diet and herbal medicine. In addition, herbalists recognise the concept of herbal tonics and adaptogens (a natural substance considered to help the body adapt to stress). Some herbs are considered to have tonic effects to the circulatory, or immune system, or the musculoskeletal system, for example, and others more broadly to our vitality and adaptive potential.

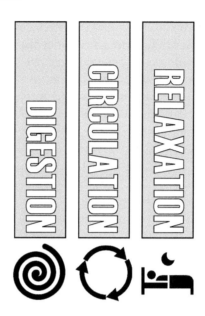

A summary of the core principles of the practical application of herbal medicines

To relieve suffering by addressing the following fundamentals of health:

- Positively influence digestive health (tissues, secretions, organs, microbiome)
- Assess and enhance elimination of metabolic waste products (at the tissue level, and via the organs of excretion)
- Assess and restore circulation (central and peripheral)
- Consider all aspects of the nervous system, its health and function
- Application of trophic herbs where needed
- Support adaptive potential with adaptogens
- Apply vulnerary and healing plants wherever needed[18]

The framework of the book

We will take a deeper look into the plants themselves and the compounds associated with them in Chapter 2. This book then dives into the study of our physical body and its interconnectedness. We have attempted to draw attention here to some of the fundamental differences between conventional and herbal medicine. Join us after this for an exploration of 15 key medicinal plants from the Western tradition (Chapters 4, 6 and 8). See how practical and helpful these herbal allies are, and observe how they have been examined in modern times to increase our understanding of how they can uniquely help us. We have included recipes and self-help measures so that you can experience each of these fantastic plants in a practical way. Herbal medicine, specifically the utilisation of whole plants such as bramble, nettle and oats, is often described as occupying the grey area between food and medicine. In Chapter 5 we will look more closely at this from the perspective of food, and how we can use the foods we eat to keep us healthy. Most of us will experience some form of health complaint at some time. Chapters 7, 9, 10 and 11 examine some of the commonest health issues that people might see their doctor for, and considers the herbalists' perspective. This is illustrated throughout with case histories from our own practices. We consider research, safety and the role of herbal medicine in our modern technological (anthropocene) world. Finally we will draw together the key points from the book in Chapter 12, which summarises our thoughts and experiences, and our hopes for the future of this vibrant and supportive form of medicine.

But first, we would like to outline some key concepts from within herbal medicine about our plant allies. Once we start to look at anything in detail, we can all too easily lose the phenomenon as its true whole. We hope to retain that wholeness despite the analysis within this book.

Key concepts about medicinal plants

- Plants typically used in herbal medicine practice have multiple compounds that are of benefit to the plant, but also to human health, resilience and function.
- Plant constituents often demonstrate synergy, that is their interactions with each other produce therapeutic results beyond the merely additive.
- Co-evolution with many edible and medicinal plants has altered our genetics allowing us to tolerate medicinal plants to a greater degree than would be otherwise expected of mono-chemical drugs.

- Plants and humans have their own microbiome, or mini-ecosystem of commensal microorganisms.[19]

Definition—*Microbiome:* The microorganisms in a particular environment (including the body or a part of the body).

—Oxford English Dictionary Online

Plants can positively impact a depleted human microbiome directly and also indirectly by having active compounds that correct gut function. It stands to reason then why care of our wider ecosystem is so important for everyone's health.

Synergy

Medicinal plants have many well-researched individual therapeutic compounds. These are considered to (and have often been shown to) act synergistically.[20] The use of whole plants with their multiple compounds, and multiple herb prescriptions, can result in better results than can be demonstrated by a single herb or single 'active constituent' research. This property is closely connected with the potential for herbal medicines to have properties beyond what can be described by solely looking at their compounds or pharmacology. A 'greater than the sum of parts' effect, known as synergy, is an example of a recognition of the dynamic nature of nature.

Examples of synergistic interactions would include the ability of one constituent to maximize the absorption of another constituent across the gut wall (pharmacokinetic synergy), or the multiple differing pathways by which the constituents of a plant exert their effects, coming together to provide broad based support for a system, and therefore resulting in better than expected outcomes (pharmacodynamic synergy).

This dynamic nature of nature can also be exemplified in the energetic approach of Ayurvedic and Traditional Chinese Medicine systems, and other traditions of the world. Many Western herbalists still consider this way of thinking as vital to the practice, some still refer to the humoral approach, the original 'energetic' approach of Western herbal medicine. We will revisit and expand this theme in later chapters.

A summary of the extra characteristics that herbalists recognise within plants:
Each characteristic has multiple potential layers of meaning.

Stimulating	Relaxing
Sedating	Astringing/condensing
Trophic	Adaptogenic
Nervine	Vulnerary

Key concepts of the approach of the Western medical herbalist

> [Today, medical herbalists] *critically evaluate both historical documentation and the latest empirical findings underpinning herbal prescribing.*
>
> —G. Tobyn, A. Denham and M. Whitelegg[21]

Modern Western medical herbalists (phytotherapists) value a detailed consultation and case history taking, allowing the person time to speak, to be heard, and time for the herbalist to ask about information concerning each and every body system, not just the current symptom or focus of primary diagnosis.

An emphasis is placed on the interconnectedness of all parts of our physiology, and the inherent vitality that can be suppressed in some people or some situations, and can therefore be supported and nourished with certain herbal interventions.

A timeline and chronology of events from wellness to un-wellness is mapped out, and areas of weakness, fragility or lack of function are identified. The aim is to direct focus and treatment to the perceived root causes, and to apply herbal medicines (and any other valued activity such as nutrition, exercise, lifestyle advice) to areas that need attention.

Each medicinal plant has multiple capacities, and so care in the selection of plants to suit the person and the situation is taken by the herbalist. Herbal therapy therefore may be, for example, 'anti-inflammatory', but *also* stimulating, relaxing or tonifying in nature. These actions may be attributed to plant compounds and our current pharmacological understanding of them, and also to traditional understanding or empirical sources from centuries of use.

Herbalists value a deep connection with the plants they enrol as medicines. Being a herbalist often results in a glorious life-long relationship with plants and nature.

Herbal therapy can be applied internally and/or externally and in a huge variety of forms—tea, tincture, capsule, syrup, pessary, ointment and so on, and thus individualised to the situation and/or to the patient and their requirements. We shall explore some home pharmacy recipes later in this book.

Evidence

One fairly common and misguided comment made concerning herbal medicine is the lack of research underpinning practice. Although there is undeniably a lack of well-structured quality human research specifically designed for the purpose of investigating whole plant remedies, it is untrue to say that there is no relevant research.

This is a misconception that we have striven to address where possible in the writing of this book. Research is out there; fragmented at times, but out there none the less. One aspect of this, however, is the thorny question of animal research. We do not believe that animal research involving the wilful harming of living creatures should be supported. This has in places led to us deliberately not quoting what could be seen by some as 'relevant' supportive research. We feel such research is profoundly in conflict with the spirit of a healing profession for which we both care deeply and strive to practice with integrity and love. The tenet of 'do no harm' should be adhered to at all times, and this includes all living creatures that come under the auspices of herbal medicine (which is to say—all living creatures).

What is evidence, particularly where any medicine is concerned? This often depends partly on whom the evidence is intended to inform. The research that produces evidence can be qualitative or quantitative, or even a mixture of the two.

The originators of the concept of evidence-based medicine defined it as:

> The integration of best research evidence with clinical expertise and patient values.
>
> —D. L. Sackett et al., 1996[22]

There is a perceived hierarchy of evidence recognised today, that could be said to have developed because of its intrinsic link to the development and manufacture of drugs by companies looking for a market, and potential validation by government organisations. Any patient-centred intervention is likely to fall short of criteria designed to fit mono-chemical therapy applied to disease labels. A gradual realisation of the significance of more qualitative data, case reports and patient-centred medicine is growing within the medical community.

Levels of evidence include:

- *Patients*: often bring evidence in anecdotal form from previous cases that they have heard about that reflect their own.
- *Clinicians*: are interested in evidence that gives a probability of success or adverse effects, to guide their prescribing.
- *Clinical researchers*: want a comparison of one group against another with blinding and randomisation to eliminate placebo and nocebo effects. The randomised, placebo controlled trial (RCT's).
- *Laboratory researchers*: use experiments to identify causative factors and mechanism of action.
- *Office-based researchers/clinical analysts*: the highest regarded research currently for analysing clinical effectiveness is the meta-analysis and systematic reviews of groups of trials. This is the basis of government recommendations to clinicians. As we shall see, however, this is not always applied evenly.

Herbal medicine has been criticised for having a lack of RCT's, but, despite significant stumbling blocks such as lack of financial backing, some do exist. Conversely, despite a lack of RCT data showing efficacy for paracetamol (acetaminophen/tylenol) for clinical effectiveness for the pain of osteo-arthritis (OA), it continues to be the most prescribed medication by conventional UK practitioners for OA and is NHS funded.

Meta-analysis has been championed by the Cochrane review, but poorly designed trials on herbal medicines such as those on echinacea have produced results that suggest no clinical effectiveness. Concerns have been raised about the poor quality or quantity of plant material used in these RCT's.[23]

Lack of evidence for efficacy is not the same as evidence for lack of efficacy.
—S. E. Edwards et al.[23]

This short and seemingly simple statement belies a massive lack of understanding on the part of many people. If something has not been proved by accepted scientific methodology, this does not signify that it has actually been disproved. The confusion caused by the statement. *'there is no scientific evidence for this'* or words to that effect are regularly taken as evidence of disproof. This misconception often lies at the heart of perfectly sound interventions being discarded or maligned.

It is important to be observant when herbal medicine research is being presented in the media, because often research trial data is discussed but 'opinion' pieces are tacked on to the end of the discussion, and presented as if they are as factual as the research itself. So even a positive herbal medicine outcome might also have the researcher comment that the public should still be wary of herbal medicine safety, for example. An alternative statement such as 'refer to a qualified herbal practitioner' would be more balanced reporting, and would be the equivalent to 'seek advice from your doctor'.

Confusion about (or wilful muddling of) the distinction between herbal medicine and other complementary and alternative medicine (CAM) modalities also occurs, and can be used to ridicule herbal medicine as part of CAM. This is due to ideological beliefs that in order to further 'rational science', an opinion should be held that all past forms of medicine are based on flawed scientific thinking and must therefore be eradicated.

> *Complementary medicine is a misleading umbrella term for this cluster of unconnected theories and methods.*
>
> *Osteopathy, chiropractic, acupuncture, herbal medicine, nutritional therapy, hypnotherapy? Their most obvious shared feature is their being absent from the medical curriculum.*
>
> —Professor David Peters

There are many conventional clinicians who find they have effectiveness gaps in terms of the treatment they can offer their patients in a real-life setting, and interest in complementary approaches and integrated medicine is growing among this sector.

There is inconsistency in terms of implementation of herbal medicine by governments, and dissemination of correct information to doctors about herbal medicine. Despite a Cochrane review demonstrating that St John's wort (*Hypericum perforatum* L.) was equivalent in efficacy to selective serotonin reuptake inhibitors (SSRI antidepressant drugs) in the UK, health claims for herbal medicines can only be based on 'traditional use', and so the efficacy data for St John's wort cannot be used as advice for doctors. It could be argued that this set up keeps herbal medicine in a 'traditional use' straight-jacket.[24]

A large amount of pharmacological evidence for herbal medicine and its compounds exists, as does some clinical evidence. Although plants contain multiple compounds, and traditional use often mixes multiple plants, pharmacological evidence will often support traditional use. An example of this would be the growing body of research confirming improved bio-availability of phytochemicals resulting from the use of complex plant mixtures (a form of synergy in whole plant medicines).[25]

Research data on herbal medicines can be found in journals such as:

The Journal of Herbal Medicine (Elsevier)
Phytotherapy Research
Planta Medica
Journal of Ethnopharmacology
Fitoterapia
Phytomedicine

Online searches via Pubmed/Medline and Google Scholar may also prove fruitful.

Herbal safety

Some examination of what we mean by safety, what we mean by adverse events and the case to answer is needed. Clarification of what is meant by placebo, and in terms of herbal safety what is meant by nocebo, is also required.

The common refrain 'just because it is natural doesn't mean it is safe' is often applied to herbal medicine. To some extent this is true. Plant identification by those wishing to harvest a herbal medicine from the wild has, and can, result in potentially dangerous misidentification. Unscrupulous companies marketing herbal products have and can sell defective, adulterated and occasionally poisonous 'herbal' products. Issues of quality have been and continue to be a very real problem, which means it can be difficult for those wishing to self-medicate for minor ailments with herbal medicine to do so effectively. Each European country has its own rules about quality, but companies based outside of the EU may have little or no regulation or pharmaco-vigilance.

In the UK, herbal products provided to practitioners of Western herbal medicine have the highest standard of good management practice ensuring the quality of the end product. A licensing scheme for over-the-counter products exists for herbal products in the UK not provided via a practitioner and these products clearly state they are licensed and contain a public information leaflet.

Once again reporting of herbal safety is not conducted using the same criteria applied to conventional medicine. Many adverse herbal medicine events occur as the result of excessive ingestion of a plant.

> **Definition—*Adverse reaction*:** A response to a drug that is noxious and unintended and which occurs at normal doses for human use.

Even in the instance of such a plant being medicinal, most reported adverse reactions have occurred when significant overdoses were taken.

That does not mean that all herbs are safe, and herbalists are, and should be, hyper-vigilant. Medical herbalists have a yellow-card reporting scheme for herbal medicines, as exists for conventional medicines. We should always work from the assumption that any herbal remedy consumed is done so respectfully, and for a targeted purpose—to relieve suffering, to promote healing and wellbeing, and with an aim to restore resilience and function.

Particular care should be taken when people are taking conventional medicine, and/or mixing herbal medicines or taking herbs with vitamins and mineral supplements.

Medical herbalists are trained in pharmacology and are the experts in using plant medicines in a modern context of conventional drugs and over-the-counter remedies.

It has become increasingly clear that the UK government and the MHRA (Medicines and Healthcare Regulatory Agency) do not have any great concerns about safety with regard to the practice of herbal medicine by registered practitioners. Statutory regulation for herbal practitioners in the UK has been rejected several times, and lack of public risk is repeatedly given as a key reason for this.

Things to consider with regard to herbal safety:

a) Be aware of rare but known adverse reactions to some herbs (e.g., *Actaea racemosa* L. has been known to cause self-limiting but unwanted headaches in rare cases.)
b) Remain alert to issues of safety and observe any signs for potential harm to liver, kidney, heart or other body systems.
c) There are rare but occasional risks of phototoxicity or allergy with any substance.
d) Be mindful of vulnerable sectors of the population.
e) Be mindful of the small number of conventional medicines which are genuinely vulnerable to herb/drug interactions (this includes drugs that operate within a narrow therapeutic dose such as anticoagulants or immune-suppressant drugs).[25]

Actaea racemosa (L.) was previously, and more commonly, known as *Cimicifuga racemosa, or black cohosh*. Concerns have been raised about this herb in connection with serious liver damage. Research into this issue has not, to date, been able to prove conclusively that the small number of cases of liver damage recorded are definitely attributable to *Aceta racemosa* (L.) and were in fact products made with a non-medicinal plant wrongly identified as *Actea racemosa*.

Another implication of herbal safety has arisen from plants that contain unsaturated pyrrolizidine alkaloids (PA's) such as comfrey (*Symphytum officinale* L.), coltsfoot (*Tussilago farfara* L.) and borage (*Borago officinalis* L.). Use of these herbs has been restricted or banned in some countries, despite concern that the animal and human case-study data used to inform and legislate may have been flawed. There are numerous PA's found in plants, they undergo complex metabolic change via liver pathways, and range from dangerous unsaturated PA's to the least toxic forms. Small amounts of the most toxic can be found in coltsfoot, large amounts of the least toxic in comfrey, while borage, (eaten widely as a vegetable in Europe) appears relatively benign all round. A person's liver health, drug and alcohol use, and nutritional deficiencies (such as anti-oxidants) that can impact on liver metabolism are therefore all essential factors in the safe use of these traditionally used herbs. PA's are not absorbed through the skin, so external use is safe. Internal use of these herbs should be avoided in pregnancy, as this is one situation where evidence of rare harm has been found.

Systematic reviews and multifaced case analysis studies were commissioned by the National Institute of Medical Herbalists in 2016. The findings are now published and show that although establishing directly causality of poisoning by PAs, could not be established, adverse events arising from ingestion of these plants is a rare harm, and that a patient-specific risk: benefit analysis should always be conducted before these plants are prescribed.[26]

By far the most common feature of herbal medicine adverse reactions we have observed in our practice setting is when a patient reports a (self-limiting) change to bowel movements early on in the treatment. Sometimes there can be temporarily increased diuresis, or other idiosyncratic reactions related to normal healing responses. Sometimes patients will report an increase in coughing, and expulsion of mucous from the nose when being treated for a cold for example. Mucous is produced by the body to both protect the membranes of the body and also as a vehicle to eliminate pathogens or the results of successful infection reactions. Producing more mucous more easily is exactly what the body needs to do to clear the respiratory tract of debris so that healing can occur. Here is a real case history showing the sort of thing that can happen.

Case history

Background

A 38-year-old woman presents with depression, recurrent colds and rhinitis following several miscarriages in the last 18 months. She is exhausted, and feels cold and miserable. She has a regular menstrual cycle but experiences heavy, painful periods. She eats a varied diet but is slightly overweight for her height. She has difficulty sleeping through the night, waking frequently, and feels anxious with occasional palpitations. She is pale, her tongue is pale, and she has a full 'jumpy' pulse despite a 'normal' blood pressure of 120/80 mmHg.

Herbal intervention

Herbal medicines included chamomile flowers (*Matricaria chamomilla* L.), ginger root (*Zingiber officinale* Roscoe), nettle leaf (*Urtica dioica* L.), yarrow herb (*Achillea millefolium* L.), echinacea root (*Echinacea purpurea* (L.) Moench) and raspberry leaf (*Rubus ideaeus* L.). She also had a night-time herbal medicine containing passionflower herb (*Passiflora incarnata* L.) and motherwort (*Leonurus cardiaca* L.). She was happy to include other herbal teas, especially chamomile and fennel, cinnamon and ginger, and oat flower and lemon balm.

Dietary advice

She was advised to try to avoid bread in her diet (she tended to eat bread for breakfast and lunch), and to try to find a non-wheat alternative. This was partly to create more variety in her diet. A multi-grain, seed, nut and fruit muesli with live plain yoghurt was suggested for breakfast, and a buckwheat and lentil tabbouleh with handfuls of green herbs (parsley, mint, coriander) with a tahini sauce was suggested as a possible lunch.

What happened next

The patient telephoned within a week of starting the herbal medicine feeling she was experiencing palpitations. On questioning, she was experiencing them mornings and evenings when going to bed and waking from sleep. She had reported palpitations at her first visit, and was reminded of this. She agreed that she had been anxious about allowing herself to sleep more, when she was already very tired during the day. The herbalist encouraged her to embrace the sleep, and allow her body to rest and re-charge.

The review consultation

The patient returned for a follow-up consultation 3 weeks later, reporting she was sleeping very well. So well, in fact, that the herbal medicine was now making her feel 'drowsy'. She had begun to make changes to her diet, and was enjoying the new foods. The rhinitis was gone. She had had another menstrual period, this time heavy but much less painful than usual. She was encouraged to continue with the daytime and night-time herbs for another month/cycle.

Another review

Within that time her sleep continued to be good, the drowsiness gradually disappeared and her next menstrual cycle was moderately heavy with no pain. The palpitations had gone, except for some on the day of her period (a disappointment for this lady who wanted desperately to conceive). Her pulse was strong but less 'jumpy', and her tongue was more pink rather than pale. She felt less 'depressed' although she continued to suffer from a propensity to low mood. She went on to have two full-term pregnancies.

It can be seen from this complex but typical case history, that it is difficult to put all of the presenting symptoms into a single conventional diagnosis, or to conclude that improvements were down to any single intervention introduced by the herbalist, whether dietary or herbal. This case does illustrate the ideas of the perceived importance by the herbalist of restoring sleep, in this case by using herbal medicine (passionflower and motherwort), of improving circulation (yarrow and ginger), and the concept of 'tonics' (nettle, oat flowers, raspberry leaf). The extra nutrition achieved through dietary change and through the nourishing herbs can be delivered by the improved circulation, and improved digestive function. The tongue and pulse can be monitored and give extra information to what the patient reports in terms of symptoms. The patient reported mild 'adverse effects' (possibly nocebo effects), early in treatment, but was persuaded to continue, and the symptoms disappeared.

Placebo and nocebo

The placebo effect

> *Be enthusiastic. Remember the placebo effect—30% of medicine is showbiz.*
> —Ronald Spark

It is very likely that over the years you will find people who claim that all complementary medicine, including herbal medicine, works mainly by the placebo effect. Well, before we dismiss that, let's take a closer look at just what the placebo effect is.

The word placebo is derived from the Latin for 'I shall please'. If you were living in medieval England a placebo would be someone who tells you what you want to hear, rather than telling you the truth: a sycophant.

Moving forward into the 1800s, a dictionary from 1811 defined placebo as a medicine designed more to please than benefit the patient. In the 20th century, placebos were thought of as a medicine that the doctor thought was beneficial, but which turned out to be ineffective or inert.

Of course doctors have (and still do in some parts of the world) given placebo medicines deliberately, and their beneficial effects have been documented in many cultures. So currently we view the placebo effect as a positive response to an inert medication.

If there can be positive responses to inert medications, there can also be negative ones. When a patient responds negatively to a medicine that subsequently turns out to be inert, this is termed a nocebo response.

Modern-day medicine has had the placebo effect on its radar for quite a few years now, as it is regarded as an irritating and confounding effect in drug trials of new pharmaceutical medicines that needs to be screened out as far as possible.

> *You are a placebo responder. Your body plays tricks on your mind. You cannot be trusted.*
>
> —Ben Goldacre

A lot of research has gone into trying to identify 'placebo responders' so that they can be excluded from clinical trials. This has turned out to be impossible, however. In the real world the meanings we ascribe to all sorts of things can play into healing and our responses to medicines. The term 'placebo effect' is quite correct when we are dealing with clinical drug trials, but in the real world what we are really talking about is meaning responses.

The anthropologist Daniel Moerman has studied this area for many years. In his book *Meaning, Medicine and the Placebo Effect*, Moerman states that:

> *A human being is simultaneously a cultural and a biological creature … what we think, say and know about the world can have a dramatic influence on our biology, as culture and biology overlap in powerful and important ways.*
>
> —Daniel Moermann[27]

In our Western culture, the practice of medicine is very firmly rooted in a specific 'cause and effect' paradigm. We also operate in what may be described as a reductionist way of thinking.

Definition—Reductionist: The practice of analysing and describing a complex phenomenon in terms of its simple or fundamental constituents, especially when this is said to provide a sufficient explanation.

—Oxford English Dictionary

Breaking things down into their simplest parts so that we can understand them is at the root of Western medicine (think about the study of things like anatomy, microbiology, endocrinology etc). This has brought a fantastic understanding of human physiology on many levels, but is not very good at seeing the big picture, the phenomenon. Also, what about the things we cannot see?

Moerman lists three ways in which the human body responds to injury:

- *Autonomous responses*: Known biological mechanisms mobilized by the body for healing to take place (i.e. clot formation, white blood cell recruitment etc.).
- *Specific responses*: Interactions with medications (i.e. anti-inflammatories etc.)
- *Meaning responses*: Interactions within the context in which the healing takes place (i.e., blue pills are calming; the use of medical instruments and machines is viewed as very powerful). We ascribe certain meanings to the world around us and respond accordingly. Our world is full of meaning to us, some of it we are consciously aware of, and some of it is so ingrained that we are not aware of it.

Meaning responses are not just confined to medicines. Many other factors play significant roles in our response to healing. Consider the patient/therapist consultation. In consultation a) the doctor/therapist is very enthusiastic about the medicine she is prescribing. She has listened carefully to all of the patients' concerns, offered explanations and advice where necessary and is very confident that the medicine she is prescribing will be helpful.

In consultation b) the doctor/therapist is apathetic in attitude, spends half her time typing on a computer, does not give any information about the medicine itself or how it will benefit the patient and does not appear to be actively listening to the patient. Both doctors/therapists prescribe the same medicine at the same dosage. Which one do you think will be more successful? Why? The patients' faith in the practitioner and the practitioners' faith in their remedies can be crucial to outcomes. Meaning responses are not confined to inert medicines: active medicines are also affected by them.

The act of diagnosing a condition is an intervention of a kind and can be filled with meaning. When a diagnosis (and prognosis) is good, it is most likely that things will improve. How does this compare with the psychological significances of a charm? If the diagnosis (and prognosis) is bad, things are more likely to deteriorate. How does this compare with the psychological significances of a curse? Where does 'self-fulfilling prophecy' come into all this? There are hard facts and there are also meaning responses. Untangling them may be harder than we think.

One thing that we can take from all this is that things that please us psychologically have a knock-on effect on our physiological responses. Conversely, things that worry or displease us can do the opposite. This is an excellent example of the mind-body connection.

It is important for us to acknowledge that there is no form of treatment (up to and including surgery) that is not affected by a meaning response. Therefore to claim that the placebo effect is the only reason that some interventions work is to show a lack of understanding of how ubiquitous meaning responses are. The advent of the clinical drug trial has put a negative spin on what is a positive and very powerful influence on therapeutic outcomes. Meaning responses are a natural corollary of being human and interacting with the world around us according to the facts as we see them.

> *Biology and culture interact. To turn ones eye away from such powerful human interactions is not only short sighted and foolish, but utterly unethical.*
>
> —Daniel Moermann[27]

The nocebo effect

Although it was popularly accepted that approximately 30% of all patients treated would get better even with a 'dummy' treatment (intervention), it has now been shown that placebo benefits can occur in any proportion of a treatment group from almost none, to almost all, depending on the condition and circumstances.

It is not surprising therefore that such potency can also generate the opposite of a placebo—the adverse reaction, (even when a dummy pill has been given)—known as the nocebo phenomenon.

Most extraordinary of all is that adverse-placebo (nocebo) has been demonstrated in measurable physiological signs (altered blood test results) from the patients, not just reported symptoms!

In 1999 the liver enzyme alanine transaminase (ALT) was measured in a study monitoring 93 healthy volunteers all of whom were given a placebo (dummy) medicine over 14 days. During this time approximately 20% of them developed elevated ALT levels.

ALT is commonly used as a marker for liver damage, so this would have raised considerable concern if a real drug or herb was being tested.[28]

The power of adverse suggestibility occurs when the patient expects adverse events, or when patients learn from previous experiences to expect adverse events. Anxiety, among other conditions, increases the likelihood of nocebo response. So under certain conditions patients are more likely to report, and sometimes more likely to actually experience, adverse reactions.

In our own practices, patients have self-selected themselves and probably thought long and hard about whether to invest their time, trust and money in seeing a medical herbalist instead of their doctor. In that scenario, we have found that people are prepared to 'put up' with some transient discomfort to achieve their aims. They may not have instant results and may have to spend more money with us 'in faith' that given time, improvements will be seen. They also may notice discomforts ranging from the nasty taste of the 'unfamiliar' medicine, mild indigestion sensations on using it, or even the occasional transient 'healing crisis' where symptoms may appear that show that the body is responding to treatment and mobilising the immune response. For example a cough may become more productive before clearing altogether.

But patients who have self-selected themselves for complementary medicine have probably already committed themselves and have a more positive and benevolent attitude to this unconventional treatment. This is a regular criticism we receive from doctors when we give presentations on herbal medicine—self-selection is thought to induce a more powerful placebo response. Conversely however anxiety about the possible dangers of stepping outside of the doctor's advice may elicit a nocebo response.

A mini case history

A patient seen for a first follow-up consultation was delighted at the significant improvements to their mood (they had presented with depression), improvements to energy levels, headaches and digestive symptoms but also wanted to report that they had experienced an adverse event. They reported that they had been repeatedly woken from their sleep at around 3am since using the herbal prescription, but they were prepared to continue the herbs because so many other symptoms had been relieved.

However, recorded in the notes from their first visit, one of their original symptoms was waking at 3am on a regular basis. The patient was amazed, and admitted they had forgotten that this symptom had been present before starting treatment. They also admitted that they could not conceive of a drug (even a herbal one) having no side effects—if it works, there must be adverse events—by definition.

Quick checklist for clinicians advising patients about the use of herbal medicine

These groups of people should seek the advice of a qualified medical herbalist rather than buy over-the-counter herbal medicines.

- Patients who are at higher risk of herb–drug interaction or idiosyncratic drug reactions.
- Patients using drugs that are within a high-risk therapeutic area.
- Patients who are self-medicating with herbal medicines without success.
- Patients who are using herbal medicines long term rather than for short-term or minor ailments.
- Patients who may be pregnant or be medically compromised through frailty, age or health.

The future

This introductory chapter places herbal medicine as practised in the UK within its own unique historical context. The ecological viewpoint of the modern herbalist is a unique lens through which to apply herbs therapeutically. Although the development of modern phytotherapy has run parallel with that of conventional biomedicine, it remains unique and different to it. The core principles of person-centred, individualised symptomatology and recognition of the complexity and synergy of plants as medicines make the herbalist also unique.

It has potentially made it all the more challenging in conveying to the public, the media, other health care professionals and researchers, what herbal medicine is. It places herbal medicines outside the normal scope for gold-standard research as is currently practised, and also makes it difficult therefore for governments and institutions to legislate for herbal medicine alongside conventional funded care. Nevertheless evidence in the areas of efficacy, quality and safety has matured, and progress continues.

> time has allowed an evolution from a traditional medicine for coping with life-threatening illnesses, before ambulances, powerful modern synthetic medicines and hospitals, to one that can live alongside these services and meet their shortfalls.
>
> —Simon Mills

We hope that you have enjoyed this brief introduction to what is a very complex and absorbing subject area. We have attempted to address some of the more poorly understood 'thorny' issues surrounding the practice of Western herbal medicine. In the following chapters we will look more closely at 'how herbalists think', and give you examples of how this thinking bears fruit.

Useful websites

https://www.henriettes-herb.com/
www.healthyhildegarde.com
https://pfaf.org
Greive, M. 1st edition, 1931. *A Modern Herbal*. Also available, in part, online: http://www.botanical.com/botanical/mgmh/mgmh.html

Professional organisations of medical herbalists:
The National Institute of Medical Herbalists
(est. 1864) www.nimh.org.uk
Other UK based herbal professions are listed at:
www.herbalist.org.uk

Where to train in the UK to be a medical herbalist:
Find out up to date information at:
https://www.nimh.org.uk/becoming-a-herbalist

Heartwood
heartwood-uk.net

Lincoln College, UK
https://www.lincolncollege.ac.uk/courses/
bsc-hons-clinical-herbalism/

References

1. Manniche and Lise., *An Ancient Egyptian Herbal*. 1999: British Museum Press.
2. Sinead Spearing. A History of Women in Medicine. 2019: Pen & Sword Books.
3. Pollington, S., *Leechcraft: Early English Charms, Plantlore, and Healing*. 2000: Anglo-Saxon Books.
4. Van Arsdall, A., *Medieval Herbal Remedies: The Old English Herbarium and Anglo-Saxon Medicine*. 2002: Routledge.
5. Green, M., *The Trotula: A Medieval Compendium of Women's Medicine*. 2001: University of Pennsylvania Press.
6. Francia, S. and A. Stobart, *Critical Approaches to the History of Western Herbal Medicine: From Classical Antiquity to the Early Modern Period*. 2014: Bloomsbury Press.
7. Sinclair and E. Rohde, *The Old English Herbals*. 1922: Minerva Press.
8. Pughe, J., *The Physician's of Myddfai: The Medical Practice of the Celebrated Rhiwallon and His Sons, of Myddfai, in Camarthenshire*. 1993.
9. Allen, D. and G. Hatfield, *Medicinal Plants in Folk Tradition: An Ethnobotany of Britain and Ireland*. 2004: Timber Press.
10. Grigson, G., *The Englishman's Flora*. 1975: Paladin Books.
11. Milliken, W. and S. Bridgewater, *Flora Celtica: Plants and People in Scotland*. 2004: Berlinn Ltd.
12. Haller J. S. Jr, *The People's Doctors: The American Botanical Movement 1790–1860*. 2000: Southern Illinois University Press.
13. Wood, M., *The Magical Staff: Essential Doctrines of Western Vitalist Medicine*. 1993: North Atlantic Books.
14. Romm, A., *Botanical Medicine for Women's Health*. 2010: Churchill Livingstone.
15. Wood, M., *The Practice of Traditional Western Herbalism*. 2004: North Atlantic Books.

16. West, V. and A. Denham, *The clinical reasoning of Western herbal practitioners: a feasibility study*. Journal of Herbal Medicine, 2017. 8: pp. 52–61.

17. Barker, J., *Notes toward a therapeutic model of phytotherapy in Britain*. British Journal of Phytotherapy, 1991. 2(Spring): pp. 38–46.

18. Priest, A. W. and L. R. Priest, *Herbal Medication: A Clinical and Dispensary Handbook*. 2nd ed. 2000. ed. 1983: C.W. Daniel Company Ltd.

19. Köberl, et al., *The microbiome of medicinal plants: diversity and importance for plant growth, quality and health*. Frontiers in Microbiology, 2013. 4: p. 400.

20. Nahrstedt, A., *Pharmakokinetic synergy of constituents in Herbal Medicine Products*. Planta Medica, 2008. 74(3).

21. Tobyn, G., A. Denham and M. Whitelegg, *The Western Herbal Tradition*. 2011: Churchill Livingstone.

22. Sackett, D. L. et al., *Evidence based medicine: what it is and what it isn't*. BMJ, 1996. 312(7023): pp. 71–72.

23. Edwards, S. E. et al., *Phytopharmacy: An Evidence-Based Guide to Herbal Medicinal Products*. 2015: Wiley Blackwell.

24. Bone, K. and S. Mills, *Principles and Practice of Phytotherapy: Modern Herbal Medicine*. 2nd ed. 2013: Churchill Livingstone.

25. Bone, K. and S. Mills, *The Essential Guide to Herbal Safety*. 2005: Elsevier, Churchill Livingstone.

26. Sue Evans PhD, Catharine Avila PhD, Ian Breakspear MHerbMed, Jason Hawrelak PhD, Ses Salmond PhD. *Report on the safety of the oral consumption of the pyrrolizidine alkaloid containing herbs Symphytum officinale, Tussilago farfara and Borago officinalis*. Report to the National Institute of Medical Herbalists, September 2018.

27. Moerman, D., *Meaning, Medicine and the Placebo Effect*. 2002: Cambridge University Press.

28. Rosenzweig, P., N. Miget and S. Brohier, *Transaminase elevation on placebo during phase I trials: prevalence and significance*. British Journal of Clinical Pharmacology, 1999. 48(1): pp. 19–23. https://doi.org/10.1046/j.1365-2125.1999.00952.x

CHAPTER TWO

Developing knowledge of plants: an introduction to plant science

Introduction

For many embarking on a study of herbal medicine, it is the plants themselves that are so attractive and interesting. Their extraordinary diversity and beauty combined with their manifold usefulness provokes wonder and fascination. Plants have formed a major role as food, as medicine and as comfort at key stages of our lives since the earliest humans walked this Earth; plant medicines are also used by other-than-human species including other primates. Many cultural applications of plants are so embedded as to form part of language and ritual, even in the most modern of societies.

This chapter explores some fundamentals of plants as living organisms, in the same way that we look at human anatomy and physiology. Building our knowledge in the accurate identification and classification of plants and their families helps create a sound basis for expanding this learning. Using this information to sensorially deepen your knowledge of plants will continue your study and learning well beyond this introduction, and the scope of this book. In three of the following chapters

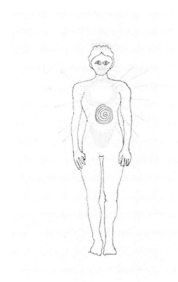
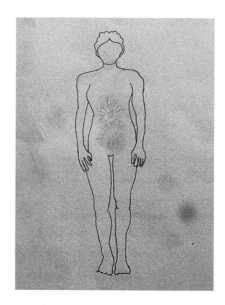

Tea tasting Exercise: Mary and Anita independently taste fennel seed. Drawing of 'how it feels'.

of this book we will look in more depth at 15 key medicinal plants used in Western herbal medicine. We can all read and research in great detail about each of these magnificent healing herbs. We would invite you, however, to first consider them as the living beings that they are, and to explore your own interaction with them.

In this chapter we will teach you a simple tasting technique to introduce the concept of using our senses to gain information about plants. You can then compare this to what others have written about those medicinal plants and their effects.

We begin however, by looking closely at four key medicinal plant families. We will explore similarities within those families, whether in terms of structure, or in terms of compounds and medicinal uses, and we will introduce some of the compounds created by plants that are of particular use to the herbalist.

The scientific naming of plants

Plant families included in this chapter include the rose family, the carrot or parsley family, the mint or deadnettle family and the sunflower or daisy family. In botanical science, plants are given scientific names, and are grouped then into scientific families.

Each scientific family name ends in 'aceae':

Carrot family: Apiaceae
Mint family: Lamiaceae
Sunflower or daisy family: Asteraceae
Rose family: Rosaceae

All these four families are dicotyledonous plants (see definition below), and many will be familiar to you. For example, in the Rosaceae we have apple, pear, cherry, apricot, almond, as well as roses of all types. Of the two main divisions of plants—dicotyledons and monocotyledons, the dicots form by far the largest group.

> **Definition—*Dicotyledons*:** Dicotyledons are plants that grow from the embryo within the seed with a pair of first leaves, or seed leaves, known as cotyledons.
>
> Alliums or members of the onion and garlic family are **monocotyledons** having a single seed leaf. Other well-known monocotyledenous plants include ginger (*Zingiber officinale* Roscoe.), and turmeric (*Curcuma longa* L.).

These families can be further divided into tribes and sub-tribes, and eventually into genera (*singular = genus*). The genus is important because it is the first name of the *two* scientific Latin names given to individual plants. The second name refers to the species of that plant genus. Whenever we refer to the scientific name of a plant, we will use the genus name followed by the species name.

So let's take thyme as an example. You may know that there are many different types of thyme, such as common or garden thyme (*Thymus vulgaris* L.), and wild creeping thyme (*Thymus serpyllum* L.).

Each one is in the genus *Thymus*, in the mint family (*Lamiaceae* family), and we can be sure which thyme we are talking about by adding the name of the species of thyme to the genus name to create the scientific name e.g., *vulgaris*.

Thus, as you can see from these examples, using the scientific name avoids confusion:

Alchemilla vulgaris aggr. auct. = Lady's mantle
Alchemilla arvensis (L.) Scop. = parsley piert
Petroselinum crispum (Mill.) Fuss = garden parsley

This format of genus + species is called binomial nomenclature, and was first developed into formal taxonomy by Carl Linnaeus. Note that the genus name carries a capital letter, the species name does not, and both are usually written in italics. Humans, for example, are classified as *Homo sapiens*, European green woodpeckers are *Picus viridis*. The name of the particular variety of the species can also be added after the species name to make the classification even more exact (e.g., *Thymus vulgaris* Argenteus (silver thyme)). Note that the variety is not written in italics. You can also see, at the end of the latin names the initial of the botanist who named that plant. For example *Curcuma longa* L. where the L stands for Linnaeus. Another custom to note relates to how the latin name changes over time. If a plant is re-named, the initials of the botanist who originally named the plant are then put in brackets and the initials of the botanist who supplied the new name are put after this. You can see an example of this on the previous page where *Petroselenium crispum* (Mill.) *Fuss.* was originally named by the botanist Philip Miller, and later renamed by Johann Fuss.

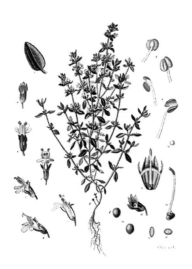
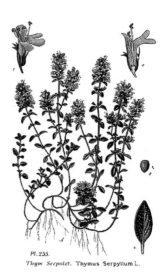

Common thyme (*Thymus vulgaris* L.)   Creeping thyme (*Thymus serpyllum* L.)

Common names and scientific names

It can seem intimidating to learn the scientific name for each plant. Common names often seem easier to remember than scientific names, but they are not as precise and do not reflect modern scientific taxonomy.

Not only can a common name refer to many different plants, but a single species can have more than one common name; there may be lots of common names for the same plant! This can lead to confusion, and potentially to serious problems if people confuse poisonous species or varieties with harmless ones. The scientific name is truly international and so also forms a shared language across the world.

Here in the UK, a record of local names for the same plant was recorded by Geoffrey Grigson in his book *An Englishman's Flora* first published in 1975 by Paladin Books. His list of names used for St John's wort, *Hypericum perforatum* L. include:

Amber	Balm of the warrior's wound
Cammock	St John's wort
Penny John	Rosin rose
Touch-and-heal	

The names often hint at earlier uses.[1]

Common and botanical names are often interesting as a record of social history and may also contain information about the plant itself.

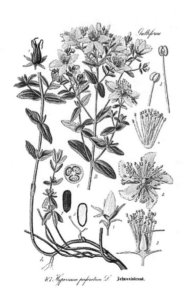

St. John's wort
(*Hypericum perforatum* L.)

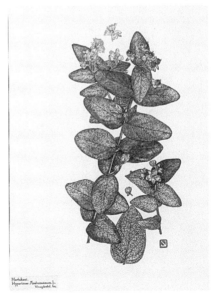

Shrubby St. John's Wort
(*Hypericum androsaemum* L.)

Hypericum perforatum L., and a related plant *Hypericum androsaemum* L. were both sometimes referred to as 'Amber'. This name was supposedly because of the dried leaves when crushed smelled like ambergris. One explanation of the name Hypericum is from a corruption of the name 'park' by which this plant was known to ancient herbalists. Before scientific nomenclature had properly catalogued *Hypericum androsaemum* L. it was incorrectly thought to be the *agnus-castus* described by Pliny (*Vitex agnus-castus* L.). This is an example from antiquity of why standardising names for plants is very important and helpful.

> **Definition—*Authority citation*:** In scientific botanical nomenclature, an author citation refers to the person or group of people who first published the scientific name of a plant as specified by the international code of nomenclature. Standardisation of author names has been achieved for almost all plants, so that for example, a plant classified by Carl Linnaeus (1707–1778), is now cited as L. So—*Alchemilla vulgaris* L. refers to Lady's mantle, as classified by Linnaeus.

Scientific names can give you important information about a plant.

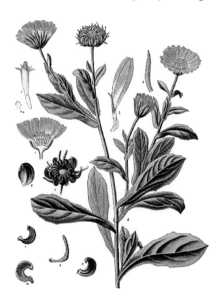 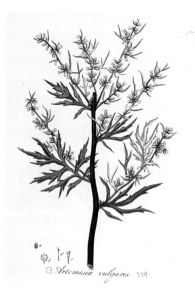

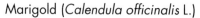

Marigold (*Calendula officinalis* L.)   Mugwort (*Artemisia vulgaris* L.)

For example, the use of the variety name 'officinalis', meaning 'of the office', tells us that it was once an officially recognised medicinal plant. An example is marigold, *Calendula officinalis* L.

Also, the use of the variety name, as in 'vulgaris', meaning 'used commonly by people', signifies the traditional use in folk traditions as a medicinal plant. An example is mugwort, *Artemisia vulgaris* L.

Four important medicinal plant families

One of the (many) magnificent things about herbal medicine is that you can meet the agents of healing, the plants themselves, in their natural environment. You can interact closely with plants on many levels, including being out in nature, and observing the changes with the seasons. It is interesting to reflect on what happens through the cycle of the year, noticing the changes all living beings need to make in summer heat or winter cold.

Members of particular plant families are often recognisable by similarities of form, for example similarities between their flowers, stems, seeds and fruits. We now look in more detail at the Apiaceae, Lamiaceae, Asteraceae and Rosaceae plant families as used in herbal medicine. What features do plants share within the same family, and are there compounds and medicinal actions that are shared too?

It is great to learn about wonderful plants growing near where you live. Perhaps you have a plant from one of these families you can get to know more, over the coming year? Correct plant identification is the place to start, and is essential if you intend to use a herb collected from the wild, or even from your garden. Using a plant identification guide-book is complicated at first but becomes easier with practice. Identification of plants is often easiest when the plant is flowering and sometimes impossible when it is not. Learning a new plant in your locality, and revisiting it throughout the year will help you notice it in other locations and commit it to memory. Buying species-correct plants from a nursery, and then growing them in your garden is another way to really get to know a plant in more depth. You may then notice all sorts of features that are not necessarily recorded in popular plant manuals.

Using a hand lens, smelling, tasting, feeling, growing and harvesting plants are all ways we can use our senses to enrich our plant knowledge through observation, just as we use observation techniques in the practice of herbal medicine.[2]

Foraging guidelines

When foraging or out trying to identify a plant for edible/medicinal purposes, it is very important that you are absolutely certain you have identified it correctly before tasting it, and sometimes even before picking it, as some plants have an irritant sap.

- Mid-spring is a good time of year to start identification.
- If in doubt, ask someone, and never eat anything about which you are not 100% certain.
- Always ask permission of the landowner before picking. Take care not to trespass.
- Check you are not picking a rare protected plant species.
- Avoid contaminated sites (industrial, commercial, canine) where possible.
- Do not over-pick nor take all of a plant from one site.
- Only harvest from abundant populations.
- Leave plenty for other wild creatures.
- Do not take more than you need.
- Avoid or minimise damage to habitat—do not trample!
- Remember the Countryside Code.

Some checks to ensure correct identification:

Location does the plant grow in the location specified in your wildflower guide?

Time of year is this plant flowering at the expected time of year? If not, it may be something else.

Height does your plant fit within the height range given?

Stems stems can rise from the base of the plant or branch out from a main stem. Stems can be rough or smooth, ridged, hollow, coloured or hairy.

Leaves take your time to really observe. Leaves are remarkably variable even on one plant. Look for leaf shape, leaf margin, leaf veining, the upper surface and underneath of the leaf, and whether the leaf is smooth (glabrous) or hairy (hirsute).

Petals or sepals check for shape, number, the colour of petals and sepals.

Flowers check not just colour, but flowering time and shape. Stamens and stigma are the male and female reproductive organs, and also usually occur in a specific number, and arrangement.

Seed how does your plant manage seed dispersal? Use a hand lens to see the seed more clearly.

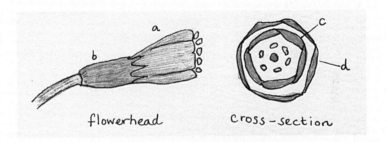

flowerhead   Cross-section

Definitions—Petals (a) are modified leaves that surround the reproductive parts of flowers. They are often brightly coloured or unusually shaped to attract pollinators. They are usually accompanied by another set of specialized leaves called **sepals (b)**. The group of petals in one flower are collectively called the **corolla (c)**, a group of sepals collectively form a **calyx (d)**.

Carrot family (Apiaceae)

(Known as the carrot, celery or cow parsley family).

This family consists of plants that can be annual, biennial or perennial.

Definition—Annual, perennial, biennial: Annuals germinate, blossom, produce seed and die in one growing season. Perennials flower reliably every year. Their leaves may die back, but the roots do not, the plant re-emerges from this root. Biennials take 2 years to complete their biological lifecycle. They develop their leaves (often in a rosette), stem (often very short) and roots in the first year, then produce flowers and seed in the second. In doing so, they usually use up their root storage and die. This is particularly important for medicinal plant harvesting of biennials, like *Angelica archangelica* L. The roots will ideally be harvested at the end of the first year, and before the start of the growth in the second.

A central characteristic of this family is that their flowers can often be grouped in broad or tight heads known as umbels. All the flowers are borne on stalks arising from one point on the main stem, a), rather like the spokes of an umbrella. Each main spoke can be further divided into secondary umbels b).

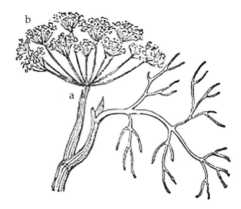

The mass of numerous small flowers held closely together in broad, flat or rounded heads is ideal for insects to land on, thus promoting pollination.

The leaves of members of this family are alternate. Alternate leaves occur when leaves are arranged singly, in an ascending spiral arrangement along a branch or stem.

Leaves are large and generally pinnately divided (feather like), often with inflated and sheathing leaf bases.

Flowers of the Apiaceae are generally made up of five sepals and five petals separate, usually notched with an incurve.[3]

This family can be difficult to correctly identify out in the field. Be very careful to avoid picking (due to skin reactions), or ingesting (due to poisonous compounds) certain members of this family such as giant

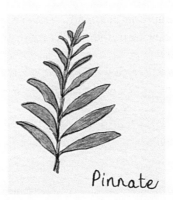

Pinnate

Definition—*Pinnate*: feather-like. Pinnate leaves of yarrow or elder show different types of pinnate leaf forms.

hogweed *Heracleum mantegazzianum* Sommier & Levier., hemlock water dropwort *Oenanthe crocata* L. or fool's parsley *Aethusa cynapium* L.

Despite these more poisonous family members, this family also contains some of the most fantastic, useful and important medicinal plants for herbalists including:

- Celery, *Apium graveolens* L.
- Chervil, *Anthriscus cerefolium* Hoffm.
- Sweet cicely, *Myrrhis odorata* (L.) Scop
- Alexanders, *Smyrnium olusatrum* L.
- Aniseed, *Pimpinella anisum* L.
- Fennel, *Foeniculum vulgare* Mill.
- Dill, *Anethum graveolens* L.
- Garden parsley, *Petroselinium crispum* (Mill.) Nyman.
- Caraway, *Carum carvi* L.
- Coriander, *Coriandrum sativum* L.
- Lovage, *Ligusticum levisticum* L.
- Garden angelica, *Angelica archangelica* L.
- Wild angelica, *Angelica sylvestris* L.

Plant compounds of this family, other than aromatic volatile oils and resins, include coumarins (e.g., umbelliferone), furo-coumarins, chromono-coumarins, terpenes and sesquiterpenes, triterpenoid saponins and acetylenic compounds. Alkaloids occur rarely in Apiaceae plants, although hemlock *Conium maculatum* L. contains the alkaloid coniine.[4]

We examine the important plant constituents called saponins, later in this chapter.

Mint family (Lamiaceae)

(Known as the mint or deadnettle family).

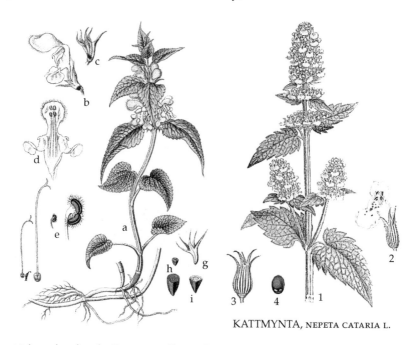

KATTMYNTA, NEPETA CATARIA L.

White deadnettle (*Lamium album* L.)   Catnip (*Nepeta cataria* L.)

This family is made up of herbs or shrubs, generally with square stems, often with glandular and aromatic trichomes (hair-like projections) on their surfaces. It includes plants such as mints, thymes and woundworts, all of which have a recognisable scent.[5]

Leaves are opposite, and usually simple. Opposite leaves occur when two leaves grow at the same position on the stem on opposite sides. Often the next pair of leaves will grow higher up the stem at right angles to the pair below, and so on up the stem towards the flower clusters.

The flowers of plants in this family are referred to as irregular or zygomorphic and are found on the stem in distinct lateral clusters or verticillasters. These often whorl around the stem, making a leafy spike known as a panicle.

If you look at white dead nettle, *Lamium album* L. flowers or catnip, *Nepeta cataria* L. you will recognise the distinct shape of the flowers of this family.

Definition—*Zygomorphic*: Botanical adjective (of a flower) having only one plane of symmetry, as in a pea or snapdragon. Bilaterally symmetrical.

In botanical classification, flowers of the Lamiaceae family are described thus:

The calyx has five teeth, sometimes two-lipped. The corolla is two-lipped with a couple of exceptions, and the lower lip is three-lobed, the upper lip is two-lobed.[3]

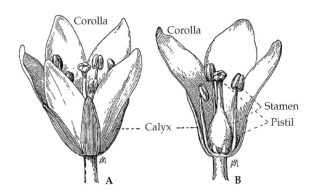

This botanical 'shorthand' conveys a lot of information and can be difficult to follow at first. We can use books on wildflowers to help us identify plants, both by using the pictures and this botanical shorthand. It gets easier with practice.

There are over 3000 species of Lamiaceae worldwide, including many familiar aromatic medicinal herbs such as:

- Lemon balm, *Melissa officinalis* L.
- Basil, *Ocimum basilicum* L.
- Thyme, *Thymus vulgaris* L.
- Rosemary, *Rosmarinus officinalis* L.
- Lavender, *Lavandula officinalis* L.

- Motherwort, *Leonurus cardiaca* L.
- Sage, *Salvia officinalis* L.
- White horehound, *Marrubium vulgare* L.
- Catnip, *Nepeta cataria* L.

Many of the species of the Lamiaceae are used as ornamentals, garden and culinary herbs as well as medicinal or aromatic herbs in cosmetics, foods, hygiene products and perfumery. The secondary metabolites made by this family include terpenoids and flavonoids, although alkaloids, iridoids and ursolic acid have been found. Many of the medicinal uses are assumed to be connected to the terpenic constituents of the essential oils of these plants, which are fungicidal, antispasmodic and prebiotic.[6]

> **Definition—*Secondary metabolites:*** Secondary metabolites are specialised organic compounds produced by plants that are not required for normal growth, photosynthesis, development or reproduction. They are made and broken down in response to environmental factors, and may be essential for protection from insect or microbial attack for example.
>
> It is these secondary compounds that are of particular use to the herbal medicine user over and above the proteins and carbohydrates, vitamins and minerals made by plants that we might use for food.

A discussion of the properties of essential oils will be made later in this chapter.

Daisy family (Asteraceae)

(Known as the daisy or sunflower family).

The daisy, like the sunflower, is easily recognisable; but what appears to be the flower of the daisy is in fact an inflorescence—a head of many, many tiny flowers or tubular florets, grouped together in a head or capitulum, often with lingulate (strap-shaped) ray florets looking like petals around the outer edge.

In the case of common daisy, *Bellis perennis* L., this arrangement gives the appearance of white petals around a yellow centre, but what we are actually seeing is white strap-like ray florets a), arranged around like rays of the sun, around a capitulum or head, of many tiny individual yellow flowers, b).

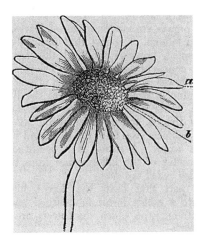

This head, known as a disc floret, may be flattened or domed. The disc florets of the sunflower, *Helianthus annuus* L. can appear quite flattened, whereas the daisy is often more domed.

If you have a small hand lens with 5X or 10X magnification, it is fascinating to look at plants in the daisy family and see in magnification all the tiny flowers that make up the head or capitulum.

Interesting Fact: Daisies

The name 'daisy' is from the words 'days-eye', meaning the flowers move on their stems and follow the sun rising in the East and setting in the West.

Members of the daisy family have either all strap or ligulate florets, like a dandelion, *Taraxacum officinale* F.H.Wigg. or they have all *tubular* florets, like common tansy, *Tanacetum vulgare* L.

Moreover, not all members of the Asteraceae have florets sitting on a flat capitulum like a daisy. One such example is the wonderful wild mugwort, *Artemisia vulgaris* L., and another is the equally charismatic, wild yarrow, *Achillea millefolium* L.

The *Echinacea* species belong to the Asteraceae family, and demonstrate firm florets in the centre of the capitulum, giving rise to their name meaning 'like a hedgehog', from the Greek 'Ekhinos'.

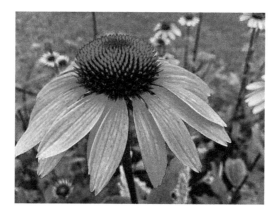

Other important medicinal plants found within the Asteraceae family include:

- Burdock, *Arctium lappa* L.
- Milk thistle, *Silybum marianum* (L.) Gaertn
- Goldenrod, *Solidago virguarea* L.
- Elecampane, *Inula helenium* L.
- German chamomile, *Matricaria chamomilla* (L.) Rauschert
- Pot marigold, *Calendula officinalis* L.
- Feverfew, *Tanacetum parthenium* (L.) Sch.Bip
- Arnica, *Arnica montana* L.
- Roman chamomile, *Anthemis nobilis* L.
- Boneset, *Eupatorium perfoliatum* L.
- Wormwood, *Artemisia absinthium* L.
- Gumweed, *Grindelia camporum* Greene
- Coltsfoot, *Tussilago farfara* L.
- Tansy, *Tanacetum vulgare* L.

Ethnopharmacological studies have identified the Asteraceae family of plants as containing some members with notable healing properties.[7] Our common daisy (*Bellis perennis* L.) has a long history of use in the treatment of wounds and bruises. Marigold (*Calendula officinalis* L.) is also a supreme healer from this family, and we will be looking at this more closely in Chapter 6.

Many Asteraceae members feature as food plants (sunflower *Helianthus annus* L. and artichoke, *Cynara cardunculus* L.), and they have many useful medicinal compounds including lipids, flavonoids, terpenoids, alkaloids, sesquiterpene lactones, essential oils and mucilages.[4]

We shall take a more in-depth look at the wonderful world of mucilages later in this chapter.

Rose family (Rosaceae)

(Known universally as the rose family).

A diverse family of trees, shrubs and herbs, this family includes well-known fruit-bearing plants such as apples, pears, almonds, peaches, apricots, strawberries, raspberries, cherries and sloes.

Their leaves are alternate, with either simple or compound leaf shapes.

The flowers are terminal and solitary, or appear in racemes, cymes or panicles.

Definition—Raceme, cyme and panicle: *These are all botanical words to describe variations in the structure of flower heads.*

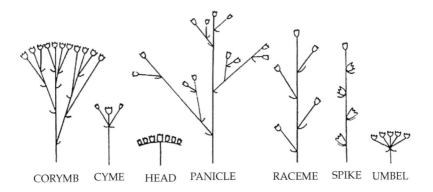

CORYMB   CYME   HEAD   PANICLE   RACEME   SPIKE   UMBEL

The flowers are usually composed of five sepals and five petals, but with numerous stamens.

The seeds can be few or many, and are highly variable—as are the fruits, which can vary from a collection of achenes as in meadowsweet, a drupe as in plum and cherry, druplets as in raspberry and blackberry or a pome in apples and pears.

Definition—*Drupe, drupelets and pomes:* These are all botanical words to describe variations in the structure of seeds.

Some of the wonderful medicinal plants in the Rosaceae family:

- Dog rose, *Rosa canina* L.
- Agrimony, *Agrimonia eupatoria* L.
- Meadowsweet, *Filipendula ulmaria* (L.) Maxim.
- Tormentil, *Potentilla erecta* (L.) Raeusch
- Raspberry, *Rubus ideaus* L.
- Blackberry, *Rubus fructicosus* L.
- Parsley piert, *Alchemilla arvensis* (L.) Scop. *Note: see how common names can be confusing—this is not a parsley!*
- Lady's mantle, *Alchemilla vulgaris* L.
- Hawthorn, *Crataegus monogyna* Jacq.

Rosaceae family plants contain a large number of useful medicinal compounds such as phenolic acids and polysaccharide compounds, flavonoid glycosides, procyanidins, xanthines, therapeutic tannins, as well as useful minerals and pectins.[5]

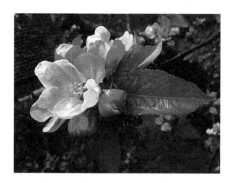

Bramley apple blossom
(*Malus domestica* L.)

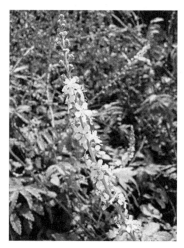

Agrimony
(*Agrimonia eupatoria* L.)

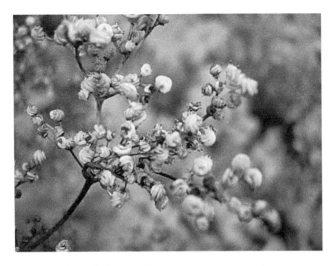

Spiral shape of meadowsweet seeds.

In the next section, we look at the plant compounds, the tannins, in more detail.

Plant constituents

In this section, we consider the chemical compounds found in plants in more detail, and review four plant constituents of particular relevance to herbal medicine—mucilages, tannins, saponins and essential oils.

Herbal medicine (phytotherapy) uses whole plants with their array of medicinal compounds, acknowledging synergy between them. Herbal medicine operates in that interesting greeny-grey area somewhere between food and drugs. This is not to be confused with homoeopathy, a completely different system and philosophy, that uses minute dilutions and vibrations of minerals, plants and animal extracts.

Many of the major dietary compounds found in plants beyond basic proteins, carbohydrates and fats, are classed as vitamins and minerals. Examples include the vitamin C found in berries and fruits of the Rosaceae, such as rosehip (*Rosa canina* L. fructus) or Blackcurrant (*Ribes nigrum* L. fructus). It is increasingly understood that many edible plants and herbs contain different types of antioxidant compounds (including vitamin C), and contribute to preventing cell damage around the body.[8]

The red and blue pigments synthesised by plants into red-blue coloured fruits and vegetables is a signature for the presence of anthocyanins, a secondary metabolite belonging to the class of compounds known as flavonoids. In plants, they may act as an attractor for pollinators or for attracting animals for seed dispersal. In the human body, flavonoids are known to have certain health benefits, rather than providing a direct food source. Flavonoids are mildly astringent, and contribute to the health and integrity of the membranes on the surfaces of our body, for example, in periodontal health and hygiene.[9] Flavonoids have also been investigated as one potentially anti-inflammatory constituent of willow bark working in synergy with other compounds. It is now recognised that the anti-inflammatory effects of willow are not entirely the result of salicylates.[10]

Fibre is another obvious dietary compound that is a potential contributor to health such as the soluble fibre found in linseed, or flax (*Linum usitatissimum* L.). Soluble fibre has an important *pre*biotic role as well as contributing to hormone balance and regulation.

Herbal medicine recognises that plant foods can have beneficial wellbeing outcomes, and many 'kitchen herbs' are positively medicinal. For example we can take therapeutic quantities (antibacterial quantities) of raw or powdered garlic (*Allium sativum* L.).

The herbalist may make recommendations about diet to utilise the helpful benefits of certain foods, but is also focussed on the therapeutic application of plant medicines to restore resilience and function. An assessment of the person's constitution and condition may also result in recommendations of eating certain foods. This is more than just about phytochemicals, in that it is also an 'energetic' assessment.[11]

Choosing a plant for an individual may involve interpretation of numerous beneficial compounds, so that a just a few herbs can formulate a prescription, yet have multiple therapeutic benefits.

> The drug (herbal medicine) changes the physis of the body, while on the other hand the food increases its substance.
>
> —Manfred Ullman[12]

Case history

A woman in her late 60s presented with a long history of digestive discomfort. She had persistent abdominal pain and bloating, with episodes or 'flare-ups' of frequent bowel motions—up to 20 per day. Between 'flare-ups' her bowel movements were twice daily but felt incomplete, and she had observed a corresponding urinary irritation if her bowels were very upset.

Diagnosed with coeliac disease, she also suspected she was lactose intolerant, and she successfully avoided those foods, whilst eating a balanced diet. She found that eating this way and taking probiotics had helped slightly.

She was motivated to see a medical herbalist after a prolonged 'flare-up' of her symptoms following a recent viral infection.

Using plants as a deliberate medicine to restore digestive function was discussed, and a herbal combination was suggested alongside the probiotic capsules and dietary care she had already introduced herself.

Her medicine contained agrimony herb (*Agrimonia eupatoria* L.), German chamomile flowers (*Chamomilla recutita* L.), lemon balm herb (*Melissa officinalis* L.), lavender herb (*Lavandula officinalis* L.) and Black walnut hull (*Juglans nigra* L.).

These plants were chosen for a variety of potential effects including antispasmodic, anti-inflammatory, increasing digestive enzymes, prebiotic, antiviral and relaxing and healing (vulnerary). The herbs used are gently warming (often useful for older people), and a balance between drying and moistening was also important.

The patient took a small dose of the combined herbal tincture at each meal to try to improve digestive capacity. She reported that within 24 hours she felt less bloated and thought some of the pains had subsided.

Within a week her bowel movements had regulated to two or three per day but were much more comfortable. After 12 weeks she had had no flare-ups, which had occurred at least monthly prior to starting treatment.

Changing her diet and taking probiotics had helped this lady, but the herbal medicines were specifically selected to address insufficiencies in the function of the gut and gently stimulate them to work.

Although identifying and testing secondary plant metabolites and compounds is a major focus of research, it is important that we should resist any temptation to assume that the action of any plant relies solely on the action of any *single* chemical or compound. The action of the whole plant *is always more than* the action of its parts. Synergy is increasingly seen as being a fundamental component of plant medicines in the biological sciences.[6]

Just as the human body can be broken down into parts in order to study its complexity, medicinal plants can be examined through their compounds, but the plant then needs to be reassembled whole for us to have completeness of understanding.

It is useful to look at plant compounds and constituents nevertheless as they can help to provide:

- Possible explanations for traditional use.
- Possible mechanisms for the medicinal actions of forgotten/un-investigated plants.
- Clarity about possible benefits or negative effects of medicinal plants.
- Illustrate the scope and diversity of plant pharmacology.

Secondary metabolites within a plant form part of an array of constituents, and here we look at four archetypal ones:

- Mucilages
- Tannins
- Saponins
- Essential oils

Mucilages

Mucilages are normal products of metabolism formed within plant cells, and may act as storage material, especially for germinating seeds where they act as a water reservoir.

Mucilages can be found in quantity in the epidermal cells of leaves, as well as inside seeds including psyllium, *Plantago ovata* Phil. (*formerly known as Plantago psyllium and isphagula*) and linseed, *Linum usitatissimum* L. Mucilages are also found in the roots of marshmallow, *Althaea officinalis* L. and in tree bark, for example slippery elm, *Ulmus fulva* Michx.[13]

Though extremely common in plants, gums and mucilages seem to be rather disregarded by pharmacologists. Their action in the human body is largely physical rather than chemical, and they are often capable of reaching the large intestine because they are not completely broken down by the stomach and small intestine in the digestive system. So they can have their demulcent healing effects all of their slippery way down the tubing.

Many well-known herbal medicines that are mucilage-containing have predictable effects on the digestive, respiratory and urinary systems, despite the fact that there will have been no direct contact with the mucilaginous compound beyond the digestive system; that is they do not come into physical contact with the lung or the bladder. This phenomenon raises an important pharmacological question often discussed in plant medicine—how do some medicinal plants manage to affect parts of the body, on a mechanical level, that they physically cannot reach?

It has been acknowledged that some body tissues—such as those found in the respiratory, urinary and digestive systems, share a common embryological root. Even after the embryo has developed and tissues have diversified, they may remain responsive to the same stimuli, and also respond similarly via reflex nerve pathways.[11]

Actions

Here are some of the potential medicinal actions of mucilages in humans:

- Demulcent (soothing, cooling, anti-inflammatory)
- Emollient (moistening, especially to mucous membranes)
- Nutritive (nourishing, improving tissue integrity)
- Emulsifying (making nutrients available for digestion)
- Prebiotic (encouraging microbiome establishment and diversity)
- Vulnerary (accelerating regeneration of tissues—healing)
- Aiding pharmaco-kinesis (helping with the movement of medicinal constituents into the body).

Traditional Western herbal medicine classifies mucilages as neutral in temperature and moistening. They are considered to be mild and agreeable, even to the most delicate patient. This traditional classification is recognised in addition to more recently discovered pharmacological properties. In Western herbal medicine, there is often a fusion of science with traditional or 'energetic' observations. For example, all medicinal herbs can be classified as being either Warm, Neutral or Cool.

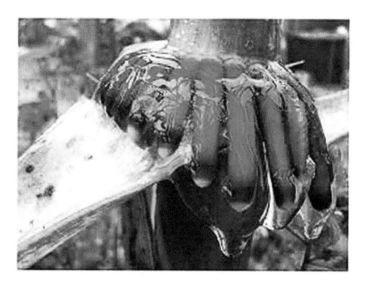

Mucilage dripping from a plant.

Medicinal plants containing significant quantities of mucilages include marshmallow, *Althaea officinalis* L.; comfrey, *Symphytum officinale* L.; linseed, *Linum usitatissimum* L.; psyllium seed, *Plantago ovata* Phil.; and slippery elm, *Ulmus fulva* Michx.

Mucilages are graded by the 'swelling index', that is, by their ability to swell and increase their surface area.[13] An alternative word would be gloop!

In the picture above, we can see a perfect example of a mucilage produced from a plant. The Sierra Mixe maize has aerial roots, which produce large quantities of mucilage, which it gives to bacteria for food in return for nitrogen. This is a fine example of 'gloop'.

Linseed, also known as flax seed, and psyllium seed are often left in water to swell before drinking. The product can then coat and soothe the linings of the digestive system. These herbs tend to taste very mild, and pleasant. It is usually the texture that initially offends some people. However, they are a really great way to explore our sensory interaction with plants!

Tannins

The term 'tannin' was first applied to substances present in plants able to combine with the proteins contained in animal hides, preventing their putrefaction and converting them into leather.

Two main groups of tannins are usually recognised—hydrolysable and condensed.

Hydrolysable tannins

If something is hydrolysable, it means it can be broken down by water. Plants that contain large quantities of hydrolysable tannins are not suitable for use internally, nor are they suitable for use on open wounds.

Condensed tannins

Condensed tannins are so named because they are formed from a condensation of molecules called *flavans*, related to the flavonoids, a group of compounds highly beneficial to health.[8] Unlike hydrolysable tannins, condensed tannins cannot be broken down by water, and tend to form red, insoluble substances and are largely responsible for the brownish colour of so many herbal tinctures! There is little evidence of ill-effects and much evidence of benefit from condensed tannins, so they are considered suitable for both internal use, and for application to open wounds.

One example of a very useful plant in the Rosaceae family is tormentil, *Potentilla erecta* (L.) Raeusch, which has condensed tannins in its reddish-brown roots. Tormentil was traditionally used to stop diarrhoea, and the positive effects of the tannins it contains are as follows:

- Dries up excessive watery secretions
- Heals digestive membranes
- Increases resilience of membranes against invading infection
- Potentially destroys invading organisms by their ability to precipitate proteins

From the beneficial effects of tannins listed above it is easy to see how and why tannins have a strong history of use externally in the treatment of burns. When a tannin solution comes into contact with tissue it interacts with the tissue proteins to form a tough, leathery structure called an eschar. The formation of this eschar acts to seal the wound, thus preventing subsequent infection and allowing new tissue to form.

Use of tannins for this purpose was practised during World War I, and was thought to be responsible for saving many lives.

Recent research published in the *Malawi Medical Journal* in 2005 revisited this technique and concluded that;

> *This study was not blinded. However, results of this pilot study suggest that the use of tannins may provide benefit by reducing colonisation of Staphylococcus aureus with better quality of healing and at the same time not increasing toxicity.*
>
> —L. Chokotho and E. van Hasselt[7]

(*We would like to stress here that any serious burn should be treated by a healthcare professional as a matter of urgency.*)

It has been observed that some plants increase their production of tannins in response to grazing by animals. This causes the animals to move on, and not over-graze a particular tree or shrub. Interestingly, the response to produce more tannins also occurs simultaneously in neighbouring plants, suggesting that some communication between plants is happening and the plants are helping each other out!

Many tannins have beneficial effects in small to moderate doses by sealing wounds and strengthening mucous membranes. Improvement to the resilience of any epithelial tissue will increase the immunity to infection there.[11] Taken in excess, tannins can inhibit nutrient absorption, so that excessive black tea consumption can lead to iron deficiency for this reason.

Interesting Fact: Tea

Incidentally, the plant in the UK we call 'tea' is in fact *Camellia sinensis* L. The word 'tea' actually refers to the method of preparation of an infusion or 'tisane'.

One traditional use of tannin-rich herbs is in mouthwashes to prevent or treat gum disease. Tannin-rich plants were traditionally used as snuff to treat nasal polyps. In barber's shops they were used to stop bleeding from shaving cuts.

You may already be familiar with witch hazel water, prepared from the medicinal plant *Hamamelis virginiana* L. This distilled water can be applied externally to bruises, helping to seal up the internally broken blood vessels that lead to bleeding under the skin, as in a bruise. Witch hazel water has been a common first aid box ingredient for bruises and sprains. It is prepared from the leaf of the witch hazel tree, and contains hydrolysable tannins that should be used externally only, and on unbroken skin. The bark of witch hazel contains only condensed tannins, and can therefore be used internally.

The sensation we associate with tannins is known as astringent, and the taste is described as Sour. Use of the word Sour with a capital S, suggests an energetic property. Western herbal medicine embraces modern science, but also honours the rational aspects of a more traditional or energetic approach.

Note: **Western herbal medicine perspective on 'sour' taste.** Small amounts of Sour tasting herbs are traditionally considered to increase digestive vigour and tone. They stop the membranes of the body from becoming too flaccid or floppy, and by doing so improve function. They stop 'leakage' and loss of vital reserves or nutrients and increase resilience and dynamic strength. These are qualities observed by our forebears that can be explained today in more scientific terms—endothelial resilience.

Saponins

Saponins are glycosides, characterised by their ability to produce frothy foam in water. Their molecular structure allows them to bind to water-soluble (hydrophilic) sugars at one end and fat-soluble (lipophilic) aglycones at the other end.

Taken by mouth, they are relatively harmless, absorbed poorly from the gut following interaction with bacteria in the colon and are regularly consumed in everyday foods. Tomatoes, *Solanum lycopersicum* L. contain saponins as do many grains.

Note: Plants in the Solanaceae (deadly nightshade) family, such as tomatoes, potatoes, peppers and chilli, contain a distinct sub-group of steroidal saponins known as steroidal-alkaloids that are possibly responsible for lowering plasma cholesterol concentrations.

Medicinal herbs that contain beneficial saponins include sarsaparilla, *Smilax ornata* Lem., a medicinal herb from the Americas used in non-alcoholic beverages. It was, and still is, used as a therapeutically valuable and safe saponin containing plant.

Saponins have a high molecular weight, and according to their structure are divided into two main groups: steroidal saponins (tetracyclic triterpenoids) and triterpenoid saponins (pentacyclic triterpenoids).

The systemic effects of different saponins include:

- Immunomodulatory, cytotoxic, anti-tumour and anti-mutagenic.
- Anti-inflammatory, anti-allergic, antiviral and antifungal.
- Anti-hepatotoxic and improves nutrient absorption.
- Anti-stress effects, expectorant and adaptogenic effects.

Steroidal saponins

Steroidal saponins are less common in the plant world than other types of saponin, but they are of great pharmacological importance. This is because of their relationship to important compounds in human physiology such as sex hormones, cortisone, diuretic steroids, vitamin D and cardiac glycosides.

Scientific understanding of plant steroidal saponins led to the development and manufacture of drugs such as the contraceptive pill, and a plant that played a crucial role in this development was the edible yam, *Dioscorea villosa* L., although the plant itself does not contain hormones comparable to the contraceptive pill. Interestingly, wild yam has a long traditional use in the relief of problems associated with sex hormone imbalance.

Plant steroidal saponins have the capacity to block or stimulate receptor sites in our body cells, producing an amphoteric effect.

> **Definition—*Amphoteric*:** Like a terracotta pot with two handles, it has a capacity to balance in either direction.

Another well-known plant containing steroidal saponins is fenugreek, *Trigonella foenum-graecum* L. which has a long history of use helping balance blood sugar levels.[14] In modern times, it has been shown to have an effect in reducing cholesterol levels and having a positive effect on hormones called androgens.[15]

Soya beans and ginsengs are other examples of plants containing steroidal saponins.

Triterpenoid (pentacyclic) saponins

This group of saponin compounds can be found in a wide range of dicotyledonous plants including liquorice, *Glycyrrhiza glabra* L., primrose, *Primula veris* L., marigold, *Calendula officinalis* L. and horse chestnut, *Aesculus hippocastanum* L. The saponins found in these plants have an array of therapeutic benefits, including anti-inflammatory and expectorant effects.

> **Definition—Expectorant:** An expectorant is a compound that makes coughing more effective by promoting the expulsion of mucous/phlegm. Mucous is produced by the body as a natural response to inflammation, in an effort to reduce that inflammation. A build-up of mucous can become a problem in its own right however, especially in the lungs.

Essential oils

Some of the most fascinating and complex of herbal constituents, essential oils (also referred to as volatile oils) are made up of several constituents.

The word volatile comes from the Latin *Volare,* meaning 'to fly', and refers to the fact that the fragrant oil is easily vaporised into the atmosphere where we can detect it with our olfactory cells, the smell receptors of our nose.

Poor quality, badly stored, badly prepared or old herbs can lose their essential oils, and thus lose a key component of their potential medicinal effect.

Curiously, essential oils are barely recognised as therapeutic agents by conventional medicine, excepting perhaps peppermint oil.

Mint family

The mint family contains a number of species that contain relatively large amounts of essential oil.

Fresh peppermint, *Mentha x piperita* L. contains 1% essential oil, and when you make an infusion of healthy peppermint leaves, the array of beneficial compounds in the tea includes essential oil of peppermint.

Note: Colpermin—a medical drug made of peppermint essential (volatile) oil in a capsule—is prescribed for the relief of IBS symptoms.

Using a distillation method, it is possible to isolate an essential oil and extract it from the other compounds found in the leaf. Peppermint pure essential oil is a highly aromatic volatile oil made up of a number of compounds including menthol. Isolated menthol is a highly irritant substance capable of burning the skin.

Definition—Menthol: An organic compound made synthetically or obtained from corn mint, peppermint or other mint oils. It is a waxy, crystalline substance, clear or white in colour, which is solid at room temperature.

The focus by the pharmaceutical industry on individual compounds within plants and their extraction leads to the isolation of substances that are markedly different from, and have different applications to, the original whole plant. They may not even be extracted from a plant at all. Drinking peppermint tea is a different experience from the use of peppermint essential oil in, say, a peppermint sweet, which is different again from using menthol, or mentholated products, which have been manufactured and need to be used with much more care.

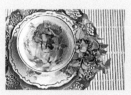 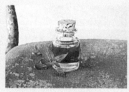 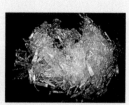

Peppermint tea   Peppermint oil   Menthol crystals

Compounds within essential oils

Naturally occurring essential oils are, chemically speaking, mixtures of hydrocarbons and oxygenated compounds including terpenes, monoterpenes and sesquiterpenes. Menthol is an example of a monoterpene, as is camphor. You may recognise these two monoterpenes from common decongestant lozenges and inhalants for blocked nasal passages.

Monoterpenes have antiseptic properties, increase blood flow and act on the nervous system to relax muscles via nerve reflexes. They can therefore help relax painful digestive spasm. They have also been shown to reduce nervous excitability, and there is current research investigating potential beneficial effects of monoterpenes on period pain and childbirth, echoing traditional use of these aromatic compounds in some cultures.[16,17]

Sensorial tasting of medicinal plants

Our knowledge about plant compounds is nowadays confirmed by technologies not available to our forebears. For ancient peoples it was the sensory clues that gave rise to understanding the usefulness of plants. We still have these highly accurate senses: sight, smell, taste, touch, sound, which can be utilised to help us recognise some of the key qualities that a plant may have.

It is popularly thought that knowledge about the medicinal usefulness of certain plants was gained by trial and error. Whilst to some extent and in certain circumstances this may be true, a number of alternative theories also have credibility.

When asked about how people learned about the medicinal or toxic qualities of the native botanicals, botanist, zoologist and author of the bestselling book *Supernature* Lyall Watson tells us he was told that they asked the plant, and the plant spoke to them. When pushed for exact details of this, he was told that a leaf or part of the plant was placed on the tongue and information was transmitted.

Although this may sound a rather esoteric explanation of learning, it is an explanation repeated in other traditional cultures around the world. It is a record of some form of communication between human and plant and vice versa.

A young German poet and 17th-century scientist Johann Wolfgang von Goethe explored and systematised a method of plant exploration and 'communication' and this method was taken up and recorded by Rudolf Steiner in the early 20th century. He was keen to *sensorially* experience *the phenomenon* (in our case a plant), as a whole, not as dissected parts. Their work offers a more qualitative approach to plant study but both authors were keen to emphasise rigour in the application of the process.

For Goethe, it was the use of our senses without the confounding factor of our intellect that would give us an insight into the signature or essence of a living plant being. It allows the phenomenon to be felt by the researcher, perhaps in the same way as an artist captures the essence of a thing, so that we can recognise an oak tree in a painting made of only a few brush strokes.

The contemplation and use of our own 'scientific instruments'—our senses, can allow profound recognition of inner laws, patterns and relationships that then facilitate the experience of a moment of 'intuition' and of the wholeness of the phenomenon as itself, or the 'ur-phenomenon' as Goethe called it.

Steiner developed this approach into anthroposophical medicine, and other authors and researchers have applied his methodology to plant study—such as Wilhelm Pelikan (*Healing Plants I* and *II*). Goethean methodology has also been used in architecture and other areas of life and is promoted by the Goethe Institute in Germany. The science of phenomenology continues to be used in other areas of research.

Goethean methodology was also taken forwards by two pioneering medical herbalists in the 1990s, Keith and Maureen Robertson. Keith and Maureen ran a School of Herbal Medicine in Glasgow, Scotland. They worked with Goethean practitioner Dr Margaret Colquhoun, founder of the Pishwanton Project, and developed the Goethean method for use by students of herbal medicine. They utilised this method to gain insight and deepen relationships with the medicinal plants they were studying and would eventually go on to use in practice.

We would like to acknowledge the source of some of the plant exercises we have included here as being from Keith and Maureen Robertson, medical herbalists, and their fabulous experimental work with Goethean scientist Margaret Colquhoun. Other herbalists have used sensory plant communication and developed techniques similar to this and we wish to acknowledge, Elisabeth Brooke, Hildegarde of Bingen, Juliet de Bairacli-Levi, Stephen Harrod Buhner, Carole Guyette and Christopher Hedley.

Speaking about how physicists strive to discover universal, elementary laws, Einstein once said;

> *There is no logical path to these laws; only intuition, resting on sympathetic understanding of experience, can reach them. The state of feeling which makes one capable of such achievement is akin to that of the religious worshiper or one who is in love.*
>
> —Albert Einstein

A sympathetic understanding of contemplation and experience is at the core of this, and is central to the practice of Goethean methodology.

Here we would like to introduce you to a simple tea tasting exercise involving the leaves of the magnificent nettle plant. This is a sensorial or organoleptic tasting and is used as a key component of plant study in the Heartwood Foundation Course. We reproduce a simplified version of the method here for your use if you wish to conduct your own contemplative sensory plant tastings as we look at more magnificent plants throughout this book. We recommend that you read through the next section thoroughly before embarking on a tea tasting so that you have a good sense of what is needed.

Definition—*Organoleptic*: acting on, or involving the use of, the sense organs.

Organoleptic tea tasting

We recommend you read through these notes on tea tasting once before you begin.

Preparation

- Make an infusion using 2 tablespoons of fresh nettle leaves, or 1 tablespoon of dried loose-leaf nettle.
- Pour freshly boiling water (approximately 200–300 ml) over the leaves and leave covered for 8–10 minutes.
- Whilst you are waiting, prepare yourself. Be in a comfortable place, with writing and/or drawing materials to hand. Maybe close your eyes for a moment. Take a few slightly deeper breaths. Notice, how

you feel. What sounds are around you? Relax. Be present in this moment, right now.

- We would like you to enter into this tasting experience with an open-hearted, innocent, child-like wonder. It is our intention that you enter into this exercise with a sense of humble excitement and anticipation—as if you are meeting a person for the first time. In a way—you are!

Step 1a

- Strain some of the infusion into a clean mug and begin by smelling the tea. Record your observations on the sheet provided.

Notes

You may feel the tea smells 'fruity', 'dry', 'moist', 'spicy', 'mineral-rich' or 'lemony', these are examples of good descriptive words to use. There may be more than just one or two words because of the complexity of compounds within a single plant. It is okay to have only one or two words.

You may also note that smell brings a feeling with it. Observing it is 'warm' 'comforting' or that it 'reminds you of something' are useful observations to make.

It is important not to slip into brain-led value-judgements here. We are using our hearts not our heads. We are enquiring with a completely open mind, and without trying to be clever or to derive a medicinal property. So, try not to say things like 'I feel this plant may be good for the liver' as this sort of comment has leapt well beyond observing that you per-haps have an awareness of your abdomen—even just from the smell, or perhaps an awareness of the ears or eyes—just from the smell.

By the way—these notes apply to when you are tasting, as well as when you are smelling, the infusion of the plant. Goethe emphasised that we should try to capture the brief moment as we experience a phe-nomenon, and immediately before our brains kick in to construct ideas around the experience. He said that *our senses are true, our brains and thinking are often not.* Also Goethe acknowledged that it is impossible to un-learn everything you know up to this point. So—tasting the infusion of a plant you are already familiar with will inevitably influence you consciously but also unconsciously.

Modern authors who are interested in this technique such as Stephen Buhner, Pamela Montgomery, and others, note that by employing a child-like, but enthusiastic or 'euphoric' state we secrete different hormones that affect our ability to allow information past our neural 'gating' channels. We induce a hormonal change that allows us to perceive more richly. It is that feeling you get when you are out in nature and filled with a deep sense of joy and harmony and possibly have a flash of insight or inspiration. Trying to feel this way also helps silence the critic in your head who is telling you that you are being silly!

Despite our tendency to allow prior knowledge to influence our senses—it is still worthwhile pursuing this practice. With practice, you will deepen your experience and you will expand your capacity to notice and then verbalise that experience. Maybe you do not feel anything at all at first. Don't try to force it, just keep going, observing, listening. After you have recorded everything you have noticed about the 'smell' (approximately 1–3 minutes), it is now time to taste the infusion that you have made.

Step 1b

- Begin by writing down all of the actual taste/tastes that you can. What does it taste like?
- You may at any point in smelling or tasting, experience a sense of colour or movement that is difficult to express in words. Use coloured pencils, pens or crayons to record these colours and movements.
- Re-taste the infusion as you consider the questions below.

Step 2

- As you taste the infusion, where does it go in your body?
- Does it stay in your mouth? Move to your pelvis or evaporate through your skin or none of these!? Suspend disbelief.

Step 3

- How does this plant feel like it moves around your body? Is it slow, sliding and syrupy? Is it tingly and active? Is it strong, fast or gentle in its movement and effect?

Step 4

- What is the infusion doing now you have observed where it is going?
- What is its effect now it is there? Again, be careful not to choose medical words, refrain from using your intellect to describe these active effects. Choose simple descriptive words, try to get right back to the feeling, rather than trying to interpret that feeling.

This tea-testing exercise is only one part of a whole methodology that is beyond the scope of this book to reproduce here.

Keep your tasting (and smelling) notes in a way that you can reference them again at a later date. Make a note of the date and time, the herb tasted and the method used to prepare it. You may taste this plant again and it would be interesting to compare experiences as you do more tastings through your training, and on into practice.

Here are some of our tasting notes from tasting nettle to give you an idea the process.

Nettle tea tasting notes: Example A

What does it smell like?
Slightly chewy. Green. Mild. A hint of citrus but more complex.

What does it taste like?
Warming and drying. Slightly sweet and slightly salty. Tastes like it has a lot of body. Supportive. Cleansing. Softer after 5 minutes. Reminds me of a very thin syrup.

Where is it going?
Pelvis and eyes.

How is it getting there?
Diffusing. Like smoke.

Nettle tea tasting notes: Example B

What does it smell like?
Warm, nutrient, spicy, cooking potatoes, apple-sharp notes, dark, earthy.

What does it taste like?
Soft smooth, pleasant, food-like, mineral, earthy, cooked/boiled vegetables.

Where is it going?
Everywhere! Very slowly works its way everywhere. I am aware of all parts of my physical body that help with balance, my ears, shoulders, hips, hands and feet. Also aware of my skin and my internal organs especially in my mid-back.

How is it getting there?
Still, solid, strong but light (not heavy), calm, balanced.

Note: Nettle. Nettles have adapted their leaves to create hairs known as trichomes that are modified epidermal cells consisting of a bulb filled with formic acid. This is the irritant we all recognise from handling *Urtica dioica* L.

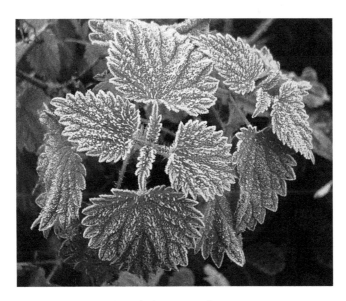

Nettle leaves in frost.

Nettles need no description, they may be found by feeling, on the darkest night.

—Nicholas Culpeper[18]

Conclusion

Many herbalists use this sensorial method, or something similar when dispensing their tinctures or making a medicine for a patient. It forms part of our pharmacognosy—the ability to confirm the identity of the commercial product as it arrives, macroscopically, and microscopically. It may be that a dried herb looks a little pale, or brownish on delivery, but using a trusted sense of smell or taste will alert you to any problems with your herbal material, as well as remind you why you love a particular herb.

We hope you have enjoyed this introduction to plants, their anatomy and compounds. Please see the book listed under Further Recommended Reading, which you will find under the Bibliography at the end of this chapter, if you would like to find out more about botany via an easy to use text. We intended to have set the scene for how plants form such a fundamental place as food and also as medicine. The compounds they contain can, and have been, studied independently because medicinal plants have so many identifiable compounds that have profoundly positive activity in human physiology. We also hope to bring you back to the whole. After looking at some of the key components such as tannins, mucilages, oils and saponins, we wish to keep hold of that interconnectedness between us, and nature: how we might trust our experience and our senses to explore and get to know common medicinal plants as wholes. We hope you have enjoyed trying out our tea tasting with one of the plants suggested. May this develop your own capacity to deepen your relationship with yourself and with herbal medicine. The feeling is the medicine!

Bibliography

Abraham, David, *The Spell of the Sensuous*. Penguin, 1996: Random House.

Brooke, Elisabeth, *Women Healers Through History*. 1993: The Women's Press.

Buhner, S. H., *The Secret Teachings of Plants: In the Direct Perception of Nature*. 2004: Bear and Company.

Mills, S., *Out of the Earth: The Essential Book of Herbal Medicine*. 1991: Penguin Books.

Pelikan, Wilhelm, *Healing Plants I and II Insights Through Spiritual Science*. 2012: Mercury Press.

Sutton, D., *Kingfisher Field Guide to the Wild Flowers of Britain and Northern Europe*. 1992: Kingfisher Books (cost effective quick guide).

Streeter, D., C. Hart-Davies, A. Hardcastle and L. Harper, *Collins Wild Flower Guide*. 2nd ed. 2016: William Collins (ideal for committed naturalists).

Watson, Lyall, *Supernature: A Natural History of the Supernatural*. 1993: Hodder & Stoughton.

Young, P., *The Botany Coloring Book*. 1999: Collins Reference.

Further Recommended Reading

Botany in a Day: The patterns method of plant identification. Thomas J. Elpel. 6.1 Edition. Jan 2018. MT, Hops Press.

References

1. Grigson, G., *The Englishman's Flora*. 1975: Paladin Books.
2. Colquhoun, M. and A. Ewald, *New Eyes For Plants: A Workbook for Observing and Drawing Plants*. 2002: Hawthorn Press.
3. Blamey, M. and C. Grey-Wilson, *Wild Flowers of Britain and Northern Europe*. 2003: Cassell.
4. Trease, G. E. and W. C. Evans, *Pharmacognosy*. 14th ed. 1989: WB Saunders Company.
5. Barker, J., *The Medicinal Flora of Britain and Northwestern Europe*. 2001: Winter Press.
6. Edwards, S. E. et al., *Phytopharmacy: An Evidence-Based Guide to Herbal Medicinal Products*. 2015: Wiley Blackwell.
7. Chokotho, L. and E. van Hasselt, *The use of tannins in the local treatment of burn wounds—a pilot study*. Malawi Med J, 2005. 17(1): pp. 19–20.
8. Pengelly, A., *The Constituents of Medicinal Plants: An Introduction to the Chemistry and Therapeutics of Herbal Medicine*. 2nd ed. 2004: CABI Publishing.
9. Odongo, C. O. et al., *Chewing-stick practices using plants with anti-streptococcal activity in a Ugandan rural community*. Front Pharmacol, 2011. 2: p. 13.
10. Untergehrer, M. et al., *Identification of phase-II metabolites from human serum samples after oral intake of a willow bark extract*. Phytomedicine, 2018. 57: pp. 396–402.
11. Mills, S., *Out Of The Earth: The Essential Book of Herbal Medicine*. 1991: Penguin Books.

12. Ullman, M., *Islamic Medicine*. 1997: Edinburgh University Press.
13. Evans, W. C., *Trease and Evans' Pharmacognosy*. 14th ed. 1999: W. B. Saunders.
14. Gaddam, A. et al., *Role of Fenugreek in the prevention of type 2 diabetes mellitus in prediabetes*. Journal of Diabetes & Metabolic Disorders, 2015. 14(74).
15. Rao, A. et al., *Testofen, a specialised Trigonella foenum-graecum seed extract reduces age-related symptoms of androgen decrease, increases testosterone levels and improves sexual function in healthy aging males in a double-blind randomised clinical study*. Aging Male, 2016. 19(2).
16. Fazel, N. et al., *Effects of Anethum graveolens L. (Dill) essential oil on the intensity of retained intestinal gas, flatulence and pain after cesarean section: A randomized, double-blind placebo-controlled trial*. Journal of Herbal Medicine, 2017. 8: pp. 8–13.
17. Mirmolaeea, S. T. et al., *Evaluating the effects of Dill (Anethum graveolens) seed on the duration of active phase and intensity of labour pain*. Journal of Herbal Medicine., 2014. 5(1): pp. 26–29.
18. Culpeper, N., *Culpeper's Complete Herbal*. 1995: Wordsworth Press.

The human body: a herbalist's eye view

Chapter 3: some suggestions for use

The human body provides us with a brilliant example of a complex, interactive ecosystem. Treatment and ultimate resolution of the many and various illnesses and injuries to which it can be exposed requires a good sound understanding of physiological principles, alongside knowledge of the healing art being practised.

Professional practising herbalists will have gained a very in-depth knowledge of anatomy and physiology (A&P) and, for those of you who are using this book as a companion text for the Heartwood Foundation Course, you will also be provided with more material than is represented here.

Ultimately though, to hope to achieve resolution of health issues arising amid the complexity that is the human body, a more ecological, rounded and complete overview of how physiological dysregulations affect the whole being is necessary. Therefore, although practising herbalists learn and understand anatomy and physiology in quite some depth, we specifically apply this knowledge using a more ecological approach to health and illness.

We have included this section on A&P, both to provide basic knowledge in this area, and to give some examples of how that knowledge is used on the more ecological level that underpins the basics of our practice.

We would like to recommend that, rather than reading this chapter from one end to the other, you just read the introduction and key concepts sections, and after this, use it as a handy guide to the basics of A&P that will complement information given in other chapters. Feel free to dip in and out of this particular stream of information at will, and where you feel that it is useful to you in terms of the overall flow of this book. We will provide suggestions, both in this chapter, and in subsequent ones, concerning what sections in this chapter will complement what sections in others. Take what you need.

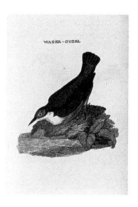

Happy Dipping

Introduction

It would not take any person long to figure out that looking at the structure and function of the human body, even on a simple level is a major proposition. The human body becomes more complex the more we look into it, much like a fractal. In fact the concept of fractals and of non-linearity is a whole area of study with regard to the calculus involved in medicine. You see? We are already getting complex!

Historically the mammoth task of the study of anatomy and physiology has been broken down into seemingly obvious sub-categories, such as the cardiovascular system, the musculoskeletal system etc. Modern-day medicine consequently is organised in this way, so that people specialise in certain body systems or areas. This approach has the advantage of developing a very in-depth understanding of well-defined areas of medicine, but also lends itself to fragmentation and isolation in our view of how the body works. Nonetheless, it is a very manageable way of dealing effectively with the vast amount of information involved. We just need to remind ourselves from time to time, that ultimately, everything is connected to everything else!

It makes good sense to look at anatomy and physiology together as they are natural dancing partners. The structures (anatomy) of our organs and organ systems have evolved to optimally facilitate their functions (physiology). If you were to design a toasting fork for example, you would probably put a good long handle on it so that you don't have to stand too close to the fire and risk getting burnt. The walls of the alveoli in the lungs are only one cell thick, to maximise the exchange of gases across their surface. 'Fit for purpose' is the phrase that may spring to mind, and all of the systems we will be looking at are magnificent examples of this.

All systems of the body interact to form a cohesive whole, and this integrated functioning unit is far superior to the sum of its parts: in fact, it is an example of *synergy* in action. In this chapter we will use the basic format of looking at systems of the body in a traditionally structured way, but we will also endeavour to link this in with the over-arching concepts of interconnectedness and complexity, giving relevant examples for each system. It is not our intention to provide a comprehensive A&P guide. Neither do we wish to re-invent the wheel. For those of you who are engaged on the Heartwood Foundation Course in Western herbal medicine, you will find more information in the coursework than is covered here on a basic A&P level. We do wish, however, to provide those of you who have general interest in herbal medicine with some basic information, coupled with an expansion of the underlying concepts of interconnectivity and complexity. Whole plant medicines are complex, and therefore often flexible in terms of their application. To optimise this precious feature, we often need to take a step back from the lens of specialised focus on body systems and look at where connections and inter-relations lie.

Henri Matisse is quoted as having said:

I don't paint things. I only paint the difference between things.

As herbalists we do not simply 'fix' organs or organ systems. We also provide support for the space between things, for flow to become optimised, and for inter-communications between things to become robust and healthy. We do not treat illness as an entity; rather we focus on the whole person as an entity.

This chapter will be divided into ten short sections. Each section will contain a brief overview of the system in question in terms of its individual A&P, followed by examples of interconnectivity with other systems. Some examples of interconnectivity have presented themselves obviously via their observed physiological interactions; other links between systems and how they inter-relate have been revealed as a result of the study of disease states (pathophysiology) and how, when things go wrong in one system, effects ripple out to others. These examples of interconnectivity are by no means comprehensive, but they do serve (we hope) to remind us of the whole beings that we are. We will mention a plant at the end of each section, to bring us back to the healing focus of this book. You may wish to read about certain body systems in conjunction with other chapters that deal more closely with the herbs or conditions associated with them (for example, read the cardiovascular system A&P before reading Chapter 6, which deals with herbs relating to this system). This may help to break up the A&P into more digestible chunks if you are struggling with a lot of new information. We will give suggestions for you to do this where relevant.

Let's start now with some simple key concepts.

Key concepts

Building blocks: building the body from scratch

If you took a lump of gold and cut it in half, then cut it in half again (etc.), ultimately you would get down to the smallest single unit of gold, the gold atom. Atoms are the smallest unit of any element. Elements are composed of atoms that have identical structures. Currently, 118 elements have been identified, although a few of these can only be produced synthetically. Examples of elements include sodium, potassium, calcium and carbon. Some of these elements are vital to our health and wellbeing and you will meet them in later sections (and in more detail in the Heartwood Foundation Course).

The smallest independent unit of living matter, the cell, is composed of elements and their compounds. Current estimates state that we are composed of approximately 37 trillion cells (give or take a few million); that's an awful lot of cells![1]

The human body is composed of many different cell types, which have become specialised to carry out specific functions. Cells with specific functions are often found together, forming tissues, which represent the next level of complexity. From there tissues come together to form organs. Organ systems consist of organs and tissues that work together to achieve the same goal. Organ systems ultimately work cohesively together to create the human body. So there we have it:

Chemicals → Cells → Tissues → Organs → Organ systems → The body.

The cell

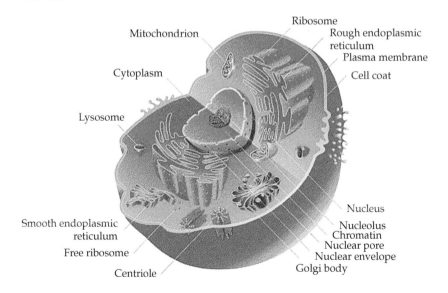

The cell membrane surrounding and enclosing the cell has a number of ingenious ways by which it can control the transport of substances into and out of the cell. This is important for the movement of therapeutic substances into and out of all the cells of our bodies.

Imagine a bouncer at the door of a nightclub. He can decide who comes in or who leaves by one of three mechanisms:

a) Anyone weighing under 14 stone can come in. There are no differentiating, criteria other than size. In terms of the cell, small molecules can just diffuse in to or out of the cell across the cell membrane.
b) Anyone wanting to enter or exit the nightclub will wander up to the bouncer and ask to be let in or out. The bouncer will only let in people who have dark hair and blue eyes, and can sing. This is a lot more specific. There are channels in the plasma membrane that are designed to only allow specific types of molecules entrance. This is a much more selective process.
c) The bouncers actively look for specific types of people, grab them off the street and pull them into (or throw them out of) the nightclub. Pumps are situated on the cell surface, which need energy to work and are very specific. Because the cell needs to expend energy for this process it will only do it where the molecule is valuable to it, or it is vital that something is removed from the cell's internal environment.

Important organelles inside the cell include:

The nucleus	Where our genetic material is stored
Mitochondria	Provide us with energy
Endoplasmic reticulum	A bit of a mouthful! There are two types, rough and smooth, and they are responsible for making all sorts of compounds for us (such as hormones and enzymes)

Much like an embryo is enclosed in the amniotic fluid of its mother's womb, cells are also enveloped in a fluid called interstitial fluid (tissue fluid). This fluid contains nutrients and oxygen absorbed from the capillary bed, which can then be taken up by cells. *The flow of this fluid is considered to be highly significant in herbal medicine practice, and certain herbs are thought to improve the flow of interstitial fluid.*

The terrain and homeostasis

Just as DNA is useless unless it has contact with the right balance of the right chemical substances in the right medium, cells cannot function effectively in isolation. The terrain in which cells exist is crucial to their survival.

Think of yourself right now as you are. What do you need to survive? You might think of the following things:

- Clean air to breathe
- Clean water to drink
- Food
- The right temperature to live in; not too hot, not too cold (like porridge)
- A way of getting rid of waste products effectively

Cells are just the same. If you were a muscle cell say, or a nerve cell, nestling quietly within the spinal cord, your basic concerns would be pretty much the same. Good health is not just about the tissues and organs of our bodies but about the internal environment that we create in which these things can function effectively. Right now I am able to write these words because my external environment is conducive to me doing so. I am warm, well hydrated and nourished and it is not too noisy. The individual cells of the body also need quite specific conditions within which to function. These include:

- pH (the measurement of acidity or alkalinity)
- Core temperature
- Blood sugar
- Blood gases
- Blood pressure

Some of these things have quite narrow margins within which they operate. The body therefore has a number of mechanisms and fail-safes to ensure that things don't get too far out of balance. These involve a complex network of sensors and feedback mechanisms, and it is these checks and balances that we collectively call homeostasis. Homeostatic mechanisms in the body keep the internal environment within certain parameters essential for life, but certain factors do fluctuate all the time within these parameters. It is a *dynamic* system. So, a simple definition of homeostasis is:

Close control of the composition of the body's internal environment.

The nervous system, the endocrine system and the immune system all work in very close co-operation to maintain homeostasis for us. They are the three major players in this enterprise, and the molecules with which they to speak to each other are often difficult to pin down as belonging to one system or another. In the following sections we will talk about all of the major body systems in turn, and at the end of each section you will find a mind map of examples of how each body system connects with others to form the integrated whole. As the immune, nervous and endocrine systems underpin the operations of all other body systems, providing mind maps of their interactions proved to be too big a task. Looking at these key systems, however, would be a great place to start on our magical journey into the complexity of the human body.

The immune system

Every day our bodies have to deal with a vast array of potentially dangerous substances, from the things we eat and drink, the things we breathe and the things that we touch and smell. To deal with this varied problem, our bodies have a number of strategies with which we protect ourselves.

Structure

The immune system operates chiefly via a number of very specific cells, which monitor our internal environment and remove dangerous substances from it.

Bone marrow, lymph nodes, the thymus gland, the spleen and various patches of tissues with the magnificent name Mucosa Associated Lymphoid Tissue (MALT for short) are all components of the immune system.

ORGANS OF THE
IMMUNE SYSTEM

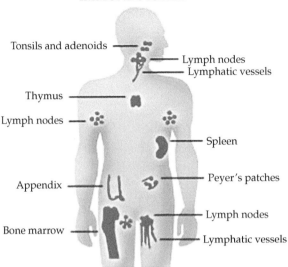

Tonsils and adenoids

Lymph nodes
Lymphatic vessels

Thymus

Lymph nodes

Spleen

Appendix

Peyer's patches

Lymph nodes

Bone marrow

Lymphatic vessels

Bone marrow

Lymphocytes (T and B cells) are manufactured here (more about lymphocytes shortly).

Thymus gland

This small butterfly-shaped gland lies behind your sternum and extends up into your neck. It grows from birth to puberty, but then begins to atrophy, and return to its birth weight by middle age. It is responsible for maturation of lymphocytes called T cells, which teach the body to differentiate between self and non-self. These T cells then either enter the bloodstream or settle in lymphoid tissue.

Mucosa Associated Lymphoid Tissue (MALT)

Just like the endocrine system, the lymphatic system has patches of tissue scattered all around the body. These patches of tissue do not filter lymph. They contain lymphocytes produced by the thymus or from bone marrow. MALT is usually found in areas vulnerable to infection such as the mucosa—the lining of the gut, the throat etc. The tonsils in the throat are an example of MALT. Peyer's patches found in the small intestine are another example.

Lymphocytes are a type of white blood cell, the commonest type of white blood cell found in the lymph. There are three major types of lymphocytes, which we shall meet later when we look at specific defence mechanisms.

Summary

Components of the immune system comprise of:

- Specialised cells such as lymphocytes (and others).
- Specialised tissues such as MALT that exist in crucial or vulnerable places in our body, and bone marrow tissues responsible for making specialised immune cells.
- We also have specialised organs, such as the thymus gland, that have a role maturing lymphocytes in early life.

We can divide the way that our immune system protects us into two main categories, non-specific and specific defence mechanisms.

Let's look at non-specific defence mechanisms first.

Non-specific defence mechanisms

Our non-specific defence mechanisms are designed to defend us from pathogens on a very general level. They include such things as our skin, mucous membranes, nose hairs, eyebrows and eyelashes, forming an active barrier.

One such barrier is the fantastic mechanism in the bronchi of the lungs called the mucociliary escalator. This ensures that, via the wave-like movement of tiny very fine hairs lining the bronchi, dust and other unwanted particles are cleared from the airways before they reach the lungs.

Saliva is slightly acidic and therefore an antibacterial non-specific defence mechanism. Saliva also contains an enzyme called lysozyme, which breaks down and destroys potentially dangerous cells. This is why we get benefits from licking our wounds! Lysozyme is also present in tears, mucous and human breast milk.

As far as our bodies are concerned, the lumen (space inside) the digestive tract is still the outside world. We carry some of the outside world around with us all the time. This means that the whole, and not inconsiderable length of the digestive tract contains a number of defensive mechanisms to stop undesirable substances from 'getting in'.

The most well-known substance produced by the stomach for this purpose is hydrochloric acid (HCL), which serves as a good non-specific defence mechanism. It sterilises our food for us, and keeps the pH of the stomach nice and low so that invading organisms, such as *Helicobacter pylori*, cannot get established. At this point it's probably a good idea to give you a few definitions for some useful words in the world of immunology of things that are innate to our non-specific defence mechanisms.

Pathogen: A disease-producing agent, especially a virus, bacterium or other micro-organism. This is what our non-specific immune mechanisms are trying to keep out!

Lysozyme: To lyse means to break open. This enzyme literally breaks open bacterial cell walls as a means of destroying them.

Macrophage: Macro means large and phage comes from phagos meaning to eat. So literally these are cells with a very big appetite. They will wander around the body chomping up anything they consider to be dangerous. We will meet macrophages again soon.

Phagocytosis: Phago (from phagos meaning 'to eat') and cytosis (from cyto meaning 'cell'), literally translates as cell eating. Macrophages do a lot of phagocytosis.

Chemotaxis: Chemo is derived from the word chemical, and taxis meaning movement (we get the word taxi from this). This word refers to the movement of cells towards a particular place as a result of chemicals being released. (Think of pheromones.) At a site of inflammation certain chemicals will be released into the circulation, which will attract other cells to the area. This is known as chemotaxis.

Inflammation: Inflammation starts as a positive action that forms part of our non-specific immune defences. If tissues themselves are damaged, an inflammatory process will be instigated. If you think of the symptoms of inflammation, it will help you to remember what's going on. Think of a bee sting: there is usually heat, swelling, redness, pain, loss of function. All of these symptoms perform a specific function. (There will be more information provided on our course at the Heartwood Foundation Course).

We have mentioned macrophages, but there are a number of other white blood cells that are involved in non-specific defence mechanisms. They include eosinophils, basophils and neutrophils.

- *Neutrophils*—respond most quickly to infection
- *Eosinophils*—raised levels in allergic conditions
- *Basophils*—enhance inflammatory reactions.

When you go to your General Practitioner (GP) for a full blood count (FBC) the results will include counts of all these different white blood cells.

Lymphocytes have three main types—B lymphocytes, T lymphocytes and natural killer cells. Natural killer cells. What a name! There is no mistaking what these guys do. We will mention them here because they have a foot in both camps so to speak. They perform what is called immunological surveillance duties. They are on patrol constantly, looking for abnormal cells. If all is not well with a cell (such as a viral infection, or cancerous changes) this is often shown on the cell membrane by the presence of abnormal structures or 'markers'. If a natural killer cell (NK cell) detects this it will kill it immediately.

And so, structurally, natural killer cells are classified as lymphocytes, which are normally involved in specific immunity, discussed next. However, unlike other lymphocytes, they are not very selective about how they go about things.

Specific defence mechanisms (immunity)

> *As part of a defence against a potentially dangerous environment, each individual develops their own unique immune system, which acknowledges only itself. Everything that is not recognized might be a threat.*
>
> —Lindsay B. Nicholson[6]

We can look at our non-specific defence mechanisms described above, as our first line of defence. But what happens if either a) something breaches those defences, and a pathogen gets in, or b) the enemy lies within (abnormal cells).

This is where our actual immune system comes into play.

There are three key differences between our non-specific defence system and our immune system:

- *Specificity*: An immune response is targeted against one very specific type of pathogen.

- *Memory*: Specialised cells involved in the immune response are capable of remembering specific pathogens so that they can mount a much faster response the next time the body is exposed to them.
- *Tolerance*: Immune cells are capable of differentiating between self and non-self cells so that their destructive nature is confined to abnormal cells only.

The blood cells involved in the immune response are called lymphocytes. There are three main types of lymphocyte (including natural killer cells). Two of these are involved in mounting a very specific form of defence against individual antigens. (An antigen is any substance capable of stimulating an immune response.) They are called T cells and B cells. Both of these cells are initially produced by our bone marrow. T cells and B cells are very good at recognising one particular type of antigen. For example the T cell for chickenpox (*Varicella zoster* virus) will recognise chickenpox and only chickenpox. Therefore we actually have many different T and B cells in our bodies programmed to respond to specific antigens.

T cells provide what is called cell-mediated immunity. They circulate through the body 'on patrol' and ready for trouble. They interact closely with macrophages. Macrophages re-present fragments of foreign particles that they have eaten onto their cell surface. This means that when a travelling T cell that is specific to this antigen finds the macrophage and the foreign particle fragment, it will respond, divide into four subtypes and proliferate.

B cells are involved in what we call antibody-mediated immunity. They don't travel around the body as much as T cells, but tend to stay put in lymphoid tissues located all around the body. They can also work directly on antigens without needing the help of macrophages. They are responsible for producing antibodies, which do travel out into the circulating bloodstream.

Function

Our immune system aims to protect us from all potentially harmful substances, whether they come from our external or internal environments. This includes viruses, bacteria, fungal infections, toxins, abnormal or cancerous cells etc.

Interconnectedness

The immune system, along with the nervous system and the endocrine system, is a key player in the maintenance of homeostasis in the body. These three systems work very closely together, and the nervous and endocrine systems share many of the same signalling chemicals as the immune system.

An example of this would be serotonin, which plays a role in the inflammatory process (inflammation is part of our non-specific defences) and also acts as a neurotransmitter for the nervous system. Although serotonin can be classified as a neurotransmitter, it is also classified as a hormone, and it interacts closely therefore with the hormonal or endocrine system. In a final flourish of interconnectedness, serotonin has an additional and important role in regulating intestinal movement in the gut. And so here we are back where we started—with our digestive membrane and its Mucosa Associated Lymphoid Tissue!

Herbal connections

We will take the opportunity here to look at one of the gentlest and yet most powerful of our herbal allies, marigold, *Calendula officinalis* L. See Chapter 4 for a more detailed look at marigold.

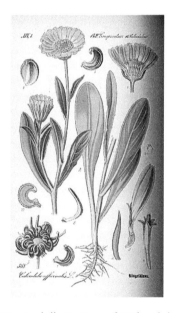

Botanical illustration of Calendula.

Marigold is still one of our 'go-to' herbs for wound healing both inside and out despite a long history of use.[2-4] In addition to its recognised healing action,[3] it has anti-inflammatory effects, and has also been proven to have modulatory effects upon the immune system via the promotion of lymphocyte production (B cells and T cells).[5] Thus it impacts both our non-specific and our specific immune systems. These qualities, combined with its mild but beneficial effects upon the lymphatic system itself, combine to present us with a formidable healing plant, with no known contra-indications. Marigold, a true healing gift, demonstrating how multiple compounds and capacities can help with the interconnectedness of our body.[6]

The endocrine system

What is the endocrine system?

The endocrine system is comprised of around seven major endocrine glands (and many more minor glands and patches of tissues scattered throughout the human body) and the hormones that they secrete. Many of our major organs also have endocrine (hormone-producing) functions.

Major endocrine glands
Male Female

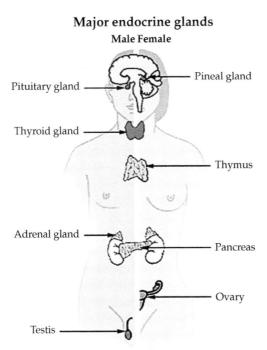

Pituitary gland

Thyroid gland

Adrenal gland

Testis

Pineal gland

Thymus

Pancreas

Ovary

Endocrine glands secrete their products directly into the extracellular fluid that bathes them, then into the bloodstream. Examples include the thyroid gland, the pituitary gland and the adrenal glands.

We also have *exo*crine glands, which secrete their products into ducts, or specialised channels. Examples of exocrine glands include sweat glands, mucous glands, and the pancreas (which is both an endocrine and exocrine glandular organ).

Here however we are dealing with *endo*crine glands.

How does the endocrine system work?

It works via the action of hormones, the chemical messengers of our body. Seven things to know about our chemical messengers are:

- Hormones are synthesised by endocrine glands.
- Hormones may be stored in those glands.
- Hormones are secreted into the bloodstream.
- Hormones travel to the site of action.
- Hormones interact with specific target cells.
- Hormones have powerful effects at low concentrations.
- Hormones may work on more than one tissue and exert more than one effect.

The cardiovascular system plays an important interconnecting role here. Endocrine glands are highly vascular (have lots of blood vessels), therefore hormones can diffuse readily into the bloodstream, and require the blood to transport them.

As mentioned above, hormones interact with specific target cells so that hormones will only bind with receptors that are specific to them. The receptors are found on the surface membranes of our cells. For example thyroid-stimulating hormone (TSH) binds to receptors on the surface of cells of the thyroid gland, but not to cells in the ovary, as they do not possess the thyroid-stimulating hormone receptors.

Cells in our body respond to a hormone when they express or show a specific receptor for that hormone. Hormone receptors are constantly being synthesised and broken down by the cell. This means a cell can decide how many receptors to have at any particular time. When a hormone is present in excess, the number of target-cell receptors decreases on the cell membrane. This is called down-regulation. When a hormone is deficient, the number of receptors expressed on the cell membrane will usually increase to maximise potential hormone binding. This is one of the body's ways of ensuring that it is not over or under-stimulated at any one time by circulating substances including hormones.

What does the endocrine system actually do for us?

Very simply it:

- alters metabolic activities
- regulates growth and development
- guides reproductive activities

Let's look a bit more closely at some of the major endocrine glands.

The thyroid gland

Our thyroid gland is located in our neck, in front of our larynx (throat) and has a sort of bow-tie shape. The thyroid gland secretes thyroxine and tri-iodothyronine (T4 and T3, respectively).

Production of T3 and T4 is stimulated by a thyroid-stimulating hormone released from another endocrine gland—the pituitary, which is, in turn, regulated by thyrotrophin releasing hormone (TRH) from the endocrine tissue of the hypothalamus. The hypothalamus is a region of the brain responsible for coordinating the nervous system and endocrine system, and some other things too! Thyroid hormones are very interesting as they regulate gene expression in the nucleus of cells, and enhance the effects of other hormones such as adrenaline. Thyroid hormones also affect the basal metabolic rate (BMR) and body heat production, and they regulate the metabolism of all food groups. The thyroid also produces a hormone called calcitonin (also known as thyrocalcitonin), which is responsible for lowering calcium levels in the blood. It works as a counter-balance to another hormone called parathyroid hormone which can increase blood calcium levels. Parathyroid hormone is made by the parathyroid glands, which are embedded within the thyroid gland tissue. We can begin to see how there are many layers of interconnectedness expressed within just the thyroid gland.

The pituitary gland

The pituitary gland and the hypothalamus act together to control the secretion of a number of hormones. The pituitary is attached to the hypothalamus by a stalk, and is situated deep and low in the skull, close to where our two optic nerves cross. The pituitary is divided into two regions, the anterior and the posterior. The anterior pituitary is composed of endocrine tissue, and hormones are produced and secreted here under the direct influence of the hypothalamus.

The posterior pituitary is composed of mainly nervous system tissue, but also produces some specific hormones.

Hormone	Function
Anterior pituitary	
Growth hormone	Stimulates growth and division of most of our cells.
Adrenocorticotrophic hormone (ACTH)	Raises the concentration and output of steroid hormones.
Thyroid stimulating hormone (TSH)	Stimulates the growth and activity of the thyroid gland, and therefore the production of T4 and T3.
Luteinising hormone (LH)	Stimulates production of testosterone in males. Regulation of ovulation and the menstrual cycle in females.
Follicle stimulating hormone (FSH)	Regulation of the menstrual cycle. Gamete (reproductive cell) production, for both sexes.
Prolactin	Initiation and maintenance of lactation (breast milk production).
Posterior pituitary	
Oxytocin	Increases force of uterine contractions and stimulates stretching of the cervix during childbirth.
Antidiuretic hormone (ADH)	Increases water reabsorption from kidney tubules.

The adrenal gland

The adrenal glands are situated on the upper pole of each kidney—most people have two kidneys, one each side of the spine, and positioned behind our ribs at our mid-back. Each is enclosed by the renal fascia; a layer of connective tissue which encapsulates the kidneys and adrenal glands.

Looking at a cross-section of an adrenal gland, you will see that there are two main areas: the cortex and the medulla, and the hormones secreted by these two areas are quite different.

The tissue of the adrenal cortex is endocrine tissue. If you look at the actions of the various hormones secreted by this endocrine gland (see below), it is easy to see how chronic stress can affect things like blood sugar levels, and also why it is important to support the adrenal glands during times like the menopause. These hormones may be significantly affected by long-term stress.

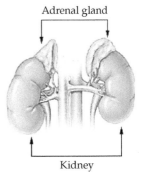

Adrenal gland

Kidney

The tissue of the adrenal medulla is comprised of nervous system tissue. There are therefore similarities between the adrenal gland and the pituitary gland in that they are both comprised of both the nervous system and endocrine system tissue.

Adrenal cortex

Hormone	Function
Glucocorticoids (i.e. cortisol, corticosterone, cortisone)	Metabolism regulators—raise blood glucose, promote the breakdown of glycogen, fats and proteins. Response to stress.
Mineralocorticoids (i.e. Aldosterone)	Reabsorption of sodium (and therefore water) from renal tubules, and excretion of potassium.
Sex hormones (i.e. testosterone/ oestrogen in small amounts)	Development of secondary male sexual characteristics. Low levels compared to testes. Raised oestrogen production in women after menopause.

Adrenal medulla

Hormone	Function
Adrenaline and noradrenaline	Neurotransmitters of the sympathetic division of the autonomic nervous system. Fight or flight reactions. Increase heart rate. Increase blood pressure. Blood diverted to essential organs. Increased basal metabolic rate. Pupil dilation.

Adrenaline and noradrenaline are neurotransmitters that are directly involved in our short-term response to stress—sometimes called the fight-or-flight response. As you can see from the table above, they act all over the body to prepare us to either fight or take flight. This is very helpful in the short term, but you can also see how chronic stress would lead to long-term issues with regard to blood pressure and disruption to our digestive 'fire' or vigour, as blood is diverted away.

The pancreas

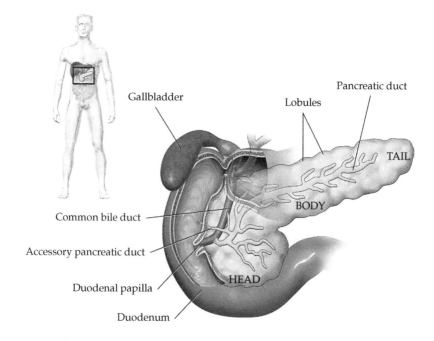

The pancreas lies posterior and inferior to the stomach. It is a leaf-shaped structure, divided into what is described as, a head, body and tail. Numerous ducts or channels collect the enzyme products of the pancreas and eventually these exit at the head of the pancreas into the small intestine. The head, body and tail of the pancreas all contain the digestive enzyme (exocrine glands) producing cells and ducts. Interspersed throughout this pancreatic tissue are also numerous tiny endocrine cells that secrete hormones directly into the bloodstream.

When people talk about the pancreas they usually think of blood sugar control. This is the role of the endocrine function of the pancreas. As we said earlier, hormones have powerful effects at low concentrations, and so the endocrine glands occupy about 1% of the total pancreatic tissue.

This leaves most of the pancreas (approximately 99%), involved in the production of digestive enzymes. This is an exocrine function of the pancreas as the digestive juices are secreted into a duct rather than directly into the bloodstream. Most of the pancreatic tissue is dedicated to the production of digestive enzymes, made by cells called acini, which are secreted into the small intestine and used to break down our food.

Back to the endocrine function of the pancreas for a moment though! The table below shows the hormones produced by the endocrine cells of the pancreas, known as the Islet's of Langerhans, and their major roles in the body.

Hormone	Action
Insulin	Increases blood glucose levels
Glucagon	Reduces blood glucose levels
Somatostatin (Growth Hormone Releasing Inhibiting Hormone GHRIH)	Inhibits glucagon, insulin and growth hormone
Pancreatic polypeptide	Regulator of endocrine and exocrine secretions

In the table above, we can already see that the situation is a lot more complex than just insulin in terms of the regulation of glucose levels.

Other regulating hormones are involved. Also, if you think about the adrenal cortex and the actions of glucocorticoids, you have another layer of complexity to deal with. Things are never about one hormone or one task.

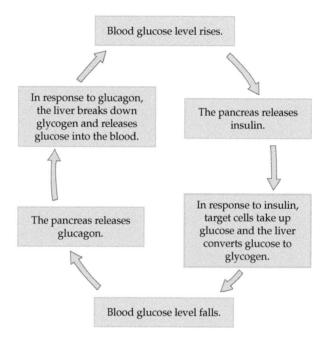

Our body usually achieves balance, stability and optimal function, by a multitude of pathways, and in this case the management and metabolism of fat, protein and glucose are managed by a variety of endocrine and exocrine glands.

In a similar way, medicinal plants work by acting at multiple sites simultaneously; complex remedies for complex situations.

Interconnectedness

We have already mentioned the close links between the endocrine system, the nervous system and the immune system. The anatomy and physiology of both the pituitary gland and the adrenal glands are an excellent example of the close partnership between endocrine and nervous tissues and systems. Our exploration of the adrenal glands and the pancreas shows the close relationship between the endocrine and nervous system, with our digestive system and cellular metabolism.

Herbal connections

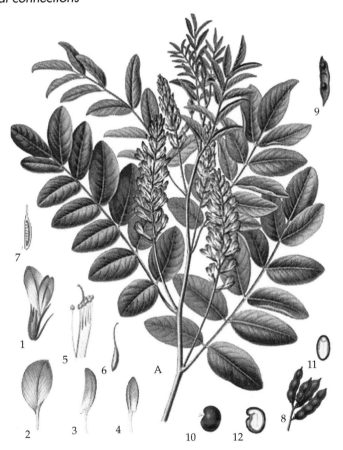

Liquorice (*Glycyrrhiza glabra* L.)

Liquorice (*Glycyrrhiza glabra* L.) is a globally wide-ranging medicinal plant from the bean family, traditionally used in support of the adrenal glands (among other capacities).

In the language of herbal medicine liquorice can act as an adaptogen, helping the body adapt to stress. Specifically it helps support cortisol levels in the system due to tonic effects to the adrenal cortex.

This traditional herb tonic is also associated with improving immune resilience,[7] having anti-inflammatory, healing, antidiabetic[8] and expectorant effects,[9] and having sex hormone-balancing actions.[10,11] Compounds we met in Chapter 2, such as triterpenoid saponins and flavonoids, have been identified in liquorice, and shown to have a major role in producing these actions.[12] Modern in-vivo research has focussed on trying to confirm these side-benefits, and to understand the mechanisms behind them.[13]

We hope that our brief introduction to the immune system and the endocrine system has demonstrated some of the links that exist between these systems. It is interesting to note that benefits from medicinal plants, like liquorice, have been observed and documented by medical systems long before modern research existed. In a final note on endocrine interconnectedness—overconsumption of liquorice extract (glyzyrretinic acid) can lead to mineral salt imbalance, and ultimately this could raise blood pressure.[14] For this reason caution is recommended when prescribing liquorice for people with high blood pressure. Liquorice has a sweet taste. Traditional medicine systems recognise that sweet foods should be consumed in moderation—we shall look at this in more depth in Chapter 5.

The nervous system

The nervous system is the system of nerve cells and groups of nerve cells that transmit impulses and messages around the body. It includes the brain, spinal cord, nerves and ganglia and serves to communicate and respond to stimuli whether that stimulus is from inside our body or externally in the environment around us.

The correct name for a nerve cell is a neuron. A neuron can either function in isolation or form bundles with other neurons or nerve cells. When they form bundles, they are known as nerves. The longest nerve in the body is the sciatic nerve, which can extend to over a metre. There are two sciatic nerves that emerge from either side of the spine, run down the back of our leg muscles and reach as far as our toes.

Surrounding the neurons are neuroglia. These are cells that form supportive tissue around neurons, as well as making the lipid-rich substance—myelin that sheaths our neurons (see below).

Let's look at the anatomy of a typical neuron.

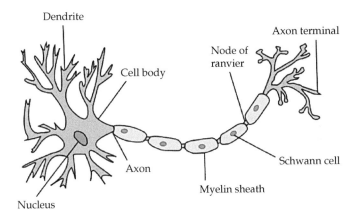

With a bit of imagination you can still see the basic cell structure that we saw at the beginning of this chapter, a cell membrane and nucleus. The nerve cell has however undergone some fairly drastic modifications.

The cell body has sprouted branch-like projections called *dendrites*, which receive electrical impulses from other cells and carry them to the cell body itself. Then there is one large long projection called an *axon*, which carries electrical impulses away from the cell body and down to the axon terminals, where they can then interact with the dendrites of other cells and transmit the impulses onwards.

The axon is surrounded and protected by a myelin sheath. We mentioned neuroglial cells a moment ago. Plasma membranes of some neuroglial cells wrap themselves around the axons of the nerve cells at periodic intervals and create a really good insulating material called *myelin*. The advantage of having myelinated nerve cells is that electrical nerve impulses can jump quickly along the neuron rather than having to travel in a slow wave. They do this by jumping between areas called *nodes of Ranvier*, where one myelin sheath ends and another begins. Nerve impulses can travel up to 130 metres per second in skeletal muscles! (That's 290.80172 miles an hour. The athlete Usain Bolt's muscles were much faster than he was.)

The transmission of a nerve impulse is known as an *action potential* and it travels in a wave. Immediately after the wave has passed along a section of an axon, that section experiences something called a refractory period (a sort of recovery period), during which re-stimulation of the nerve is not possible. The speed at which these impulses travel depends upon two things:

- The diameter of the nerve: The greater the diameter the faster the conduction
- Myelination: Myelinated nerve fibres are faster conductors than un-myelinated ones.

When the electrical impulse reaches the axon terminals, what happens next?

Well, here we enter the exciting world of the synapse.

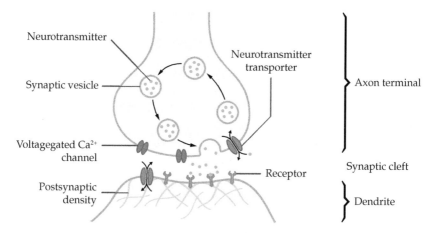

We get the word synapse from the Greek word *synapsis*, meaning conjunction. Here we are looking at the union of two neurons and there are a number of points of contact between the axon terminals of one neuron and the dendrites of the next. In reality the two neurons do not touch, there is a tiny space called the synaptic cleft between these two structures across which chemical messengers are passed in a single direction, from the axon terminals of what is called the pre-synaptic neuron to the dendrites of the post-synaptic neuron.

To summarise: Nerves are basically bundles of neurons, which are wrapped in a connective tissue coating for protection. They transmit electrical impulses along their axons, and rely on a chemical messenger to act in the cleft between individual nerve terminals. There are two types of nerves, which have two very specific functions: Sensory nerves and motor nerves.

Branches of nerve family tree

Sensory nerves (Afferent nerves)	Motor nerves (Efferent nerves)
Carry information about our environment from our skin, from other sense organs, or from internal organs.	Transmit impulses back to effector organs such as muscles or glands.
This information is then passed to the spinal cord and then either on to the brain or into a reflex arc in the spinal cord.	Effector organs may be under voluntary control (Somatic), i.e. skeletal muscles, or involuntary control (Autonomic) i.e. muscles of blood vessels.

The motor nerves over which we have no control (autonomic) are further divided into two types: sympathetic and parasympathetic nerves. We will look at these a bit more closely when we look at the peripheral nervous system.

So now we have covered the basics of nervous system tissue and how it works, let's take a closer look at the two major divisions of the nervous system, the central nervous system and the peripheral nervous system.

The central nervous system

The central nervous system (CNS) is comprised of the brain and the spinal cord.

Both of these structures are protected by specialised membranes called *meninges* and cerebrospinal fluid. Our central nervous system is absolutely vital to life, and therefore we guard and protect it well. Our spinal cord sits inside and is protected by our strong bony vertebrae that make up our spine, and of course our brain sits inside a special designer-made home called the skull. We have also installed the latest in high-tech protective headgear in the form of meninges and cerebrospinal fluid. Let's look a bit more closely at these two innovations.

The meninges

The meninges are a specialised type of protective membrane that covers both the brain and the spinal cord. There are three meninges. Named from the inside outwards they are:

1. *The pia mater*: This delicate membrane is permeated with blood vessels and completely covers the brain and all of its convolutions, and the spinal cord.
2. *The arachnoid mater*: The middle layer between the pia mater and the dura mater is called the subarachnoid space. It is filled with the arachnoid mater, which has a fine, web-like appearance, which gives it its name (*arachne* = spider in Greek) and contains cerebrospinal fluid (CSF).
3. *The dura mater*: This outer layer is formed by a durable double layer of fibrous tissue. Venous blood drains from the brain into venous sinuses in the space between the two layers of dura mater.

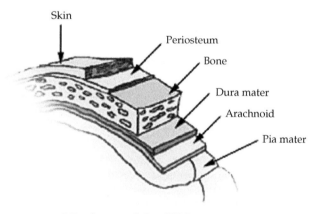

Meninges of the CNS

Cerebrospinal fluid (CSF)

Have you ever wondered where CSF comes from? Well, wonder no further! The brain contains four spaces or chambers called ventricles, and it is in the walls of these ventricles that CSF is made by a structure called choroid plexus. The choroid plexus is a highly vascular area, with a rich blood supply, which produces CSF at a rate of around 0.5 ml a minute.

CSF is then circulated with the help of blood vessel pulsations, respiration and postural changes. Research into the role of respiration and the circulation of CSF has revealed that inspiration (breathing in) in particular is very effective at enhancing the flow of CSF. Also consider that CSF actually directly bathes the area of the brain where respiratory sensors are located so it is thought to possibly influence respiration as well as respiration influencing it.[15]

If you remember, CSF is contained in the subarachnoid space. This space contains tiny villi called arachnoid villi (also called arachnoid granulations), which extend into venous sinuses. This is where CSF is reabsorbed into the bloodstream. CSF is made, and also reabsorbed—there is a turnover of the fluid.

CSF acts as a shock absorber or buffer to protect the delicate tissues of the central nervous system from damage by impacts or trauma. It also takes part in the exchange of nutrients and waste products from the brain.

The brain

The brain itself is divided into a number of functional areas. The cerebrum is probably what we think of when we visualise the brain. It is divided by a central fissure into two hemispheres, left and right. This is where complex sensory and neural data are processed and voluntary

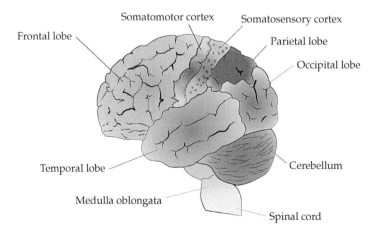

responses are co-ordinated. Other areas include the hypothalamus, which controls the secretion of hormones from the pituitary gland, and the medulla oblongata, which controls autonomic functions such as heart rate, breathing, coughing, sneezing etc. At the back of the brain below the cerebrum is the cerebellum (which means little brain). Its functions include control and maintenance of balance, co-ordination and muscle tone.

The spinal cord

There are two things that link the brain with the rest of the body: the cranial nerves, which innervate the head, and the spinal cord, which descends down the spine.

The spinal cord is like an information highway, with data passing from the body to the brain and data passing back from the brain to the body.

In some cases things are under the exclusive control of the spinal cord and the brain is not involved.

Information being passed from the body to the brain involves sensory neurons called *afferent* neurons. Sensory receptors comprised of nerve endings in the skin, muscles and joints receive information and pass it, via afferent neurons to the spinal cord and then the brain.

The brain will then send answering messages back via motor neurons, called *efferent* neurons, which will result in responses and reactions such as muscle contractions.

The peripheral nervous system

The peripheral nervous system is sub-divided into parts that divide off from specific areas of the brain or spinal cord. The main divisions of the peripheral nervous system are: the spinal nerves, the thoracic nerves, the craniosacral nerves and the autonomic nervous system.

The spinal nerves

The spinal nerves are an integral part of the peripheral nervous system and are mixed nerves, carrying different types of impulses or signals. The spinal nerves are made up of combinations of motor, sensory and autonomic nerves and are responsible for communication between the spinal cord and the body:

- There are 31 pairs of spinal nerves, which exit the spinal column.
- After emerging from the spinal column, spinal nerves divide into branches called rami.
- The nerve branches or rami unite in some places to form large masses of nerves called plexuses.
- In the plexuses, the nerves are re-arranged before continuing their journey to supply skin, muscles, joints etc.
- There are five main plexuses: Cervical, brachial, lumbar, sacral and coccygeal, each plexus provides nerves to and from particular areas of the body.
- Structures in the body are often innervated from more than one nerve supply, so damage to one nerve does not necessarily mean loss of function.

Thoracic nerves

Of the total of 31 pairs of nerves, these 12 pairs do not form plexuses when they exit the spinal cord. They exit as 12 single pairs of nerves and innervate the thorax, including ribs, intercostal muscles, posterior and anterior abdominal walls, and overlying skin.

Cranial nerves

These also consist of 12 pairs of nerves responsible for innervation of the face and major sense organs associated with the face and the head. This includes the optic nerves responsible for sight, and the olfactory nerve, for our sense of smell. They are usually numbered using Roman numerals, so that the olfactory nerve is cranial nerve I, the facial nerve is cranial nerve VII.

Autonomic nervous system

This is the section of the nervous system that controls all the things that you don't have conscious control over, but you may sometimes be aware of like our heart rate or our breathing.

It has two divisions, the sympathetic and the parasympathetic nervous systems, which work together to maintain a balance. The best way to explain how these two divisions work is to consider what the body needs when it is at rest, and what it needs when it is active.

When the body is active the sympathetic nervous system is sympathetic to this, and works to supply more blood to the heart, more oxygen to the skeletal muscles and more glucose for energy, so that we can do all the things that we want to do, like running, swimming etc. It will also help us by shutting down 'non-essential' things like digesting food or producing saliva. This all goes back to survival instincts. Where does the body need to put its energy to get away from the dirk-toothed tiger? What does it not need to do?

The parasympathetic nervous system does the opposite. When we are at rest, the parasympathetic nervous system takes charge, encouraging things like digestion of food, production of urine, calming the heart rate and breathing.

It is perhaps possible to imagine how in our lives, we might put these two systems at odds with each other, by eating and drinking whilst still trying to think and do things for example.

Interconnectedness

The nervous system plays a vital role in every other system of the body, providing stimulation, relaxation and tone. Its influence is so extensive and all-encompassing that it is difficult to single out specific examples. One area however, that should not pass without a specific mention is our digestive tract.

Often called the second brain, our digestive tract contains the second-largest amount of nervous tissue in the entire body. The main nerve that innervates the digestive tract is in fact a cranial nerve, number ten (X)—the vagus nerve! Gut feelings are in fact a real 'thing' and there are many very good reasons as to why, when we get nervous, we feel butterflies in our stomach or can be sick to our stomachs.

At the very least, when you think of the sympathetic and parasympathetic nervous systems, it becomes easier to explain why we can feel queasy just before going on stage or speaking in public. Our sympathetic nervous system has moved to shut down the digestive processes, so anything we have been working on down there, shuts down, leaving unfinished business in the gut! Further than that though, the nervous system of the gut has been shown to influence the brain, and the term 'gut–brain axis' has now been coined.[16]

Herbal connections

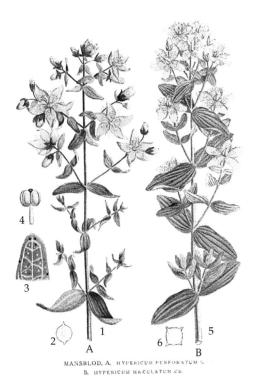

MANSBLOD. A. HYPERICUM PERFORATUM L.
B. HYPERICUM MACULATUM CR.

St. John's wort (*Hypericum perforatum* L.)

St John's wort (*Hypericum perforatum* L.) is possibly one of the most well-researched herbal remedies of our time. It is also one of the most satisfying to talk about in terms of how herbs work in our bodies.

It has proved impossible to isolate a single active constituent responsible for its actions, as there is no single constituent. The actions of the plant are dependent upon a number of different constituents acting via different biochemical pathways in the body, both directly and indirectly to exert an effect. The research has therefore made it an excellent example of synergy found in whole plant medicines.

Key constituents identified include naphthodianthrones such as hypericin and pseudo-hypericin, and flavonoids and phenolics, including hyperforin. It is also an excellent example of a tonic herb, with specific applications to the nervous system. It has a strong tradition of use as an anti-inflammatory for the skin and nerves, classically used for the pain of shingles. It is also helpful in viral conditions and some human research confirms this.[17]

Some of its actions involve the modification of the availability of neurotransmitters (the chemicals acting at the neuronal synapse) and their ability to bind at receptor sites. These include influences on serotonin and benzodiazepine, as well as influencing the enzyme monoamine oxidase. As a result of research into these actions, and research showing significantly less adverse effects at high dosage, summarised in the German Commission E Monographs,[18] this plant has been chosen over conventional antidepressant drugs by doctors in Germany.

Not only is hypericum one of the most researched herbal medicines of our time, but it was also one of the most frequently used mediaeval herbal medicines, and evidence of its extensive use was found at Soutra Aisle hospital (established 1164 CE) by medico-archaeologists working between 2010 and 2011. This healing plant has a very serious provenance indeed!

The five senses

Aristotle (384–322 BCE) is credited with the traditional classification of the five sense organs: sight, smell, taste, touch and hearing.[19,20] He considered them as representative of the five classical elements (fire, water, air, earth, quintessence or aether).

Most modern-day textbooks still follow the classic five senses classification, which we will discuss here, but the reality can be viewed as a whole lot more complex.[21] Each of the five classical senses consists of organs with specialised cellular structures that have receptors for specific stimuli. These cells are linked to the nervous system and thus to the brain via the cranial nerves and the peripheral nervous system.

Sensing is done both at a 'primitive level' in the cells and also integrated into more complex sensations in the nervous system. Each of the five sensory organs (the eye, ear, nose, mouth, skin) are integrally linked with the nervous system in order to convey any signal picked up by these sense organs to the brain. We can respond to this sensory data with both 'automatic' or physiological responses involving our autonomic nervous system, or with more consciousness-related 'meaning responses' involving the cerebrum of our brain.

In the brain, we automatically sift through all the sensory data and quickly develop ways of deciding what data is important, developing 'short-cuts' and ways of ignoring or interpreting data into our thoughts and actions. This 'sensory gating' can be enormously helpful when completing complex tasks and allows us to do much more without consciously sensing each individual thing.[22] However it might also mean we sometimes filter out data that may have been useful, or we can reject our 'intuition' our so-called sixth sense.

For our purposes, lets us take a look at each of the organs of our sensory system in a little more detail, before coming back to the overall picture of the nervous system and some herbal medicine-related thoughts on our senses.

Sight

The eye is the organ of vision. It performs optical image-collecting functions like a camera. It also has neurological apparatus for transmitting that information from the eye to the brain.

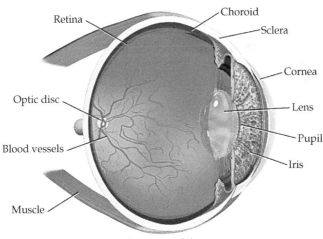

Anatomy of the eye

The eye has a complex structure consisting of a transparent lens that focuses light on the retina (specialized light-collecting cells) and an optic nerve to carry that information to the brain for interpretation.

The delicate structures of the eye are kept within the sclera (the white 'eyeball'). A transparent cornea and conjunctiva cover the aperture at the front of the eye. The eye has specialised gel-like transparent media internally, which keeps the structures in place, moist and nutrified. At the front of the eye this gel-like area is called the aqueous humour and is constantly replenished with new fluid. Behind the lens towards the back of the eye is the vitreous humour, which is thought to not be replenished with fluid, and can shrink with age causing changes in visual acuity. There is a specialised visual covering inside the back of the eye, the retina, which is covered with two basic types of light-sensitive cells: rods and cones.

The cone cells are sensitive to colour and are located in the part of the retina called the fovea, where bright daylight is normally focussed by the lens. The fovea is the centre of an area of the retina at the back of the eye called the macula. Thus macular degeneration results in the loss of central vision (as you look straight ahead).

The rod cells are not sensitive to colour, but have greater sensitivity to light than the cone cells. These cells are located around the fovea and are responsible for peripheral vision and night vision. Thus to see more clearly in darkness, we should look slightly to one side of the object.

The brain combines the input of our two eyes into a single three-dimensional image. Although our eyes are at the front of our head, optic nerves carry sensory information from our retina cells to a 'control centre' in the brain, called the thalamus. Some of the fibres cross over to the other side of the brain whilst they are doing that. From the thalamus, the information is taken further back in the brain to an area called the occipital lobe situated in the cerebrum. It is here that the complex processing of images we have perceived takes place.

Muscles that surround the eye allow us to move it without moving our head. These are operated by other cranial nerves. The iris is a specialised muscle that contracts in bright light. In bright light the iris makes the dark spot in the centre of our eye (the pupil) smaller. The iris is the blue, green, or brown coloured part of our eye and will contract in strong light protecting the delicate cells within the eye.

In low light, the iris opens, allowing more light to enter through the pupil, making our pupils dilate and become larger. The lens, inside the eye at the front, behind the pupil, focuses light by also contracting and expanding. It uses a specialised muscle to do this—the ciliary muscle. It causes light to fall on specific parts of the retina depending on the light conditions that we are in.

Interesting Fact: Reindeer eyes!!

Arctic reindeer have to cope with extreme variations in the amount of light in their environment at different times of the year.

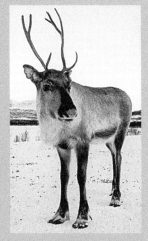

Their eyes therefore have an extra structure behind the retina called the *tapetum lucidum* (Latin for shining layer), which undergoes structural changes to its collagen layer depending upon the season. In summer, it is a golden colour, and most light is reflected out through the retina. In winter, when light is scarce, it changes to blue, trapping more light within the eye, and increasing the sensitivity of the retina.[23] (Reindeer can also see in ultraviolet!)

The eye is connected to the brain through a cranial nerve called the optic nerve. The point where this nerve penetrates the retina is called the blind spot. It is insensitive to light because it is made up of optic nerve fibres not light-sensitive cells—rods and cones.

The ciliary muscle has to work (contract) hardest when we are looking at something very close. This is one reason why *focussing on close objects can tire the eyes* and why a walk in nature can revive them!

Note: The eye and Western herbal medicine. The eye itself is regarded as giving us information about the liver in Western herbal medicine. Therefore any problems arising in the eye might be treated functionally, but also with consideration to the function of the liver.

Also, the area around the eye, the eyelid and above and below it, are seen to pertain to the health of the adrenal gland. So any problems arising in this area may be treated functionally, but also with regard to adrenal depletion for example.

Hearing

The ear is the sensory organ of hearing. It is also the sensory organ of balance. The structure of the ear can be considered to be in three parts. The external, middle and internal.

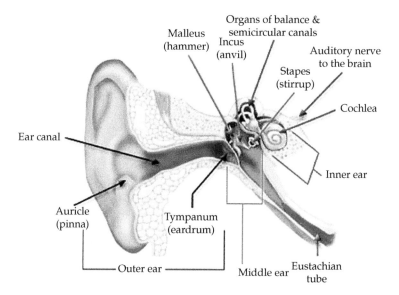

The external ear is made up of the ear pinna that protrudes away from the head and is shaped like a cup to direct sounds into the auditory canal as far as the tympanic membrane ('eardrum'). The main purpose of this external 'auditory meatus' is to provide a protective opening for the delicate inner structures of the ear. Hair and wax protect us from trauma, foreign bodies and infection and so can also be regarded as part of our non-specific immune system. Its shape is also designed to easily direct sound waves.

The middle ear is a chamber lined with respiratory epithelium (respiratory cells) containing a series of small bones called the malleus (hammer), incus (anvil) and stapes (stirrup). These ear bones (ossicles) fit together and link the eardrum with another membrane that separates the middle ear from the inner ear—the oval window. The purpose of the ossicles is to transmit sound vibrations from the eardrum (tympanic membrane) through the oval window into the cochlea of the inner ear. The inner ear develops from nervous system tissue, unlike the respiratory cells of the middle ear.

The epithelium of the middle ear is a modified respiratory epithelium or membrane with ciliated and secretory cells, including goblet cells. As such it can produce secretions and is potentially vulnerable to infection and congestion. The middle ear is joined to the nasopharynx by the eustachian tube. In adults this tube is normally closed and opened by swallowing. It helps maintain atmospheric pressure inside the ear relative to the pressure around us. Ideally the eustachian tube prevents infection from moving up from the throat and respiratory system into the ear and helps drain secretions if infection or inflammation does occur.

Note: We have met cilia before, lining the bronchial tract, the mucociliary escalator. Cilia sweep mucous out of the body via the nearest exit. They have a strong wave motion forwards, followed by a slow recovery stroke backwards. Cilia are also found in the inner ear and retina, although in both cases these cilia are adapted to function like nerve receptors.

The inner ear, or cochlea, is a spiral-shaped chamber (snail-shell-like) covered internally by nerve fibres that react to the vibrations of sound waves and transmit impulses to the brain via the auditory nerve or cochlear nerve. This nerve is one branch of a cranial nerve known as the vestibulocochlear nerve (cranial nerve VIII). You may recall that a nerve is a collection of nerve cells known as neurons, all bundled together. Our cochlear nerve has approximately 30,000 neurons. The brain combines the input of our two ears to determine the direction and distance of sounds.

The inner ear also has a vestibular system formed by three semi-circular canals that are approximately at right angles to each other and which are responsible for the sense of balance and spatial orientation. The second part of the vestibulocochlear nerve—the vestibular nerve carries information about our spatial orientation and whether we are we upside down or not?!

Both chambers of the inner ear are filled with a specialised viscous fluid and they are in communication with each other. The movement of small particles (*otoliths*) over small hair cells or cilia, in the vestibular system of the inner ear, sends signals to the brain that helps in the maintenance of our balance. The information is processed together with visual information, plus sensory information from the joints in our legs and feet and sent to a part of the brain called the cerebellum.

Note: Western herbal medicine perspective—middle ear epithelium. Herbal medicines can have positive effects on the mucous membranes, and respiratory epithelium. Many have anti-inflammatory capacities, mucolytic effects and positive effects upon cilia. Some herbs can improve the function of respiratory epithelium (mucous membranes) in many locations simultaneously. So drinking eyebright tea (*Euphrasia officinalis* L.) for example, can have potential benefits to all mucous membranes (respiratory epithelium), including the ear, eustachian tubes and the sinuses.

Smell

The nose is the organ responsible for the sense of smell known as olfaction. Olfaction is an early evolutionary sensory adaptation. Olfaction is used to help us detect food, individuals, danger, location, gender among other things and therefore can invoke strong emotions. Different smells can cause profound effects, memories and behaviours; even for us humans, who are not thought to have as keen a sense of smell like many other animals.

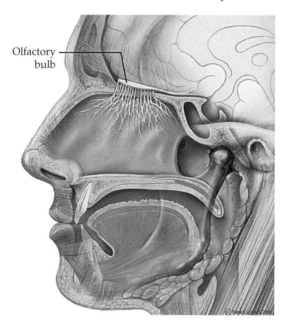

Olfactory bulb

The cavity of the nose is lined with mucous membranes that have smell receptors located in the superior nasal sinuses. The sensory receptor cells are then connected to the olfactory nerve, a cranial nerve, that enters the cranium (our skull) through the cribriform plate to the olfactory bulb in the brain. The olfactory nerve is known as the first cranial nerve (I).

The smells themselves consist of airborne vaporised molecules of various substances that enter via our nostrils. These gaseous substances need to dissolve in the moist mucous layer of the linings of the nose and sinuses in order to activate the receptor cells.

Once in the brain, olfactory bulb nerve cells (neurons) interact with higher centres in the brain. One of the targets is the primary olfactory cortex, which is the site of perception, discrimination and memories. A second target is the limbic system where smells influence behaviour and emotions. Some of these relate to instinctive behaviours, for example pheromones. Other targets are the hypothalamic centres of the brain. These regulate automatic responses, feeding, reproductive hormones, arousal and attention. Olfaction therefore has important but generally unobtrusive effects on human behaviour.

Damage to the olfactory nerve can lead to a loss of the capacity for the sense of smell, and is called anosmia. It is one type of peripheral neuropathy, affecting the peripheral nervous system. Problems within the brain itself may be a cause and should be ruled out.

The sense of smell is most commonly temporarily lost when a person has a cold or has sinusitis. This is not a neurological loss of the sense of smell, but the result of disturbances to the mucous membranes during infection and inflammation. Excess mucous and swelling of the membranes lining the nose and sinuses block the capacity for olfactory receptors to function, and the sense of smell usually returns during recovery. Incomplete recovery may occur with more chronic rhinitis and sinusitis.

Note: Western herbal medicine perspective—taste buds and sinusitis. Interestingly, research is revealing that bitter taste receptors may have a key role of listening-in to the molecules, or microbes that infect the respiratory airways.[24] This may have particular significance for chronic rhinosinusitis, where bacteria become resistant by forming a biofilm. Robust treatment for sinusitis with powerful herbs for sinus infection may have a suggested mechanism for action here as the herbs traditionally used in Western herbal medicine contain a particularly bitter alkaloid known as berberidine. We shall look at the herbal medicine approach to respiratory infection in more detail in Chapter 9.

There are some drugs or behaviours such as smoking that can lead to a reduced or abnormal sense of smell. Loss of this sense can be a feature of some dementias, Parkinson's disease and diabetes. Rarely, zinc and thiamine (vitamin B1) deficiency may produce a loss or distortion to the sense of smell.

> **Note: Western herbal medicine perspective—smell and pituitary gland.** It is perhaps no surprise that the highly effective hormone-balancing herb chaste tree—*Vitex agnus-castus* L., shown in many research studies to be safe and effective and to work via the pituitary-hypothalamic system, is also known as monk's pepper.[25] Vitex is a highly aromatic plant with a strong peppery smell that feels like it goes right up your nose into the centre of your brain!

Taste

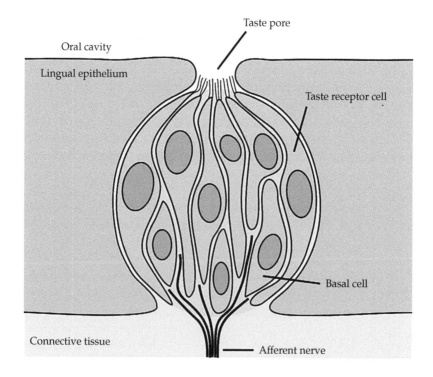

The receptors for taste (gustation), are found within taste buds, and are situated chiefly in the tongue, but they are also located in the roof of the mouth and near the pharynx. They are all able to detect four basic tastes: salty, sweet, bitter and sour. The tongue also can detect sensations such as pungent and umami (a sort of savoury taste) from taste receptors sensitive to amino acids.

Generally, the taste buds close to the tip of the tongue are more sensitive to sweet tastes, whereas those in the back of the tongue are particularly sensitive to bitter tastes. The taste buds on the side of the tongue are preferentially sensitive to salty and sour tastes. The idea that there is a clearly demarcated taste receptor tongue-map has now been disproved, as all taste buds are considered to have a capacity for all tastes.

At the base of each taste bud there is a nerve that sends the sensations to the brain. Three cranial nerves are involved in our sense of taste, transporting impulses from the anterior portion of the tongue (cranial nerve VII), and the posterior of the tongue and throat (cranial nerves IX and X).

Three areas of the brain are thought to be responsive to taste signals—firstly the medulla oblongata, where saliva production can be then stimulated. Secondly higher centres in the brain (including the hypothalamus and limbic system) contribute to hedonic (pleasant/unpleasant) responses, and hunger/satiety. The third area connected to taste is the thalamus and cortex of the brain. This serves our perception of taste recognition, and the discrimination between flavours.

The sense of taste functions in co-ordination with the sense of smell, and so a loss of the sense of smell can impact negatively on our capacity to taste. It is presumed that taste receptors have had evolutionary significance for us as foragers. The sense of taste also drives us to maintain homeostasis (balance of) of electrolytes (the taking in of salts, sugars and fluids), and protects us from potentially harmful substances.

Our ancestors will almost certainly have used taste as a major sensory input into the understanding of medicinal plants. Eventually, Ayurveda, traditional Chinese Herbal Medicine, and humoral medicine systematised plants according to tastes. Tastes were ascribed qualities that linked with elements, seasons, diseases and other active properties. Our desire for certain tastes suggests a persons' natural constitution, or an imbalance in dis-ease.

Note: **Western herbal medicine perspective—bitter.** A regular comment from users of herbal medicines is how bitter they taste! Bitters are considered highly therapeutic in all traditions of herbal medicine. They are described as having diverse and multiple effects around the body and in different body tissues, organs and systems.

Certain phytochemicals (alkaloids, triterpenoids, iridoids, di-terpenes, ketones and amino acids) are known to have a bitter taste and cause intracellular biochemical changes that lead to effects in the neurons of the digestive system, and immune system.

Bitter compound receptors are expressed on the cell membranes of our cells, and not just in the mouth and throat. It is now understood that bitter receptors can be expressed at distant sites throughout the digestive epithelium, the pancreas and the brain. Evidence now suggests that bitter and sweet taste receptors are also important in sensing bacteria and regulating innate immunity.[26]

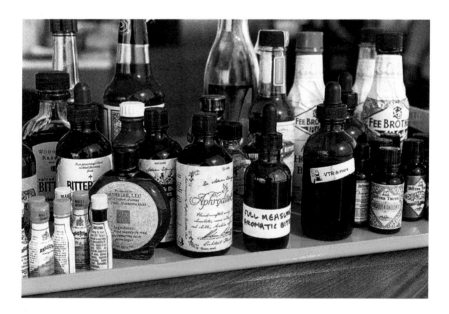

Across the world cultural practices remember a universal recognition that bitters restore wellbeing and appetite and also relieve over-indulgence of rich foods. The commonplace social norms of choosing bitterness in beverages like coffee, coffee substitutes like chicory, in digestif's, and vermouths are the result of this ancient herbal practice. Culturally, bitters were often mixed with aromatic plants such as aniseed or mint, each to a unique and popular recipe such as Campari, Cynar, and Angostura bitters (there are many more!) to induce a more carminative effect as well as mask the bitter taste!

Research shows some of the complex results of allowing bitter substances to pass over the receptors of the tongue including stimulation of the gastrointestinal hormone gastrin. Gastrin is known to result in at least a dozen diverse physiological actions including digestive enzyme production, bile flow, intrinsic factor secretion, insulin, glucagon and calcitonin secretion, changes in muscle tone of the gastric walls and associated sphincters, even cell division and repair of the lining of the small intestine and of the pancreas. Production, flow and quality of bile is enhanced, allowing better digestion of food and thus protection of the delicate membranes of the small and large intestines. We shall return to the digestive system later in this chapter.

Although not every bitter food has physiological actions, the bitter taste in many medicinal plants has unique and vital significance in herbal medicine and produces modulating effects in the gastrointestinal system. Correct functioning of the digestive system contributes to a healthy and diverse microbiome, and will in turn improve the tone, peristalsis and secretions of the digestive mucosa.

This information illustrates the diverse indications for bitters in the Western herbal tradition. The actual bitter taste is the result of many different kinds of compounds within the plant, each with its own specific action. We consider the therapeutics of taste in Chapter 5.

Touch

The sense of touch is distributed throughout the body. Nerve endings in the skin and other parts of the body transmit sensations to the brain via the sensory nervous system, part of the peripheral nervous system.

Some parts of the body have a larger number of nerve endings and, therefore, are more sensitive. The fingertips, areas around the mouth and the sexual organs have the greatest concentration of nerve endings.

Four kinds of touch sensations can be identified as having their origins in the skin: cold, heat, contact (pressure) and pain. The phenomenon of converting sensation from sensory receptors in our skin into electrical impulses that ultimately result in sensation is called sensory transduction. Hairs on the skin can magnify sensitivity and act as an early warning system for the body.

Sensory receptors in the skin transmit information through neurons that pass back to the spinal column, to the brain and on to specialised areas within the brain to interpret the sensations. These nerve pathways are called afferent nerves, and they transmit information from the skin to the brain. Physiological and mechanical responses to skin sensation (touch) are caused by efferent nerve signals passing back down the spinal column from the brain and leaving the spinal cord at the appropriate vertebrae. Fast-conduction nerve fibres transmit crude sensation so we can react very quickly— so that we might, for example, remove a hand from a very hot pan without even thinking about it—in this instance, we have used our automatic reflexes.

The skin is considered to be a physiological system in its own right. In conventional medicine, diseases of the skin are managed within the medical speciality of dermatology. The skin is often described as the largest organ of the body. It may not be immediately obvious that the skin has a number of complex functions beyond sensory ones.

1. *Protection*: It acts as a mechanical barrier between the deeper tissues and potential injury, toxicity and UV rays from the environment.
2. *Regulation*: Skin contributes to the homeostasis of body temperature by allowing sweating, raising body hairs to trap warmth, and by the blood vessels within the skin layers responding to temperature.
3. *Formation of Vitamin D*: Our skin is a major provider of Vitamin D, an essential vitamin for healthy bones, and immune function. Skin cells manufacture vitamin D in the presence of sunlight using a steroid precursor chemical, cholesterol.
4. *Sensation*: Nerve receptors in the skin are adapted to sense light, touch, deep pressure, pain and temperature. In this way, the skin can communicate to the internal tissues what is going on in the outside world.
5. *Excretion*: The skin is able to excrete unwanted substances through sweat. It is also able to secrete aromatic chemicals, which give each person a unique smell. This is part of the non-verbal communication possible between individuals.
6. *Absorption*: This function is considered conventionally to be very limited, but the skin can absorb substances from the external environment. This can be interpreted as another sensory role of the

skin—allowing the body to respond to what is happening in the outside world. The skin is particularly sensitive and able to absorb, fats and oils (especially volatile oils), but also hormones for example, hormone replacement therapy (HRT) patches.

7. *Communication*: The skin can blush when we feel embarrassed or nervous. In traditional herbal medicine systems the skin can also give information about a person's 'constitution', and via a system of facial diagnosis—the skin can indicate the healthy function of the interior.

Note: Western herbal medicine perspective—skin and routes of elimination. Problems arising on the skin are seen in Western herbal medicine as arising from within the body. Even contact reactions resulting in dermatitis can be seen as inappropriate responses by our body—overreactions by our immune system for example.

The skin is seen as being created from the blood. The blood may contain irregular amounts of stress hormones, immune factors, infective agents or waste products of metabolism.

Therefore an enduring approach within Western herbal medicine is to improve the co-ordination of elimination of normal waste products of metabolism by enhancing the function of the organs of excretion (bowel, kidney, lung, uterus, skin including lymph). Words such as depurative and alterative describe the capacity of a herb to broadly enhance this normal function of the body.

The ecosystem as the model of human physiology is demonstrated fully in the herbal approach to treating skin conditions. Herbal medicines prescribed for the skin may be simultaneously applied to the function of the gut, the microbiome, the lymphatic and immune system, the nervous system, the circulatory system, the kidney or respiratory system, and/or the endocrine (hormonal) system.

Beyond the five sense organs

Describing how many senses we have depends on how we categorise them. In addition to sight, smell, taste, touch and hearing, humans also have sensory awareness of balance (equilibrioception), pressure, temperature (thermoception), pain (nociception), vibration and motion. All senses that may involve the co-ordinated use of multiple sensory organs.

The sense of balance for example, is maintained by a complex interaction of the peripheral nervous system—visual inputs, the proprioceptive sensors (which are affected by gravity), stretch sensors found in muscles, skin and joints, the inner ear vestibular system and the central nervous system.

Disturbances occurring in any part of the balance system, or even within the brain's integration of inputs, can cause the feeling of dizziness or unsteadiness, this can include causes such as viral infections as in viral labyrinthitis (an 'itis' at the end of a word means *inflammation of*).

Stephen Harrod Buhner, in his lovely book *The Secret Teachings of Plants* speaks of the electromagnetic field of the heart as having the ability to detect and even synchronise with other electro-magnetic fields or biological oscillators, and acquire information. This can be internal or external to the person. The ability of some people to detect auras, or energy fields from living entities such as plants and trees is thought to be an example of this. Considering the heart as a sensing organ is an interesting concept! Although the senses are often portrayed as outward-looking to our external environment, our senses are also intimately related to the detection of our internal environment and the function and balance of the ecosystem of the interior.

Kinesthesia is the precise awareness of muscle and joint movement that allows us to coordinate our muscles when we walk, talk and use our hands. It is the sense of kinesthesia that enables us to touch the tip of our nose with our eyes closed or to know which part of the body we should scratch when we itch.

Some people experience a phenomenon called synesthesia in which one type of stimulation evokes the sensation of another. For example, the hearing of a sound may result in the sensation of the visualisation of a colour, or a shape may be sensed as a smell. Synesthesia is hereditary and it is estimated that it occurs in 1 out of 1000 individuals with variations of type and intensity. The most common forms of synesthesia link numbers or letters with colours.

The sixth sense?

It could be said that our brain functions most efficiently and with vested interest when its host is at risk. We often think that conscious thought is somehow better, when intuition is in fact

like soaring flight compared to the plodding of logic.
—G. De Becker[27]

What many will dismiss as a gut feeling or co-incidence is actually a cognitive process, faster than we recognise, and different from the step-by-step thinking we rely on so willingly. The root of the word intuition—*tuere*—means 'to guard, protect'.

Gavin De Becker suggests that whilst we are busy getting on with our lives, our sensory system is processing vast amounts of information. Our brains work hard filtering the huge mosaic of input and identifying any non-usual or significant data that disturbs a pattern of events, but because the sensory data is so huge, we are simply left with a feeling that something was or wasn't quite right—an intuition. Because we cannot consciously identify the cause of the 'intuition' we often defiantly disregard it.

de Becker says:

> *Can you imagine an animal reacting to the gift of fear the way some people do ... no animal in the wild... would spend any of its mental energy thinking 'It's probably nothing'.*
> —G. De Becker[27]

Another way he says that this manifests is how

> *Many experts lose the creativity and imagination of the less informed.*
> —G. De Becker[27]

The process of applying expertise is after all, an editing out of unimportant details in favour of those known (or thought) to be relevant. And so, whilst we may prefer and choose to develop expertise, there is *also* something important about truly seeing something again, with 'new eyes'.

Our precious senses are constantly informing us about the environment we inhabit, and allowing us to respond to that environment. Processing and responding to the constant flow of information we receive is unimaginably complex, and requires co-ordination and cohesion if we are to survive. It is no wonder that our senses have evolved sometimes surprising links with our internal body systems. Please see associated mind-map for a few examples.

Now let's move on to individual body systems.

The five senses

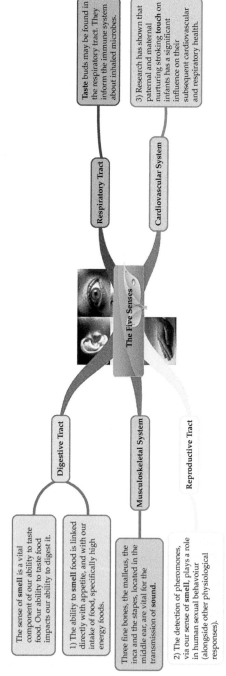

The Five Senses

Respiratory Tract

Taste buds may be found in the respiratory tract. They inform the immune system about inhaled microbes.

Cardiovascular System

3) Research has shown that paternal and maternal nurturing stroking **touch** on infants has a significant influence on their subsequent cardiovascular and respiratory health.

Digestive Tract

The sense of **smell** is a vital component of our ability to taste food. Our ability to taste food impacts our ability to digest it.

1) The ability to **smell** food is linked directly with appetite, and with our intake of food, specifically high energy foods.

Musculoskeletal System

Three fine bones, the malleus, the inca and the stapes, located in the middle ear, are vital for the transmission of **sound**.

Reproductive Tract

2) The detection of pheromones, via our sense of **smell**, plays a role in human sexual behaviour (alongside other physiological responses).

References

1) Proserpio, C., de Graaf, C., et al., *Impact of ambient odors on food intake, saliva production and appetite ratings.* Physiology & Behavior, 2017. 174: pp. 35–41.

2) Wyatt, T. D., *The search for human pheromones: the lost decades and the necessity of returning to first principles.* Proceedings of the Royal Society of Biology, 2015. 282(1804): pp. 20142994.

3) Van Puyvelde, M., et al., *Infants autonomic cardio- respiratory responses to nurturing stroking touch delivered by the mother or the father.* Frontiers in Physiology. 2019. 10: p. 1117.

The digestive system

You may wish to read this section on the digestive system in conjunction with either Chapters 4 or 5, which will be looking at herbs interacting with the digestive tract and nutrition respectively.

Gut health has historically been a key point of focus in herbal medicine and there are many good reasons for this.

- It is the interface between our body and the outside world.
- It is responsible for controlling what passes into our bodies and what remains outside of them.
- It is a major route of elimination of unwanted and potentially toxic substances.
- It is our 'second brain' containing five times more nervous tissue than our spinal cord.
- It communicates with the central nervous system but can, and does, act independently of it.
- It is the location of our gut flora (microbiota) which modern research is showing to be absolutely key to the healthy functioning of our immune systems, as well as having a significant impact on such areas as mood, weight gain/obesity and a whole raft of auto-immune based health problems.

Most practising herbalists would agree that attention to gut function and support of the digestive tract proves very beneficial in just about every situation. We are now in a stronger position than ever to understand why this is the case.

The gastrointestinal (GI) tract starts at the mouth. Much of this has been covered under the five senses and the sense of taste, but just one more thing to look at before we leave the mouth—the salivary glands.

Salivary glands

Salivary glands are examples of exocrine glands, which secrete their products into ducts. The three main pairs of salivary glands are:

- The parotid glands, which open into the mouth around the level of the second upper molar tooth.
- The submandibular glands, which open onto the floor of the mouth.
- The sublingual glands, which lie in front of the submandibular glands.

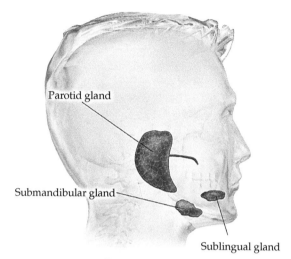

Salivary glands

We do not consciously produce saliva, rather it is an automatic response, usually to the smell or taste of food. This is controlled by the autonomic nervous system, which takes care of all the things that we do without thinking about it (such as blinking, breathing and producing saliva).

We have covered some of the functions of saliva in the section on non-specific immune system defences, but just to recap:

- Lysozyme and immunoglobulins are present in saliva as the first form of defence against anything pathogenic or toxic.
- Saliva moistens and lubricates our food, and also moistens and lubricates our mouths, helping to prevent damage to our mucous membranes by sharp or rough foods.
- Saliva helps us to taste dry foods, by making the compounds within food soluble, and therefore allowing them to interact with our taste buds.
- Saliva contains the enzyme amylase, which helps begin the process of the digestion of carbohydrates.

From the mouth we travel to the oesophagus, and then onwards on a wondrous journey through many a twist and turn, to end up again back in the outside world. Throughout this journey, the walls of the gastrointestinal tract have the same basic four-layer structure (with the exception of the stomach). These layers are a) an outer membrane, b) a smooth muscle layer, c) a sub-mucosal layer containing connective

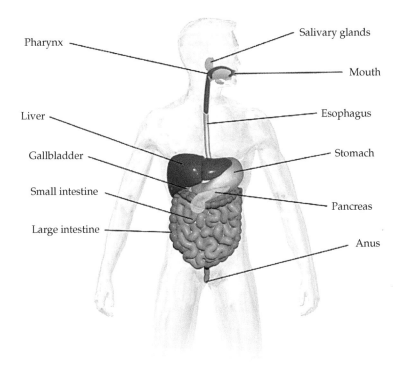

Pharynx

Salivary glands

Mouth

Liver

Esophagus

Gallbladder

Stomach

Small intestine

Large intestine

Pancreas

Anus

The components of the digestive system

tissues, blood vessels and a network of nerves and d) the mucosa, the innermost lining of the gastrointestinal tract.

The oesophagus is a muscular tube connecting the mouth to the stomach. It is the means by which food passes from mouth to stomach, and food begins its journey here, with swallowing. The oesophagus enters the abdomen through a hole in the diaphragm. The regular muscular contractions called peristalsis that move food through the digestive tract, begin in the oesophagus.

Food then enters the stomach by a sphincter called the cardiac sphincter. You can think of the stomach like a bag comprised of three layers of muscle—one more muscle layer than the rest of the GI tract. The three layers all lie in different directions and act to rhythmically squeeze the bag, thus breaking down the contents inside (yes, your stomach actually churns!). Food is not only broken down in the stomach by mechanical movement. Various secretions produced by the stomach wall also act to begin the chemical breakdown of food.

Secretion	Action
Water and mineral salts	Liquification of food
Mucous	Protection of stomach lining
Pepsinogens	Breakdown of proteins
Hydrochloric acid	Sterilisation of food
	Converts pepsinogens to pepsins
	Stops action of amylase
Intrinsic factor	Necessary for vitamin B12 absorption

These secretions together are called gastric secretions, meaning they are of the stomach sac specifically. Although we use words like *stomach* and *gastric* to mean anything *digestive*, in medicine, they have very specific meanings.

From here we will move on to the small intestine, where the bulk of the breakdown and absorption of food takes place.

The small intestine is divided into three areas:

- *The duodenum*: 25 centimetres long. Secretions from gall bladder and pancreas enter here. Pancreatic juices are alkaline, therefore they neutralise the acid from the stomach, protecting the walls of the small intestine from damage by hydrochloric acid (HCL), and providing a correct pH for pancreatic enzymes to work. Bile, secreted by the gall bladder, acts to break down fats.
- *The jejunum*: 2 metres long. Nutrients from the breakdown of food in the duodenum are absorbed here and travel (with the exception of fats) to the liver.
- *The ileum*: 3 metres long. B12 and intrinsic factor are absorbed here. Patches of immune system tissue called Peyer's patches can also be found here. Peyer's patches are key players in our response towards gut antigens and pathogenic bacteria. They are at their largest in the third decade of life.[28]

The surface area of the small intestine is estimated to be approximately half the size of a badminton court.[29] This serves to optimise the area available for digestion and absorption of food. This is achieved by the presence on its surface of structures called villi.

The villi contain blood vessels, for the absorption of nutrients and lymphatic structures called lacteals, for the absorption of fats. The villi are lined with microvilli, which increase the surface area even more.

Lumen of small intestine

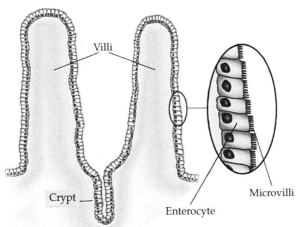

The epithelium lining the small intestine and its villi is replaced every 3 days. This fast turnover ensures that any injury heals quickly and any toxic substances absorbed by the epithelia are removed.

Next on our journey we come to the large intestine, also known as the colon. By this time nutrient and phytochemical absorption has largely taken place. We reclaim fluid in the large intestine that we originally secreted into the gut in the mouth, stomach and small intestine and haven't already reabsorbed: the fine-tuning of water balance.

A massive population of gut flora or microbiota reside here, and they are responsible for the metabolism of some hormones, production of vitamins such as B12 and folic acid, and the fermentation of insoluble fibres. Approximately half of our daily requirement of vitamin K is produced by our gut microbiota. We will be looking at the massive contribution that the gut microbiome makes to our overall health and wellbeing in other sections, but it certainly cannot be underestimated. Absorption of some drugs also takes place in the large intestine.

By the time all this processing has been completed, the outcome is of course, known to us all as faeces (or poo). Ultimately this is expelled from the body via distension of the walls of the rectum, triggered by peristaltic waves.

And there we have it—a brief journey through the digestive tract. Finally, a word about a small part of the digestive tract that has had a lot of bad press over the years: the appendix.

What, you cry, is the purpose of the appendix? (Other than to become infected and try to kill you.) Well, you will notice from the picture here,

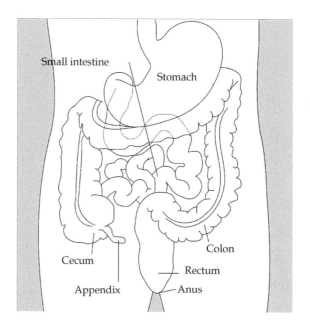

that the appendix is situated around the junction between the small and large intestine. It is formed of immune system tissue. If you are a loser in the exotic holiday tummy bug lottery and end up with a severe case of diarrhoea, the appendix is ready with a handy reservoir of good quality gut flora with which to repopulate your depleted reserves (and we all know just how important gut flora is!). The appendix has been described as possibly serving as:

> *A 'safe house' for commensal bacteria that can re-inoculate the gut at need.*
> —C. M. Guinane[30]

So it's a good guy after all!

Interconnectedness

The major systems involved in direct interactions with the digestive tract are the immune system, the nervous system and the endocrine system, all the main players in the maintenance of homeostasis in our bodies, the ability to make our interior world a wholesome and comfortable place for our organs and tissues to live. This must give us a bit of a clue about just how important this organ system is, and the profound knock-on effects it can have throughout the body when things 'aren't right down there'.

The digestive system

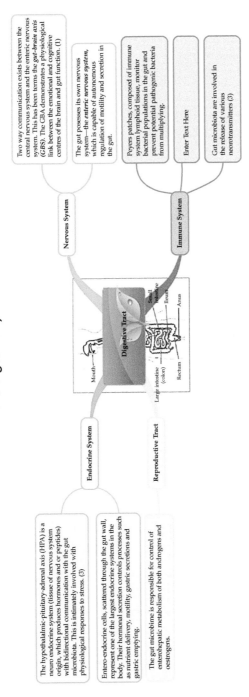

Nervous System

Two way communication exists between the central nervous system and the enteric nervous system. This has been terms the *gut-brain axis* (*GBA*). The GBA demonstrates a physiological link between the emotional and cognitive centres of the brain and gut function. (1)

The gut possesses its own nervous system—the *enteric nervous system*, which is capable of autonomous regulation of motility and secretion in the gut.

Immune System

Peyers patches, composed of immune system lymphoid tissue, monitor bacterial populations in the gut and prevent potential pathogenic bacteria from multiplying.

Enter Text Here

Gut microbiota are involved in the release of various neurotransmitters (3)

Endocrine System

The hypothalamic-pituitary-adrenal axis (HPA) is a neuro endocrine system (tissue of nervous system origin, which produces hormones and or peptides) with bidirectional communication with the gut microbiota. This is intimately involved with physiological responses to stress. (3)

Entero-endocrine cells, scattered through the gut wall, represent one of the largest endocrine systems in the body. Their hormonal secretion controls processes such as nutrient delivery, motility, gastric secretions and gastric emptying.

Reproductive Tract

The gut microbiome is responsible for control of enterohepatic metabolism of both androgens and oestrogens.

References

1) Carabotti, M., A. Scirocco, M. A. Maselli and C. Severi, *The gut-brain axis: Interactions between enteric microbiota, central and enteric nervous systems*. Annals of Gastroenterology. 2015. 28(2): pp. 203–209.

2) Altves, S., H. K. Yildiz and H. C. Vural, *Interaction of the microbiota with the human body in health and diseases*. Bioscience of Microbiota. Food and Health, 2020. 39(2): pp. 23–32. https://doi.org/10.12938/bmfh.19-023.

3) Farzi, A., E. E. Fröhlich and P. Holzer, *Gut microbiota and the neuroendocrine system*. Neurotherapeutics, 2018. 15(1): pp. 5–22. https://doi.org/10.1007/s13311-017-0600-5.

Herbal connections

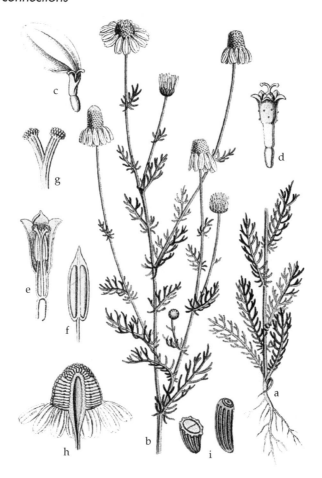

Chamomile (*Matricaria chamomilla* L., Rauschert)

Many herbs exert beneficial actions on the gut, but the one everyone is familiar with is, of course, chamomile. Chamomile species have been referred to historically as a sort of 'mother of the gut' due to its ability to soothe and calm inflamed gut tissue. Chamomile has been used extensively in the treatment of irritable bowel syndrome for its calming impact both upon the gut wall (the endothelial membrane) itself and for its soothing effects on the nervous system. The two main species of chamomile used medicinally in the West are *Matricaria chamomilla* L., known as German chamomile (synonyms include: *Chamomilla recutita* L. Rauschert and *Matricaria recutita* L.), and *Chamaemelum nobile* (L.) All., commonly known as Roman chamomile. The word *Matricaria* comes from the same source as the words matriarch or maternal, relating to mothers. When making chamomile tea, if you leave it long enough before you drink it, the tea goes quite thick and gloopy in texture, demonstrating its inherent soothing and demulcent properties.

The cardiovascular system

You may wish to read this section on the cardiovascular system in conjunction with Chapter 6, which will be looking at herbs interacting with the cardiovascular system.

Structure

The cardiovascular system is comprised of the heart and blood vessels.

The heart consists of four chambers, two atria, and two ventricles, with perfectly designed valves in between. The heart can fill with blood, and then push it out, either to the lungs or out to the rest of the body. Blood sent to the lungs can swap carbon dioxide for oxygen there, and then return straight back to the heart to be sent off, this time, to the rest of our body.

You may know that the main highway systems for the transport of blood around the body are arteries and veins. You may even also know that arteries carry oxygen-rich, or oxygenated blood and veins carry blood low in oxygen or deoxygenated blood. But is this the whole story?

Blood passes from the heart to arteries, then to smaller and more numerous arterioles, then to fine capillaries, only one cell thick, so that nutrients, food and other goodies can pass out of them into all types of body tissues. Capillaries then turn into venules, which ultimately become larger veins and return to the heart.

Arteries away!! Arteries carry blood away from the heart, whereas veins carry blood back to the heart. Of course they say there are exceptions to every rule, and there is one important exception to this one, which we will look at when we look at the heart in more detail.

The pressure in the arteries is higher than that in veins, so the arterial walls contain more elastic tissue to cope with that pressure. Arteries have a smooth lining of cells called an endothelium, surrounded by smooth muscle, vascular and elastic layers. As the arteries get smaller they become less elastic and more muscular, and it is here, in the smaller arterioles, that the fine control of blood pressure takes place, via adjustment of the diameter of these vessels. Thus we see that differing blood vessels have differing structures reflecting their functions.

Some herbal medicines exert their effects on the peripheral circulatory system, and are, where indicated, deliberately used in conjunction with others, which work as more central cardiovascular tonics.[31]

The walls of veins tend to be less elastic due to the lower pressure as blood returns to the heart. The walls of veins are thinner than arteries, but also have smooth muscle and elastic tissues. Some veins contain valves, especially those of the limbs, to prevent backflow of blood under low pressure. The valves ensure that venous blood travels in the direction of the heart. Veins can be prone to collapse or overstretching, and this can lead to varicose veins, for example. The veins rely on blood pressure itself, the movement of our skeletal muscles, and our respiration to aid venous return to the heart.

When you feel someone's pulse what is it you are actually feeling? When the heart contracts (this is called systole), blood is pushed out into the arterial circulation. Some arteries lie quite close to the surface of the body, and that surge of blood into the system can be felt as the elastic walls of the arterial blood vessels expand to accommodate it.

Let's look at the heart itself a bit more closely! When we looked at key concepts earlier in this chapter, we took a look at the basic structure of a eukaryotic cell. We also mentioned that cells become specifically structurally modified in terms of their function. The cells that make up the muscle wall of the heart are a unique type of muscle cell found only in the heart wall. Under a microscope they appear striated or striped, as do skeletal muscle cells, but they differ in that they are closely interconnected and therefore look like a sheet of muscle cells rather than individual cells. The ends of the cells are connected by structures called intercalated discs, and this means that each cell does not need its own nerve supply. When a nerve impulse is generated it efficiently spreads out over the whole sheet. This means that muscle contraction can spread like a wave (think Mexican wave!) over the surface of the heart and the atria and ventricles can contract in a flowing, coordinated manner.

Regular, smooth muscular contractions are of course a key feature to a well-functioning heart. A specialised bundle of nerve cells located in the wall of the left atria and called the sino-atrial node (SA node), sends out impulses across the surface of this unique muscle structure, to initiate contraction. First, contraction of the of the atria and then, a split second later, of the ventricles. Nerve fibres called purkinje fibres transmit this signal from the atria to the ventricles. The SA node is therefore known as the pacemaker.

Going back to the heart muscle wall for a minute; Stephen Buhner in his book *The Secret Teachings of Plants*, points out that the amount of pressure needed to force blood through the entire CV system would be equivalent to the ability to lift a 100 lb weight one mile high. Even on our worst days I don't think any of us feel that we are under that

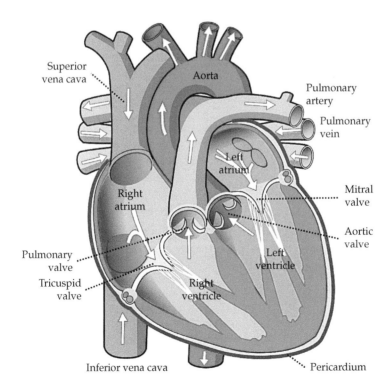

amount of pressure! The heart is not just a pump, and its role in moving blood through the body is much more subtle. Modern technology has informed anatomy and has shown that the muscles of the heart are arranged in a helical fashion.[32] This may explain why blood actually moves through major vessels in a spiral fashion, two streams spiralling around each other in the direction of flow. This is more in line with the formation of a vortex, with a vacuum at its centre.[33]

Just like any other tissue, this sheet of muscle needs oxygen and nutrients to survive, so you will see coronary arteries on the surface of the heart, which feed the heart wall itself. When these arteries get blocked or occluded, this is called a myocardial infarction, or heart attack.

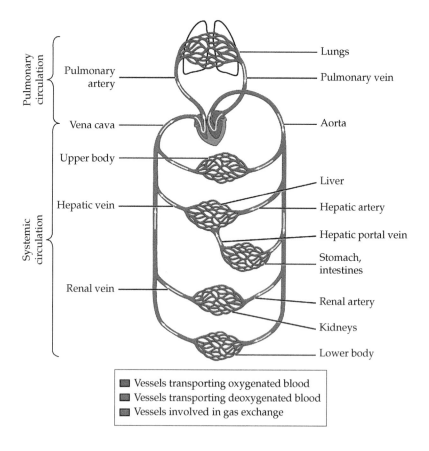

Pulmonary circulation

Systemic circulation

Lungs

Pulmonary artery

Pulmonary vein

Vena cava

Aorta

Upper body

Liver

Hepatic vein

Hepatic artery

Hepatic portal vein

Stomach, intestines

Renal vein

Renal artery

Kidneys

Lower body

■ Vessels transporting oxygenated blood
■ Vessels transporting deoxygenated blood
■ Vessels involved in gas exchange

If we go on a little journey, following the path that blood would take as it flows through the heart, we would find that the right-hand side of the heart is completely separate from the left-hand side. There is a wall of tissue running pretty much vertically through the heart, separating the two sides. Blood flow through the body can be described as a closed circular system. The scheme below shows blood flow in its simplest form.

You can see even from this simple diagram that the functions of the heart and lungs are very closely related, and it is usual in herbal practice, when treating one of these systems, to support the other also, as when one is struggling, the other may be affected.

There are two sets of valves in place in the heart, to ensure that blood flows only in the right direction. The atrioventricular valves separate the atria from the ventricles in each side of the heart, the aortic valve separates the left ventricle from the aorta, and the pulmonary valve separates the right ventricle from the pulmonary artery. The *lub dub* we hear when we use a stethoscope is the sound of these valves closing.

Function

The cardiovascular system represents the major transport system of the body, and is responsible for carrying oxygen and nutrients to all areas of the body via our blood, as well as transporting waste away, and also for circulating hormones, enzymes and a whole host of other biological compounds essential to life. This sounds like a very short explanation for a brilliantly complex and vital system, but it is also at the heart (no pun intended) of good health. As the brilliant scientist David Bohm once said, 'everything is flow'.

Interconnectedness

As you have seen, the cardiovascular system has some direct interconnections with other systems of the body. Some are more obvious than others. Here are a few examples in a mindmap:[34-36]

The cardiovascular system

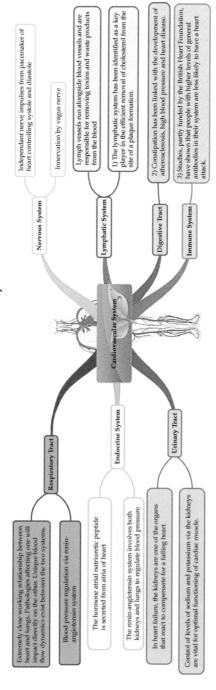

Independant nerve impulses from pacemaker of heart controlling systole and diastole

Innervation by vagus nerve

Nervous System

Lymph vessels run alongside blood vessels and are responsible for removing toxins and waste products from the blood

1) The lymphatic system has been identified as a key player in the efficient removal of cholesterol from the site of a plaque formation.

Lymphatic System

2) Constipation has been linked with the development of atherosclerosis, high blood pressure and heart disease.

Digestive Tract

3) Studies, partly funded by the British Heart Foundation, have shown that people with higher levels of general antibodies in their system are less likely to have a heart attack.

Immune System

Cardiovascular System

Extremely close working relationship between heart and lungs. Pathologies affecting one will impact directly on the other. Unique blood flow dynamics exist between the two systems.

Blood pressure regulation via renin-angiotensin system

Respiratory Tract

The hormone atrial natriuretic peptide is secreted from atria of heart

The renin-angiotensin system involves both kidneys and lungs to regulate blood pressure

Endocrine System

In heart failure, the kidneys are one of the organs that react to compensate for a failing heart

Control of levels of sodium and potassium via the kidneys are vital for optimal functioning of cardiac muscle.

Urinary Tract

References

1) Milasan, A., J. Ledoux and C. Martel, *Lymphatic network in atherosclerosis: The underestimated path.* Future Science OA. 2015. Published online.

2) Ishiyama, Y., S. Hoshide, H. Mizuno and K. Kario, *Constipation-induced pressor effects as triggers for cardiovascular events.* Journal of Clinical Hypertension, 2019. 21(3): pp. 421–425.

3) Khamis, R., et al., *High serum immunoglobulin G and M levels predict freedom from adverse cardiovascular events in hypertension: A nested case-control substudy of the anglo-scandinavian cardiac outcomes trial.* The Lancet, 2016. 9: pp. 372–380.

Herbal connections

A key herb to talk about with relation to the cardiovascular system is hawthorn (*Crataegus spp*).

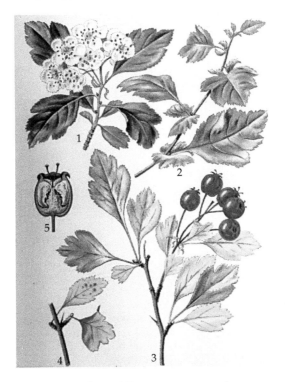

Hawthorn (*Crataegus* species)

Hawthorn's actions on the cardiovascular system are a relatively new discovery. A 19th-century Irish doctor called Green successfully used a 'secret' remedy in the treatment of cardiovascular disease. After his death in 1894, his daughter revealed his famous cure to be a tincture of ripe hawthorn berries. In 1896 Dr Jennings of Chicago wrote the first known article on hawthorn as a major heart remedy and by the early 20th-century hawthorn was gaining recognition as a cardiovascular agent.

Hawthorn's actions on the cardiovascular system include lowering the blood pressure via dilation of blood vessels, slowing the rate of con-traction of the heart itself, but strengthening the force of contraction, therefore improving the overall efficiency of the organ. The flowers, berries and young leaves can all be used medicinally, and it has an excellent track record of use with standard orthodox drugs for the cardiovascular system. We shall take a much closer examination of hawthorn in Chapter 6.

The reproductive system

You may wish to read this section on the reproductive system in conjunction with Chapter 7, which will be looking at herbal treatment for the reproductive tract.

Whilst we are in the general area of the pelvis, let's take a foray into the magical and mysterious world of the male and female reproductive systems. Adhering to tradition, let's say, 'ladies first'.

The female reproductive system

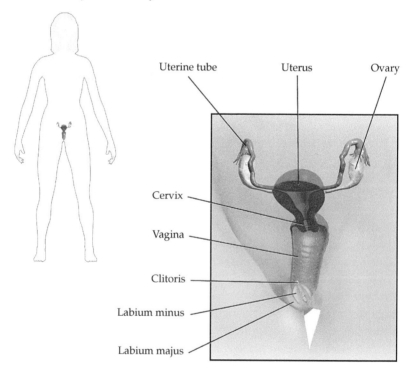

The female reproductive system

We will look at the female reproductive system in three parts:

- The external genitalia
- The internal genitalia
- The menstrual cycle

External genitalia

The labia majora comprises of two large folds or lips, that mark the boundary of the external genitalia (labia is Greek for lips). The labia minora are smaller folds of skin nestling inside the labia major (like petals in a rose). Both the vagina and the urethra open out into the labia minora. The opening inside the labia minora (into the vagina) is called the vestibule. The area between the base of the labia minora and the anus is called the perineum. The clitoris is found at the anterior end of the labia and is related to the penis in the male and, like the penis, is erectile. It rarely gets much of a mention in anatomy and physiology textbooks, despite being a very precious asset for women! Around 3/4 of the clitoris is beneath the surface. Vestibular glands (Bartholin's glands) have the important job of keeping the vagina moist. They are the size of a pea and open into the vaginal opening (the vestibule).

Internal genitalia

The vagina

The vagina is a lovely muscular tube, extending from its opening into the outside world at the vestibule of the labia minora, up to the cervix, which is the neck of the uterus. The vagina is kept moist by secretions from the cervix, and by vestibular glands and, as part of our non-specific defence system, we like to maintain a healthy population of the bacteria *lactobacillus acidophilus* here too. These helpful lactobacilli help maintain a pH of between 4.9–3.5, thus discouraging the growth of unwelcome microbes. The shape of the vagina is an excellent example of how form reflects function in terms of its ability to receive during sexual intercourse, and as an elastic passageway outward for childbirth.

The uterus

The uterus is basically an expandable, muscular organ, lying between the bladder and the rectum. Shaped rather like an inverted pear, it is lined with a velvety layer of specialised cells, the endometrium. The endometrium responds to hormones during the fertile years of a woman's' life and allows implantation of the fertilised egg in the case of conception. During pregnancy it houses the foetus and placenta, and it therefore has a comprehensive array of supportive ligaments, which help keep everything in place. It also requires its own rich blood supply, and this is achieved via a significant number of veins that sit around and below the structure.

The uterine tubes (fallopian tubes)

Fallopian tubes extend from either side of the upper part or fundus of the uterus up towards the ovaries. At their ends there are finger-like structures called fimbriae, which are in close association with the ovaries. When an ovary releases an egg it is the job of the corresponding fallopian tube to transport that egg safely to the uterus for implantation. Although we call them 'tubes' the fallopian tubes are, in cross-section, made up of numerous folds of delicate membranes along which the egg must pass. The fallopian tube does this by two mechanisms:

- By peristalsis (we also have peristalsis in the digestive system and ureters)
- By ciliary movement (we have met some cilia already)

The ovaries

Ovaries form part of the endocrine system, and each ovary is attached to the uterus via the ovarian ligament. Like the adrenal glands they have a medulla and a cortex. The cortex (outer layer) contains ovarian follicles (eggs) at various stages of maturation. The medulla is rich with blood vessels, nerves and lymphatics.

The menstrual cycle

Now we come to the complexity and elegance of the menstrual cycle. The menstrual cycle is orchestrated by a number of hormones interacting in harmony (hopefully) to produce an on-going cycle of ebb and flow during women's reproductive years. At some point during this rhythmic cycle there will be a period of time during which the rich lining of the wall of the uterus, the endometrium, is shed, exiting the uterus at the cervix, and out of the body via the vagina. This lining has been purposely built up and nourished over the preceding (usually 4) weeks to provide a safe and supportive place for a fertilised egg to take root and develop. The shedding of the endometrium is known as menstruation. Menstruation usually lasts between 3 to 5 days and is called a 'period' and it has been associated with a vast number of cultural rituals and taboos across the world.

Even today in the modern Western world it is usually regarded as at best a nuisance to be 'dealt with and endured', and at the worst a time of discomfort, emotional upset and pain. It can be hard to find people who have a positive word to say about it, and psychologically this has definitely impacted upon women's perceptions and thus experiences of the process, a definite example of a meaning response to quote Daniel Moerman.[37]

Taboos have certainly been at play in the 20th century, and older generations of women can be very reticent about discussing the whole issue, as it has been regarded as embarrassing and difficult. Modern conventional medicine certainly seems to struggle with effective tools to support the menstrual cycle, without taking it over. The treatment options are therapeutically narrow from this perspective, involving hormonal manipulation and control and/or surgery. 'Just get on and live with it' is also a common strategy. But what is actually happening?

You will see the menstrual cycle depicted in textbooks as a linear event. This is not the truth. The clue to the lie is in the name, the menstrual *cycle*. So let us step away from linear thinking for a moment and look at this more in terms of the circle dance that it is.

The dance is performed in three parts: the menstrual phase, the proliferative phase and the secretory phase. It is choreographed by the endocrine system, and a number of choreographers work together to produce it and keep natural dance partners co-ordinated.

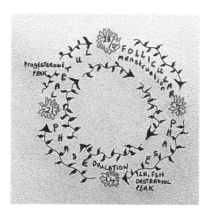

The menstrual cycle.

The menstrual phase

A circle has no beginning and no end. The first day of the period, however, is officially recognised as 'day one' of the cycle: the end is also the beginning. Day one marks the beginning of the menstrual phase of the cycle. The levels of the hormones (i.e. progesterone and oestrogen) on which the endometrium depended for support start to drop away, and thus the endometrium itself starts to deteriorate and is shed from the lining of the uterus. Negative feedback mechanisms in the body detect this fall in hormonal levels and this triggers the hypothalamus and the pituitary to kick in by starting to secrete increasing levels of the hormones Luteinising Hormone (LH) and Follicle Stimulating Hormone (FSH).

The proliferative phase

It is the job of FSH to stimulate the development of ovarian follicles so that one develops into a mature ova. The follicles start to produce oestrogen, which acts on the lining of the uterus (endometrium) so that it thickens and its blood supply and mucous secretory cells increase. The rising levels of oestrogen produced by the developing follicles also trigger a mid-cycle surge of LH, which in turn triggers ovulation (on or around day 14).

The secretory phase

Now the stage is set. LH goes on to support the development of something called the corpus luteum. Corpus luteum is Latin for the *yellow body*, and this is the area on the ovary left after ovulation. The corpus luteum acts as another endocrine gland, secreting progesterone and some oestrogen, which act on the endometrium, the vagina and the glands of the cervix to produce watery mucous which helps spermatozoa travel to the ova. It also puts a brake on the breakdown of the lining of the uterus (endometrium) and prevents bleeding (shedding of the endometrium), thus potentially allowing fertilisation of the ovum. High levels of progesterone and oestrogen inhibit the pituitary glands production of FSH and LH after ovulation, to prevent a further follicle being stimulated.

Our precious ovum is now launched out into the world, and it will only survive out there for approximately 8 hours before it is no longer fertilisable. So, one of two things can happen now:

- Fertilisation takes place. The fertilised ovum nestles happily in the wall of the endometrium and starts to produce a hormone called Human Chorionic Gonadotrophin (HCG) which continues to support the corpus luteum, thus keeping levels of progesterone and oestrogen high and inhibiting further follicle maturation. *Note: The pregnancy test is actually testing for levels of HCG.* The dominant hormones oestrogen and progesterone also start to stimulate the growth of breast tissue at this time, in preparation for childbirth and nursing. After childbirth itself, the two pituitary hormones prolactin and oxytocin are responsible for production and release of milk respectively (remember the section on the endocrine system!).
- Fertilisation does not take place. No HCG is produced, the corpus luteum degenerates, the endometrium becomes unsupported and ultimately breaks down, leading to the menstrual phase—the cycle is complete.

Menopause

Finally, a word about the menopause (although we shall cover this in more detail in Chapter 7). Usually between the ages of 45 and 55, the menopause kicks in. The ovaries gradually stop listening to the siren songs of the pituitary gland, the LH and FSH singers. Numbers of functioning follicles are now also reducing so oestrogen levels recede. This process can last anything from a few months to 10 years and requires significant adaptation. Increasingly erratic periods, changes in temperature and sleep pattern disruption are some of the symptoms experienced by women at this time, and all are amenable to support with herbs. The time of the wise woman arrives.

The male reproductive system

We will look at the male reproductive system in two parts.

- The external genitalia
- The internal genitalia

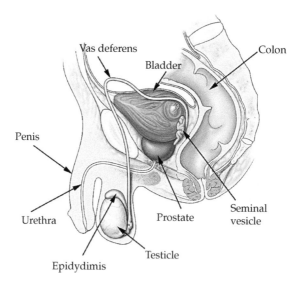

External genitalia

The external genitalia of the male consists of the penis and the scrotum, which contains the testes.

The scrotum is a specialised pouch of skin, divided into two compartments each containing testes and epididymis. There are two muscles relating to the scrotum, the cremaster muscle and the dartos muscle. The cremaster muscle pulls the scrotum up towards the body when the temperature drops, to maintain an optimal environment for sperm maturation. The dartos muscle will act to give the scrotum a wrinkled appearance when this happens, which is reversed when the scrotum descends again.

The penis creates a vehicle for the urethra, which is a common channel for both urine and semen. It is composed of both smooth muscle and specialised erectile tissue, which has a rich blood supply. The parasympathetic nervous system (involved in relaxation if you remember) controls blood flow into and out of the penis. It will allow arterial blood to flow into the penis, whilst preventing venous drainage. This allows the penis to become erect during sexual arousal.

Internal genitalia

The male internal genitalia is a masterpiece of plumbing. It consists of the testes, the epididymis, seminal vesicles and the prostate gland.

Equivalent to the ovaries, the testes are responsible for sperm production. Each testi is divided into around 200–300 lobules, and within each lobule are seminiferous tubules, specialised cells involved in the production of sperm. You may remember that FSH is responsible for the development of a mature ovum from the ovaries. This is the same arrangement, with FSH being responsible for sperm production. Between the seminiferous tubules, lie interstitial cells called Leydig cells, which secrete testosterone after puberty. The hundreds of seminiferous tubules eventually join up to form a single tubule, which folds backwards and forwards upon itself to form the epididymis.

Sperm cells produced in the seminiferous tubules mature as they pass through the epididymis. They are then stored here ready for action. From the epididymis sperm leave via the deferent duct (vas deferens) and continue on their journey to the ejaculatory duct. Here we have two pouches which open into an ejaculatory duct called the seminal vesicles. When the 'all systems go' bell is pushed, they will deliver their store of alkaline seminal fluid into the ejaculatory ducts to merge with the sperm from the epididymis. The interior of the vagina is relatively acidic (*remember the lactobacillus acidophilus, whose job it is to deter pathogens*). The seminal fluid is therefore alkaline to protect the sperm. It also contains sugars to sustain them on their long journey to glory.

The ejaculatory ducts pass through the centre of the prostate gland on their way to the outside world. The prostate gland produces a milky fluid containing a clotting enzyme designed to help thicken the semen and hold it in place close to the cervix. Finally the semen finds its way down the urethra (of urinary tract fame) and out into the big wonderful world of another person's reproductive tract. Anything between 200 million and 500 million sperm are contained in each ejaculate. That's a lot of candidates for one ovum!

Finally we will leave you with a charming poem by the well-known American herbalist Stephen Harrod Buhner.

A Poem on Pollination

Semen is latin
for a dormant, fertilised,
plant ovum-
a seed.
Men's ejaculate
is chemically more akin
to plant pollen.
See,
It is really
more accurate
to call it
mammal pollen.
To call it
semen
is to thrust
an insanity
deep inside our culture:
that men plow women
and plant their seed
when, in fact,
what they are doing
is pollinating
flowers.

—Stephen H. Buhner[22]

Interconnectedness

All life is here (potentially). All systems are involved in one way or another. Here are a few examples:

The reproductive systems

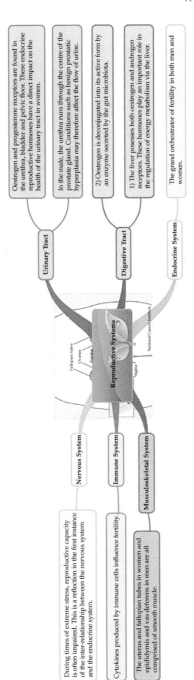

Urinary Tract

Oestrogen and progesterone receptors are found in the urethra, bladder and pelvic floor. These endocrine reproductive hormones have a direct impact on the health of the urinary tract in women.

In the male, the urethra runs through the centre of the prostate gland. Conditions such as benign prostatic hyperplasia may therefore affect the flow of urine.

Digestive Tract

2) Oestrogen is deconjugated into its active form by an enzyme secreted by the gut microbiota.

1) The liver posesses both oestrogen and androgen receptors. These hormones play an important role in the regulation of energy metabolism via the liver.

Endocrine System

The grand orchestrator of fertility in both men and women.

Nervous System

During times of extreme stress, reproductive capacity is often impaired. This is a reflection in the first instance of the inter-relationship between the nervous system and the endocrine system.

Immune System

Cytokines produced by immune cells influence fertility.

Musculoskeletal System

The uterus and fallopian tubes in women and epididymis and vas deferens in men are all comprised of smooth muscle.

References

1) Shen, M. and H. Shi, *Sex hormones and their receptors regulate liver energy homeostasis.* International Journal of Endocrinology. Published online Sept 27, 2015.

2) Baker, J. M., L. Al-Nakkash and M. M. Herbst-Kralovetz, *Estrogen-gut microbiome axis: Physiological and clinical implications.* Maturitas: The European Menopause Journal, 2017. 103: pp. 45–53.

Herbal connections

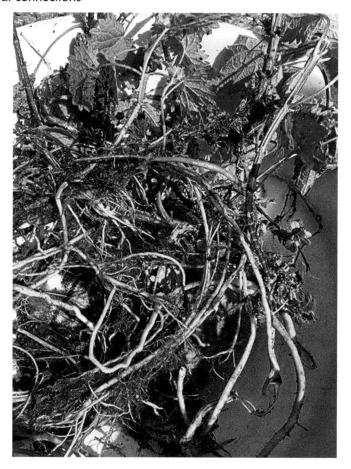

Nettle root (*Urtica dioica* L.)

This is where we get to 'sing a song of nettle'. Common nettle (*Urtica dioica* L.) has applications for both male and female reproductive systems. Nettle and raspberry leaf (*Rubus ideaus* L.) tea is an excellent tea to give pregnant women, combining as it does, the womb tonic properties of a raspberry leaf with the rich nutritional value of nettle leaf.

In terms of the male reproductive system, nettle root has proved to be of value in the treatment of benign prostatic hyperplasia (BPH).

One randomised double-blind study investigating patients with BPH and the therapeutic use of *Urtica dioica* L. concluded with the following statement:

> As a whole, nettle is recommended to be used more in treatment of BPH patients, given its beneficial effects in reducing BPH patients' symptoms and its safety in terms of its side effects and its being better accepted on the side of patients'.
>
> —A. Ghorbanibirgani, A. Khalili and L. Zamani[38]

The more we learn about the uses of the nettle the more we realise how much we owe this humble plant.

The lymphatic system

You may wish to read this section on the lymphatic system in conjunction with Chapter 8, which will be looking at herbs interacting with the lymphatic system.

The lymphatic system is perhaps one of the most overlooked systems of the body, and it is true to say that many people don't even know that it exists.

Structure

The lymphatic system consists of: Lymph, lymphatic vessels and lymph glands.

A fluid called interstitial fluid passes from capillaries into the tissues of our body and bathes all of our cells, allowing precious nutrients and oxygen to reach them. Our cells, in turn, excrete their waste products into the interstitial fluid that surrounds them, to be carried away. Think of it a bit like a house. Clean water is brought to the house via water pipes, and dirty water is removed from the house via drains and sewage pipes.

Some of this fluid returns to the bloodstream directly by way of venules, but much of it gets absorbed into the lymphatic system. The fluid contained within the lymphatic vessels is called lymph, and the lymph carries waste products away from tissues, as well as bacteria and cellular debris. Lymph also contains circulating lymphocytes, which

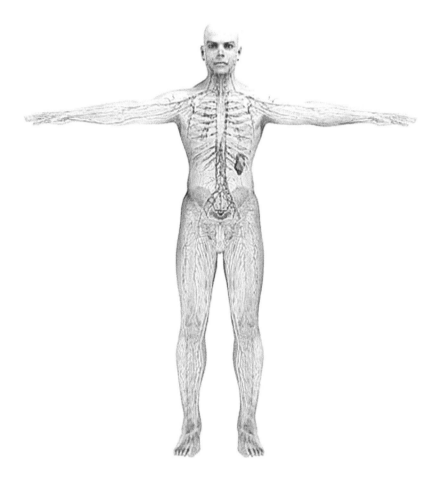

you will recall are white blood cells working as part of our immune system, keeping us safe from invading pathogens.

Lymph is generally clear, but if you looked at lymph taken from the lymphatic system in the walls of the small intestine, it would be a milky colour, because fat is absorbed into the lymphatic system first, rather than straight into our blood.

Lymphatic vessels start as tiny, blind-ended capillaries, which slowly merge to form larger vessels. Like veins, they contain valves called semi-lunar valves, which ensure that the lymph flows in one direction only. The structure of their walls is also similar to veins, including a layer of smooth muscle, which contracts rhythmically to propel lymph along. This process is also helped by the fact that lymphatic vessels often lie parallel to arteries and veins, and the pumping of blood through large arteries results in pulsations which also help to move lymph forwards. Ultimately, the multitude of lymphatic vessels from around our body, join together to form two large ducts, which empty into veins in the neck.

So, if you think about it, lymph contains waste products from cells, bacteria and cellular debris. Lymph therefore can potentially contain a variety of substances, that could be toxic or dangerous to our cells and tissues especially if we have had an infection for example—just as waste products produced in the home can potentially do us harm. For this reason structures called lymph nodes are stationed periodically along the network of lymphatic vessels, and their job is to 'clean up' and make the lymph safe before it enters the circulation.

Lymph nodes contain specialised mobile cells called lymphocytes and macrophages. Macrophages, and antibodies produced by the lymphocytes, destroy things like tumour cells, worn out or damaged tissues, invading microbes etc. By the time the lymph has reached the bloodstream it has passed through up to ten lymph nodes, and is usually clean of debris or foreign matter.

A cunning plan!

Our bodies have a cunning plan (many actually). Lymph nodes are placed very strategically around the body, and can be found in high concentrations at points of entry from the outside world. This means that anything potentially harmful entering the system can be dealt with swiftly. You may have noticed that with a head cold for example, you can get swollen glands in the neck; you feel a bit 'glandy'. This is a sign that your lymph nodes are actively engaged in defending you from infection. There is a high concentration of lymphatic tissue in the human breast to ensure that breast milk is safe for the baby to ingest.

The spleen

The spleen is the largest of the lymphatic organs and lies beneath our left ribs between the upper part of the stomach (fundus) and the diaphragm. It looks like a large lymph node, but lymph does not flow through it. It consists of red pulp containing blood and white pulp containing blood vessels surrounded by lymphocytes and macrophages. Blood passing through the spleen comes into close contact with pulp, which serves to clean the blood by removing old or damaged cells from it. Old red blood cells are broken down here and also in the liver. New red blood cells are also manufactured here, as well as in bone marrow, and the mother's spleen makes red blood cells for the foetus.

Spleen

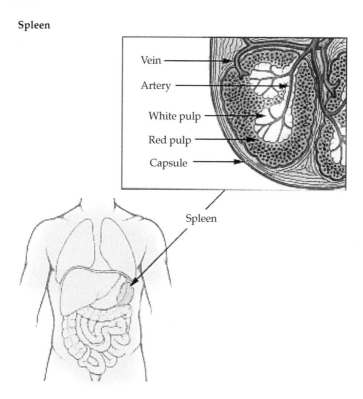

Amazing facts about the spleen

The spleen is responsible for making sure that our erythrocytes (red blood cells) are the correct shape (doughnut-shaped). It does this by making erythrocytes leave the spleen via a specially shaped exit, which reshapes them before they can go back into the circulation. If the erythrocytes aren't the right shape, they can't enter the circulation.[39] The spleen is a reservoir for blood, and can store up to a third of a litre of blood at any one time. This can be released if the body experiences sudden blood loss, as a survival mechanism. If your spleen is damaged or ruptured, it will need to be removed quickly, otherwise you may die of blood loss. You can live without your spleen.

Historically the spleen was thought to be a source of black bile, and therefore was regarded as the seat of irritability and bad temper. This is where we get the phrase venting your spleen! It is still listed today in the Oxford English Dictionary as meaning bad-tempered or spiteful (as well as an organ of the body). Interestingly though, William Harvey, who was responsible for much of our modern-day understanding of the heart and circulatory system is recorded as thinking that the spleen can make you laugh!

Function

The lymphatic system works very closely with blood vessels to serve the needs of the cells of our body. Its three main functions in life are:

- The removal of waste products from the interstitial fluid that bathes cells.
- Forming a network vital to the functioning of the immune system.
- Providing a route by which fats may be absorbed from the gut.

Therefore the lymphatic system is very closely linked with the cardiovascular system, the digestive tract and the immune system.

Interconnectedness

Much like the cardiovascular system, the lymphatic system is systemic by its nature, linking all cells and tissues. Here are a few other examples of lymphatic interconnectedness.[40]

The lymphatic systems

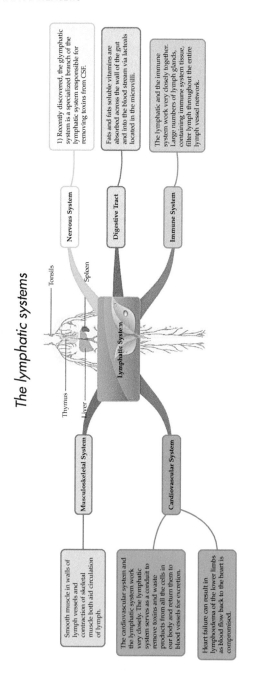

Nervous System

1) Recently discovered, the glymphatic system is a specialized branch of the lymphatic system responsible for removing toxins from CSF.

Digestive Tract

Fats and fats soluble vitamins are absorbed across the wall of the gut and into the blood stream via lactals located in the microvilli.

Immune System

The lymphatic and the immune system work very closely together. Large numbers of lymph glands, containing immune system tissue, filter lymph throughout the entire lymph vessel network.

Tonsils

Spleen

Thymus

Liver

Lymphatic System

Musculoskeletal System

Smooth muscle in walls of lymph vessels and contraction of skeletal muscle both aid circulation of lymph.

Cardiovascular System

The cardiovascular system and the lymphatic system work very closely. The lymphatic system serves as a conduit to remove toxins and waste products from all the cells in our body and return them to blood vessels for excretion.

Heart failure can result in lymphoedema of the lower limbs as blood flow back to the heart is compromised.

Reference

1) Jessen, N. A., et al., *The glymphatic system: A beginner's guide.* Neurochemical Research, 2015. 40(12): pp. 2583–2599.

Herbal connections

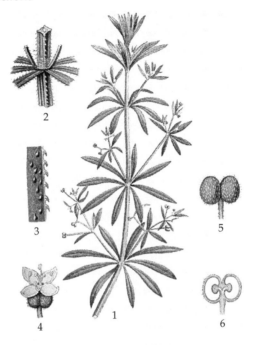

SNÄRJMÅRA, GALIUM APARINE L.

Cleavers (*Galium aparine* L.)

We are sure you will all recognise the plant cleavers (*Galium aparine* L.) when you see it even if you don't know its name (or know it by another!). It's that ubiquitous plant, which appears in spring and sticks to your clothing, hence one of its more common names 'sticky willie'. When seeds form in the autumn they tend to get stuck in dogs ears (especially spaniels).

This plant is an excellent example of a tonic, and its tonic properties are especially directed at the lymphatic system. Research has found beneficial antioxidant properties inherent in this plant,[5] and its traditional use, which goes back many centuries, is as a cleansing tonic specific to the lymphatic system.

It is a classic example of a spring tonic, being available from early spring onwards and being excellent for helping the lymphatic system in its work of shifting waste products and toxins out of the body.

A cleanser of tissues and a herb for spring cleaning of the body! Two good handfuls of fresh young cleavers in a mug, with boiling water added, will give you a cleansing tea with a green, refreshing, sweet pea taste. We revisit cleavers in Chapter 8.

The renal system (kidneys)

Our kidneys play a central role in maintaining both muscle and bone health. You may wish to read this section on the kidney and urinary system in conjunction with Chapter 10, which will be looking at the herbal treatment of the musculoskeletal system. (See also the next section on the musculoskeletal system.)

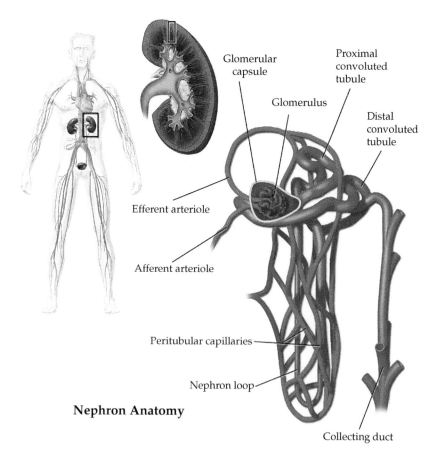

Glomerular capsule

Proximal convoluted tubule

Glomerulus

Distal convoluted tubule

Efferent arteriole

Afferent arteriole

Peritubular capillaries

Nephron loop

Nephron Anatomy

Collecting duct

The urinary or renal tract consists of the kidneys, ureters, bladder and the urethra. Primarily the kidneys act as filters for our bloodstream, and they represent a major route of elimination of toxins in the system. There are usually two of them, located on either side of the spine, behind the peritoneum, below the diaphragm and between the 12th thoracic and 3rd lumbar vertebrae.

> **Definition—*Peritoneum*:** The peritoneum is a serous membrane (fluid secreting membrane) that lines the abdominal cavity and covers most of the organs within the abdomen.

Like the adrenal glands, the kidneys have a cortex and a medulla. Each kidney also has a tube called a ureter, which connects the kidney to the bladder and is used to pass formed urine to the bladder where it is stored.

The main functions of the kidney are:

- Removing waste products and water from the blood
- Balancing important electrolytes and other substances
- Releasing hormones (an endocrine function)
- Helping to maintain blood pressure
- Helping to produce red blood cells
- Helping to produce vitamin D

Kidneys are composed of structures called nephrons, and there are approximately 1 million nephrons in each kidney. Blood is first filtered in a structure within the kidney called the glomerulus, which acts like a giant sieve, preventing large molecules such as proteins and red blood cells from passing through. The filtrate then passes along the length of the rest of the nephron (called the Loop of Henle) where other substances such as glucose, sodium and potassium are passed backwards and forwards between the filtrate and the surrounding blood, until all the waste products have been excreted and all the valuable substances have been 'salvaged'. The resultant fluid is then directed into the ureters, and on to the bladder for storage and excretion. Many hormones act on the kidney nephrons, to help balance different substances in the body and thus maintain internal homeostasis. These include:

Hormones acting on the kidney nephron

Hormone	Secreted by	Function
Atrial natriuretic hormone	Heart wall	Lowers blood pressure by reducing the reabsorption of sodium and water
Aldosterone	Adrenal cortex	Raises blood pressure by reabsorption of water and sodium
Calcitonin	Thyroid	To lower blood calcium levels
Antidiuretic hormone (ADH)	Posterior pituitary	Raise blood pressure via water retention
Parathyroid hormone (PTH)	Parathyroid glands	Raise blood calcium levels

Furthermore, the kidneys themselves possess an endocrine function as they secrete a hormone called erythropoietin, which is involved in red blood cell production. Thus we have a direct interaction between the endocrine system, the circulatory system, and the kidneys.

Interconnectedness

We have seen how the kidneys could be considered as part of the endocrine system, and have a close working relationship with red blood cell production, and they also interact with the endocrine system and the heart itself to maintain blood volume and blood pressure.

The musculoskeletal system and the nervous system are also closely associated with renal function, as the matrix of bone, and bone turnover is strongly dependent on the availability of minerals including magnesium, calcium and phosphate. The kidneys, in conjunction with the thyroid and parathyroid glands, can mobilise minerals to or from the bone.

Both muscles and nerves need a specific electrolyte balance in the body in order to function. Our kidneys and renal system are integral to the maintenance of electrolyte levels, particularly in the face of situations such as dehydration for example.

The renal system (kidneys)

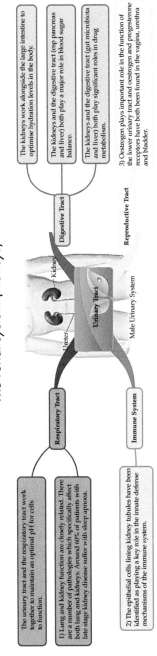

Respiratory Tract

The urinary tract and the respiratory tract work together to maintain an optimal pH for cells to function.

1) Lung and kidney function are closely related. There are a number of pathologies which specifically affect both lung and kidneys. Around 60% of patients with late stage kidney disease suffer with sleep apnoea.

Immune System

2) The epithelial cells lining kidney tubules have been identified as playing a key role in the innate defense mechanisms of the immune system.

Kidney

Ureter

Urinary Tract

Male Urinary System

Digestive Tract

The kidneys work alongside the large intestine to optimise hydration levels in the body.

The kidneys and the digestive tract (esp pancreas and liver) both play a major role in blood sugar balance.

The kidneys and the digestive tract (gut microbiota and liver) both play significant roles in drug metabolism.

Reproductive Tract

3) Oestrogen plays important role in the function of the lower urinary tract and oestrogen and progesterone receptors have both been found in the vagina, urethra and bladder.

References

1) Pierson, D. J., *Respiratory considerations in the patient with renal failure*. Respiratory Care, 2006. 51(4): pp. 413–422.

2) Hato, T. and P. C. Dagher, *How the innate immune system senses trouble and causes trouble*. Clin J Am Soc Nephrol, 2015. 10(8): pp. 1459–1469.

3) Robinson, D., et al., *The effect of hormones on the lower urinary tract*. Menopause International, 2013. 19(4): pp. 155–162.

Definition—*Electrolytes:* An electrolyte is a substance that produces an electrically conducting solution when dissolved in a polar solvent, such as water. Sodium, potassium, calcium and magnesium all act as electrolytes in our blood, tissues and cells.

Skin health is impacted by kidney function in an everyday sense, and also in more serious kidney disease where itchy dry skin and a sallow colouration of the skin can occur. Situations such as chronic dehydration can lead to constipation. This affects the digestive tract and ultimately the retention of waste products will impact most systems of the body.

Herbal connections

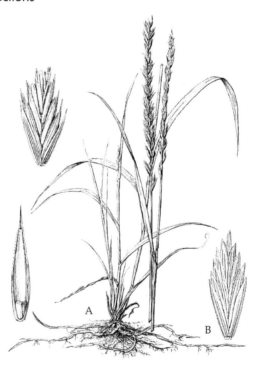

Couchgrass (*Elymus repens* (L) Gould) synonym *Agropyron repens*.

The gardeners among you may well give a weary sigh when we mention couch grass (*Elymus repens* (L.) Gould [Poaceae]). It's just one of those plants—once you have it in your garden there is virtually no way of getting rid of it. As a herbal remedy, however, it is much prized due to its calming and soothing mucilaginous rhizome.

Added to this, Elymus, once known as *Agropyron repens*, has antibiotic and diuretic properties that make it perfect as a tea for the treatment of urinary tract infections. It has the reputation, like some other herbs, of increasing resilience against recurrent infections, and there is growing evidence to support this.[41] It is traditional to treat urinary tract infections with a tea containing a combination of herbs, so that there is symptom relief and urinary antiseptic herbs combined with urinary anti-inflammatories. Couch grass is a popular choice of many herbal medicine users across Europe. An infusion ensures that a goodly amount of the herbal remedy actually reaches the kidneys where they can exert their effects, especially if the patient is compliant and drinks at least 4 cups a day.

A combination of herbs provides a broad cross-section of different pathways by which the tea can exert its actions. The combination of compounds found in each plant also exerts multiple benefits all at once. The conclusions of one study involving couchgrass concluded the benefits of this approach were the result of plant synergy:

> *Different plant extracts, traditionally used for UTI, exhibit anti-adhesive effects against UPEC under in vitro conditions. Molecular targets can be different, either on the bacterial or on the host cell surface. Combination of these medicinal plants with different targets, as observed often in phytotherapy, results in synergistic effects.*
>
> —N. L. Rafsanjany, M. Petereit and F. Hensel[42]]

Note: Abbreviations

- UPEC, Uropathogenic *Escherichia coli*
- UTI, Uncomplicated urinary tract infections.

This is a great piece of research, mentioning again, as it so often crops up in research on plant medicines nowadays, the magic word 'synergy'.

The musculoskeletal system

You may wish to read this section on the musculoskeletal system in conjunction with Chapter 10, which will be looking at the herbal treatment of the musculoskeletal system. (See also the previous section on the kidneys.)

Bones are extraordinary things. You may think of them as an inert framework, a structure upon which to hang or support all the other gubbins that make up the human body, but they are much more than that.

We have 206 bones in the human body, most of which are articulated one with another. The exception to this is the hyoid bone, located in the neck, which is not directly articulated with any other bone, nor is it considered a sesamoid bone.

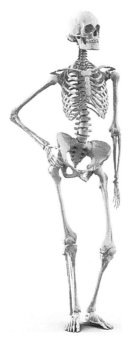

Bones can fall into five types: flat bones, long bones, short bones, irregular and sesamoid bones. The femur (a long bone) is the largest bone in the body running from our hip joint to our knee. Short bones include the carpals in the wrist, irregular bones include vertebrae, and flat bones have a protective function, and therefore do actually have a slight curve. Examples include the skull, the pelvis and the ribs. Sesamoid bones are bones embedded within a muscle or tendon. There are two sesamoid bones located in the ball of the foot, beneath the big toe joint. The kneecap is another example of a sesamoid bone.

Just like any other cells, the cells of bones require nutrients. Nutrient arteries enter the bones via openings called foramen in the bone surface. Nerve supplies usually enter via the same route. Bones are usually extensively innervated by nerves, therefore broken bones can be extremely painful. Bones are composed of calcium salts (around 65%) and collagen, a connective tissue made from protein, which gives bones their elasticity.

There are three types of bone cells:

- Osteoblasts: Build up bone tissue.
- Osteocytes: Monitor and maintain bone tissue.
- Osteoclasts: Break down bone tissue.

Osteoblasts and **osteoclasts** work together to continually remodel and repair bone.

A number of hormones are responsible for the regulation of bone growth. These include:

Name	Action
Testosterone	Influences changes at puberty and maintains structure throughout life. Influences the closure of the epiphyseal plates of the long bones, therefore influencing final height.
Oestrogen	Responsible for widening the pelvis, and maintaining bone mass in later life. Influences changes at puberty and maintains structure throughout life.
Calcitonin	Lowers blood calcium levels by increasing uptake into the bone.
Parathyroid hormone	Raises blood calcium levels by stimulating the release of calcium from bone into bloodstream.
Growth hormone	Particularly important during childhood.
Thyroid hormones	Particularly important during childhood.

Although bones stop lengthening once the epiphyseal plates (growth plates) of the long bones have fused, bones can continue to thicken, and weight-bearing exercise such as walking can help maintain healthy bones.

The axial skeleton is comprised of the skull, the vertebral column, the ribcage and the sternum. These are the core bones of the body.

The appendicular skeleton is comprised of the shoulder and pelvic girdles and the limbs.

Muscles

There are three main types of muscle in the human body, smooth muscle, skeletal muscle and cardiac muscle. Cardiac muscle is highly specialised and is found only in the wall of the heart. We have already looked at cardiac muscle earlier in this chapter. Skeletal muscle is under our conscious control—we decide when we want to move our arm or wiggle our toes. Let's look at skeletal muscle in a bit more depth.

The classic structural unit of skeletal muscle is the sarcomere. The actions of the sarcomere are responsible for the shortening, and thus contraction of skeletal muscles, and when you look at skeletal muscles under the microscope, they appear stripy, due to the presence of sarcomeres.

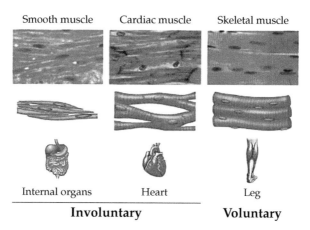

Smooth muscle	Cardiac muscle	Skeletal muscle
Internal organs	Heart	Leg
Involuntary		**Voluntary**

Skeletal muscle cells are called fibres. They are large and usually contain more than one nuclei. They also contain a large number of mitochondria, because of the amount of work that is demanded of them. A whole muscle is made up of many muscle fibres. Muscle fibres take it in turns to contract so that a muscle, that might be responsible for holding your head up, will always be partially contracted overall, but individual muscle cells do not become too fatigued. This is expressed as muscle tone. Ideally a limb at rest has muscles that are not too contracted, not too flaccid.

Muscles benefit from exercise and will improve in power and endurance as a result. With exercises such as weight lifting the individual muscle fibres actually enlarge and the result is muscular hypertrophy. Smooth muscle is found in organs and tissues under the control of the autonomic nervous system, therefore we do not have conscious control over it. Smooth muscle does not look stripy under the microscope, and some smooth muscle can initiate its own contractions independently of the nervous system—for example—peristalsis. Blood vessel walls are another example of smooth muscle.

Interconnectedness

The musculoskeletal system is, on the surface of things, the least dynamic of the systems of the body, but this is a big misconception.

The masculoskeletal systems

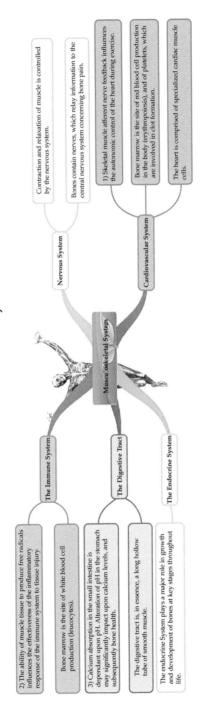

Nervous System

Contraction and relaxation of muscle is controlled by the nervous system.

Bones contain nerves, which relay information to the central nervous system concerning bone pain.

Cardiovascular System

1) Skeletal muscle afferent nerve feedback influences the autonomic control of the heart during exercise.

Bone marrow is the site of red blood cell production in the body (erythropoiesis), and of platelets, which are involved in clot formation.

The heart is comprised of specialized cardiac muscle cells.

Musculoskeletal System

The Immune System

2) The ability of muscle tissue to produce free radicals influences the effectiveness of the inflammatory response of the immune system to tissue injury.

Bone marrow is the site of white blood cell production (leucocytes).

The Digestive Tract

3) Calcium absorption in the small intestine is dependant upon pH. Alteration of pH in the stomach may significantly impact upon calcium levels, and subsequently bone health.

The digestive tract is, in essence, a long hollow tube of smooth muscle.

The Endocrine System

The endocrine System plays a major role in growth and development of bones at key stages throughout life.

References

1) Fisher, J. P., *Autonomic control of the heart during exercise in humans: role of skeletal muscle afferents*. Experimental Physiology, 2013.

2) Tidball, J. G., *Interactions between muscle and the immune system during modified musculoskeletal loading*. Clin Orthop Relat Res., 2002.

3) Yang, Y.-X., *Chronic PPI therapy and calcium metabolism*. Current Gastroenterol. Rep., 2015.

Muscle contraction depends on calcium balance, which implicates the kidneys, thyroid and parathyroid glands, the digestive tract, and of course the nervous system. Our bones likewise depend on all of the above for healthy function (including the endocrine and circulatory systems) as well as being a major centre for the production of immune system cells, and acting as a storehouse for calcium and a protective shell for all of our major organs.

Herbal connections

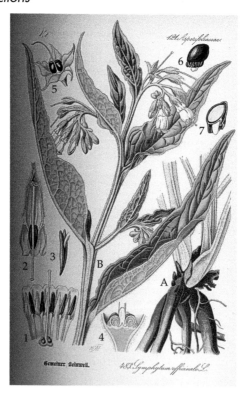

Comfrey (*Symphytum officinale* L.)

Comfrey (*Symphytum officinale* L.) is a key herb for the musculoskeletal system. The clue is in its common name, knitbone, and its scientific name (comfrey from the Latin confirm—to make stronger, and *Symphytum* from the Greek—to fuse together).

Comfrey contains significant amounts of allantoin. This is a compound produced naturally by the body as a result of protein metabolism, and is one of the compounds to which comfrey's healing and anti-inflammatory effects are therefore attributed. It has a long history of use externally as a poultice for soft tissue damage, sprains and strains, providing anti-inflammatory and tissue healing properties.

The respiratory tract

We all know that our bodies need oxygen. Our red blood cells are specifically designed to carry this precious gas around our body to reach every single one of our *millions* of cells. But exactly why do we need it?

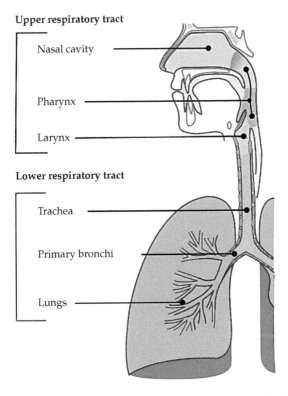

In every cell of our body we produce compounds called adenosine triphosphate (ATP). We use this ATP as a source of energy. Oxygen is vital for the formation of ATP. If we did not have oxygen we would not be able to make enough ATP. If we run out of ATP we run out of energy. It's that simple. This is where our lungs come in. Our lungs are responsible for supplying us with plentiful amounts of oxygen and also for removing carbon dioxide from our system, which would otherwise build up inside us and poison us.

Our respiratory tract is traditionally divided into the upper and lower respiratory tracts. Each part of the respiratory tract has a role to play.

Ideally, we breathe air in through our nose, where delicate structures called nasal turbinates, circulate and warm the air and nasal hairs catch any significant debris and prevent it from entering us. This is therefore part of our non-specific immune defences.

Nearly 2000 years ago Galen wrote:

> The structures of the nose, how marvellously they come next after the sponge like [ethmoid] bone ... in order that inspiration may not begin in a straight line with the artery [trachea] and that the air entering it may be bent and convoluted, so to speak. For I think this should be doubly advantageous, the parts of the lung will never be chilled ... and the particles of dust ... will not penetrate as far as the artery [trachea].
>
> —David Bohm, quoting Galen[43]

Despite their separation, the upper respiratory tract and the lungs are all part of one system, and rely on each other. Mouth breathing, and rhinitis leading to nasal passage blockage, has been linked with lung diseases and health problems such as asthma, chronic bronchitis, and emphysema.[44,45]

Moving deeper now into our respiratory tract ... known as the 'precious organs' in traditional Chinese medicine, due to their intimate relationship with the outside world. Many of us are aware of our sinuses as part of our upper respiratory tract only when we are unfortunate enough to suffer from sinusitis (We will be looking more closely at sinusitis and how to treat it in chapter nine). The biological role of the sinuses is debated, but a number of possible functions have been proposed:

- Decreasing the relative weight of the front of the skull, and especially the bones of the face
- Increasing resonance of the voice
- Providing a buffer against blows to the face

- Insulating sensitive structures like dental roots and eyes from rapid temperature fluctuations in the nasal cavity (a sort of double glazing!)
- Humidifying and heating of inhaled air

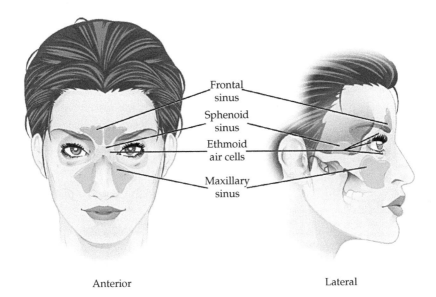

Frontal sinus

Sphenoid sinus

Ethmoid air cells

Maxillary sinus

Anterior   Lateral

Sinus cavities of the head.

The facial sinuses are paired, and grouped at the front of our skull, from our forehead to our nose. They are named for the cranial bones within which they are found, but are collectively called the paranasal sinuses. The para-nasal sinuses are joined to the nasal cavity by small channels (ostia) that pass through the bone but are lined with respiratory epithelium, which may become blocked by swelling in the nasal lining caused by allergic inflammation, or from a head cold. Normal drainage of mucous from the sinuses may then be disrupted, and sinusitis may result. All sinus configurations are unique to us, rather like fingerprints.

Air travels in past our sinuses and into the nasopharynx, pharynx and larynx—all of those spaces behind our nose and tongue—and down into the lungs via the trachea. We may use air from our lungs to expel anything that gets stuck on its way down—by coughing! The larynx is a structure made from cartilage, lined with epithelium, and houses our voice box and vocal cords. Above this is where our glottis and epiglottis fold over to prevent food from entering our trachea when we are swallowing. Food enters instead safely via the oesophagus. The oesophagus lies behind the trachea, so when a bolus of food is passed down it, the trachea can move to accommodate it. After swallowing, the epiglottis folds back into its upright resting position.

Protecting all of these important structures are cartilaginous bones that sit at the front of the larynx and are visible at the front of our neck. The most obvious of these is the semi-circular thyroid cartilage. It has a ridge at the front that tends to be more prominent in males—known as the Adam's apple. We have also already met another of these bones— the hyoid bone—you may recall it is a bone that does not articulate with any other bone.

Moving down to the lower respiratory tract, the lungs are composed of lobes, three for the right-hand lung, and two for the left lung, which is smaller due to space taken up by the heart. Lungs are composed of spongy tissue and are contained within a double membrane called the pleura. The pleura are another example of a serous membrane—just like the peritoneum in the abdominal cavity. A thin layer of fluid produced by the two layers of pleura, allows them to glide against each other without any friction.

When we breathe in, the lungs are pulled up and out by the walls of the chest, and simultaneously the bases of the lungs are pulled downwards by the diaphragm as it flattens out. When we breathe out the chest wall relaxes back, the diaphragm curves back upwards, and the air is pushed back out of the lungs.

The major muscles of respiration are therefore the intercostal muscles, which lie between the ribs, and the diaphragm. This is a good moment to practice your diaphragmatic breathing. Other muscle groups of the chest and back, will come into play when necessary.

Let's pause for a moment and look in a little more detail at the tissues of the respiratory tract. The trachea travels down from the laryngopharynx to the lungs. Its striped appearance is due to the many rings of C shaped cartilage supporting it. The lining of the trachea is composed of ciliated columnar epithelium and mucous secreting goblet cells, which act together to form the mucociliary escalator. This is another example of cilia within the body, used in this system to sweep debris up and out of the lungs. The trachea divides into bronchi then, like branches of a tree, the bronchi divide and subdivide and cartilage is gradually replaced with more flexible smooth muscle.

The bronchioles finally arrive at microscopic structures called alveoli, which under a microscope, look remarkably like bunches of grapes. It is here that oxygen is absorbed into our blood vessels and carbon dioxide is removed from it. This is a process of simple diffusion made possible by millions of tiny blood capillaries passing through the delicate sponge-like lung structure and alveoli. This gas-permeable membrane is an incredibly delicate part of our body that is in direct contact with the outside world. As you will remember, one side of our heart is constantly sending blood to the lungs and receiving it back oxygenated to then send it out to the rest of the body.

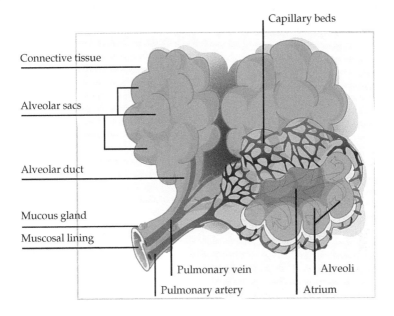

Capillary beds

Connective tissue

Alveolar sacs

Alveolar duct

Mucous gland

Muscosal lining

Pulmonary vein

Pulmonary artery

Alveoli

Atrium

Interconnectedness

So finally we have come to the respiratory tract, that which is intimately involved in breathing life into us: Prana, pneuma, the breath of life.

Definition—*Inspiration*:
- The drawing in of breath; inhalation
- A sudden brilliant, creative or timely idea
- The process of being mentally stimulated to do or feel something
- A person or thing that inspires
- In Middle English, the sense of divine guidance

The respiratory tract

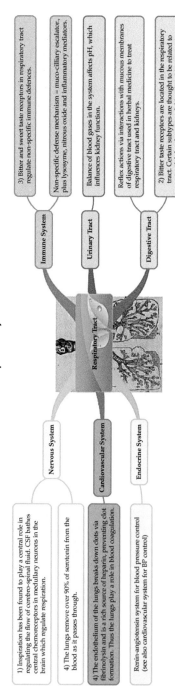

Nervous System

1) Inspiration has been found to play a central role in regulating the flow of cerebro-spinal fluid. CSF bathes central chemoreceptors in medullary neurons in the brain which regulate respiration.

4) The lungs remove over 90% of serotonin from the blood as it passes through.

Cardiovascular System

4) The endothelium of the lungs breaks down clots via fibrinolysin and is a rich source of heparin, preventing clot formation. Thus the lungs play a role in blood coagulation.

Endocrine System

Renin-angiotensin system for blood pressure control (see also cardiovascular system for BP control)

Respiratory Tract

Immune System

3) Bitter and sweet taste receptors in respiratory tract regulate non-specific immune defences.

Non-specific defense mechanism = muco-cilliary escalator, plus lysozyme, nitrous oxide and inflammatory mediators.

Urinary Tract

Balance of blood gases in the system affects pH, which influences kidney function.

Reflex actions via interactions with mucous membranes of digestive tract used in herbal medicine to treat respiratory tract and kidneys.

Digestive Tract

2) Bitter taste receptors are located in the respiratory tract. Certain subtypes are thought to be related to potential development of rhinosinusitis.

References

1) Dreha-Kulaczewski, S., et al., *Inspiration Is the Major Regulator of Human CSF Flow*. Neurobiology of Disease, 2015.

2) Cohen, N. A., *The genetics of the bitter taste receptor T2R38 in upper airway innate immunity and implications for chronic rhinosinusitis*. Laryngoscope, 2017.

3) Workman, A., et al., *The role of bitter and sweet taste receptors in upper airway immunity*. Curr Allergy Asthma Rep., 2015.

4) Joseph, D., et al., *Non-respiratory functions of the lung*. Continuing Education in Anaesthesia Critical Care and Pain, 2013.

The cardiovascular system is the most obvious link here, and this is very much taken in to account in conventional pulmonary and cardiac medicine. We also have tissues and structures familiar to us from the musculoskeletal system, especially our ribcage which articulates to allow lung function. In a traditional medicine sense, the respiratory system is an organ of elimination, along with the digestive system, the renal system, and the skin. And, of course every single cell in our body could not function without oxygen, gifted to us from our lungs.

Herbal connections

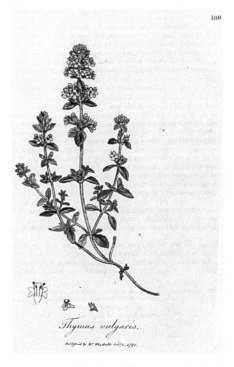

Common Garden Thyme. Medical Botany, Woodville 1790–1794.

The respiratory system is vulnerable to infection due to its close proximity to the outside world. One of the many strengths of herbal medicine lies in a large number of plants available with reliable anti-infective properties.

Common thyme (*Thymus vulgaris* L.), is a great example of this, and is definitely a 'go-to' herb when treating chest infections of any sort. Thyme species' have been found to have strong antibacterial (gram-positive and gram-negative) capacity, as well as antifungal, anti-inflammatory and antioxidant properties. This underpins their strong traditional use worldwide for treating lung infections, as well as digestive infections.[46]

The highly aromatic essential oil content makes this a great herb also for external applications such as compresses, poultices, ointments and inhalations, and it would be a great herb to include into antiseptic mouthwashes and throat gargles. As you remember from Chapter 2, essential oils form less than 10% of the plants' overall constituents. Most of these constituents have capacities and side-benefits of great use to our healing. One example is the mild astringent effect of thyme. Astringency leads to improvements in the integrity of the epithelial and mucous membranes of our body—exactly those tissues vulnerable by way of direct contact with the outside world!

Historically (and in times before microscopes and knowledge of pathogenic bacteria), people believed that thyme kept away evil spirits and purified the air. Doesn't sound so crazy now, does it? Using the essential oil to scent a room when someone has a head cold/chest infection would certainly be a modern-day interpretation of that. You could also enrol the help of the whole herb, and leave an infusion to stand where you can sit and breathe it in. What inspiration!

Conclusions

We hope that you have enjoyed this brief A&P journey. May we leave you with a few things to consider, one being the interconnectedness of all systems into a coherent and unique whole. Practising joined-up thinking in terms of how the body works can be a daunting task, particularly when things go wrong. It is a rare occurrence that only one system is involved in anything. Having at least an awareness of the reality that the whole is superior to the sum of the parts is a great step forward.

Another aspect of this is that we do march to the beat of our own individual drums. The internal rhythms of our body interact in a complex biochemical and biological dance, involving heart rate, respiratory rate, hormonal cycles, peristalsis, blinking and much, much more. There are any number of rises and falls in internal cadences coming together to create our pulse of life. A very venerable herbalist once suggested that we are drawn to certain types of music because it serves to balance us out on some level.

Maybe we need the corrective influence of certain melodies and harmonies to balance and heal us, to influence our internal rhythms somehow. Birdsong or the sound of the sea could also work. It is certainly something we have thought about on and off over the years.

In David Bohm's excellent book *Wholeness and the Implicate Order*, he considers the concept of 'measure' in ancient Greece.

> *Physical health was historically regarded as the outcome of a state, or right inward measure in all parts and processes of the body. That the essential reason or ratio of a thing being the totality of inner proportions in its structure, and the process in which it forms, maintains itself, and ultimately dissolves.*
>
> *To understand such a ratio is to understand the innermost being of that thing. Thus the words I have your measure would have referred to a deep understanding of the individual in terms of inner function.*
>
> —David Bohm[43]

Everything is flow.

Bibliography

Barker, Julian., *The Medicinal Flora of Britain and Northwestern Europe*. 2001: Winter Press.

Mills, Simon, *Out Of The Earth: The Essential Book of Herbal Medicine*. 1991: Viking.

Stephenson, Clare, *The Complementary Therapists Guide to Conventional Medicine*. 2011: Churchill Livingstone.

Waugh, A. and Grant A., *Ross and Wilson, Anatomy and Physiology in Health and Illness*. 2014: Churchill Livingstone. Elsevier.

Waugh, A. and Grant A., *Anatomy and Physiology Colouring and Workbook*. 2014: Churchill Livingstone. Elsevier.

Waller, P., *Holistic Anatomy: An Integrative Guide to the Human Body*. 2010: North Atlantic Books.

References

1. Bianconi, E. et al., *An estimation of the number of cells in the human body*. Ann Hum Biol, 2013. 40(6): pp. 463–471 doi: 10.3109/03014460.2013.807878.

2. Pranskuniene, Z. et al., *Ethnopharmaceutical knowledge in Samogitia region of Lithuania: where old traditions overlap with modern medicine.* J Ethnobiol Ethnomed, 2018. 14(1): p. 70.
3. Jahdi, F. et al., *The impact of calendula ointment on cesarean wound healing: A randomized controlled clinical trial.* J Family Med Prim Care, 2018. 7(5): pp. 893–897.
4. Stucki, K. et al., *Ethnoveterinary contemporary knowledge of farmers in pre-alpine and alpine regions of the Swiss cantons of Bern and Lucerne compared to ancient and recent literature—Is there a tradition?* J Ethnopharmacol, 2019. 234: pp. 225–244.
5. Amirghofran, Z., M. Azadbakht and M. H. Karimi, *Evaluation of the immunomodulatory effects of five herbal plants.* J Ethnopharmacol, 2000. 72: pp. 167–172.
6. Nicholson, L. B., *The immune system.* Essays Biochem, 2016. 60(3): pp. 275–301.
7. Sedighinia, F. et al., *Antibacterial activity of Glycyrrhiza glabra against oral pathogens: an in vitro study.* Avicenna J Phytomed, 2012. 2(3): pp. 118–124.
8. Wang, H., S. Shi and S. Wang, *Can highly cited herbs in ancient Traditional Chinese medicine formulas and modern publications predict therapeutic targets for diabetes mellitus?* J Ethnopharmacol, 2018. 213: pp. 101–110.
9. Gulati, K. et al., *Nutraceuticals in Respiratory Disorders.* Nutraceuticals, Academic Press., 2016: pp. 75–86.
10. Rooney, S. and B. Pendry, *Phytotherapy for Polycystic Ovarian Syndrome: A review of the literature and evaluation of practitioners' experiences.* Journal of Herbal Medicine, 2014. 4(3): pp. 159–171.
11. Denham, et al., *What's in the bottle? Prescriptions formulated by medical herbalists in a clinical trial of treatment during the menopause.* Journal of Herbal Medicine, 2011. 1: pp. 95–101.
12. Siracusa, L. et al., *Phytocomplexes from liquorice (Glycyrrhiza glabra L.) leaves— Chemical characterization and evaluation of their antioxidant, anti-genotoxic and anti-inflammatory activity.* Fitoterapia, 2011. 82(4): pp. 546–556.
13. Jiang, Y. X. et al., *Screening Five Qi-Tonifying Herbs on M2 Phenotype Macrophages.* Evid Based Complement Alternat Med, 2019. 2019: p. 9549315.
14. Luís, Â., F. Domingues and L. Pereira, *Metabolic changes after licorice consumption: A systematic review with meta-analysis and trial sequential analysis of clinical trials.* Phytomedicine, 2018. 39: pp. 17–24.
15. Dreha-Kulaczewski, S. et al., *Inspiration is the major regulator of human CSF flow.* J Neurosci, 2015. 35(6): pp. 2485–2491.
16. Hadhazy, A. *Think Twice: How the Gut's 'Second Brain' Influences Mood and Well-Being.* 2010: Scientific American.

17. Axarlis, S. et al., *Antiviral In vitro activity of Hypericum perforatum l. extract on the human cytomegalovirus (HCMV)*. Phytotherapy Research, 1998. 12: pp. 507–511.

18. Blumenthal, M. et al., *The Complete German Commission E Monographs: therapeutic guide to herbal medicines*. 2000: Integrative Medicine Communications.

19. Everson, S., *Everson, S*. 1999: Oxford University Press.

20. Sorabji, R., *Aristotle on demarcating the five senses*. Philosophical Review, 1971. 80: p. 55–79.

21. Gordon, M. S., *Looking Back: Finding the senses*. The Psychologist, 2012. 25: pp. 908–909.

22. Buhner and S. Harrod, *Plant Intelligence and the Imaginary Realm: Beyond the Doors of Perception Into the Dreaming of Earth*. 2014: Inner Traditions/ Bear & Co.

23. Stokkan, K. A. et al., *Shifting mirrors: adaptive changes in retinal reflections to winter darkness in Arctic reindeer*. Proc Biol Sci, 2013. 280(1773): pp. 2013–2451.

24. Cohen, N. A., *The genetics of the bitter taste receptor T2R38 in upper airway innate immunity and implications for chronic rhinosinusitis*. Laryngoscope, 2017. 127(1): pp. 44–51.

25. Böhnert, K.-J. and G. Hahn, *Phytotherapy in Gynecology and Obstetrics– Vitex agnus-castus (Chaste Tree)*. Acta Medica Empírica, 1990. 9: pp. 494–502.

26. Lee, R. J. and N. A. Cohen, *Bitter and sweet taste receptors in the respiratory epithelium in health and disease*. J Mol Med (Berl), 2014. 92(12): pp. 1235–1244.

27. De Becker, G., *The Gift of Fear: Survival Signals That Protect us From Violence*. 1997: Bloomsbury.

28. Jung, C., J. P. Hugot and F. Barreau, *Peyer's Patches: The Immune Sensors of the Intestine*. Int J Inflam, 2010: p. 823710.

29. Helander, H. F. and L. Fändriks, *Surface area of the digestive tract— revisited*. Scand J Gastroenterol, 2014. 49(6): pp. 681–689.

30. Guinane, C. M. et al., *Microbial composition of human appendices from patients following appendectomy*. MBio, 2013. 4(1).

31. Priest, A. W. and L. R. Priest, *Herbal Medication: A Clinical and Dispensary Handbook*. 2nd ed. 2000. ed. 1983: C.W. Daniel Company Ltd.

32. Buckberg, G. D. et al., *What Is the heart? Anatomy, function, pathophysiology, and misconceptions*. J Cardiovasc Dev Dis, 2018. 5(2).

33. Stonebridge, P. A. et al., *Spiral laminar flow in vivo*. Clin Sci (Lond), 1996. 91(1): pp. 17–21.

34. Noble, K. *Immune System linked to lower heart attack risk, study suggests*. 2016: Imperial College London. Sourced online. https://www.imperial.ac.uk/news/173046/immune-system-linked-lower-heart-attack/

35. Krack, A. et al., *The importance of the gastrointestinal system in the pathogenesis of heart failure. European Heart Journal*, 2005. 26(22): pp. 2368–2374.
36. Khamis, R. et al., *High Serum Immunoglobulin G and M Levels Predict Freedom From Adverse Cardiovascular Events in Hypertension: A Nested Case-Control Subsidy of the Anglo-Scandinavian Cardiac Outcomes Trial.* EBioMed, July 2016. 9: pp. 372–380.
37. Moerman, D., *Meaning, Medicine and the Placebo Effect*. 2002: Cambridge University Press.
38. Ghorbanibirgani, A., A. Khalili and L. Zamani, *The efficacy of stinging nettle (Urtica dioica) in patients with benign prostatic hyperplasia: a randomized double-blind study in 100 patients.* Iran Red Crescent Med J, 2013. 15(1): pp. 9–10.
39. Technology, M.I.o. *How the spleen filters blood.* 2016.
40. Schnaufnagel, D. E. and https://www.atsjournals.org/doi/full/10.1513/AnnalsATS.201302-029ED, *Lung Lymphatics: Why should a clinician care?*, in *ATS Journals*. 2013.
41. Hautmann, C. and K. Scheithe, *Fluid extract of Agropyron repens for the treatment of urinary tract infections or irritable bladder. Results of multicentric post-marketing surveillance.* Zeitschrift für Phytotherapie, 2000. 21(5): pp. 252–255.
42. Rafsanjany, N. L., M. Petereit and F. Hensel, A. *Anti-adhesion as a functional concept for protection against uropathogenic Escherichia coli: in vitro studies with traditionally used plants with anti-adhesive activity against uropathognic Escherichia coli.* J. Ethnopharmacol, 2013. 145: pp. 591–597.
43. Bohm, D., *Wholeness and the Implicate Order*. 2002: Routledge.
44. Proctor, D. F., *The Upper Airways: Nasal physiology and the defence of the lungs.* American Review of Respiratory Disease, 1977. 115(1).
45. Montnémery, P. et al., *Prevalence of nasal symptoms and their relation to self-reported asthma and chronic bronchitis/emphysema.* Eur Respir J, 2001. 17(4): pp. 596–603.
46. Prasanth, R. V. et al., *Review on Thymus vulgaris traditional uses and Pharmacological Properties.* Med Aromat Plants, 2014.

CHAPTER FOUR

Native healers: five key plants from the Western herbal tradition

Introduction

In this chapter we consider and contemplate five key and essential medicinal plants from the European tradition.

We will learn about their identifying botanical features, the parts of the plant used for medicine, and their uses in both home and clinical settings. We also look at some of the scientific research available for the safety and efficacy of each of these medicinal plants. Some real case examples have been provided to help illustrate how each medicinal plant has been and can be used in modern phytotherapeutic practice.

In exploring these five plants in more detail we shall also be able to explore some central concepts within Western herbal medicine. In particular these plants raise our awareness of the function and treatment of the digestive system, the mucous membranes and the nervous system. These five medicinal plants are also ideally suited to children's medicine as well as care of those who are vulnerable or frail.

Following on from the theory, we will provide recipes for some straightforward, but effective medicinal preparations that you can create and use at home. Some of them incorporate herbal medicines in a food-like way, others are slightly more 'pharmaceutical' in their preparation and application.

As we have seen in previous chapters, the use of foods and simple herbs in the home has ancient roots across all cultures. We will explore some of the practical history associated with the individual herbs presented here. Therefore we shall look at the simplicity but universality of preparing a tisane, infusion or 'tea', and also explore capturing some of the wonderful aromatic and volatile compounds in infused oils. Finally we look at the wonderful world of medicinal electuaries and how these ancient, semi-solid nutritive medicines can be fun to make, and to take!

> Herbal medicine is the oldest form of therapy practiced by mankind, and much of this medicinal use of plants seems to have been based on a highly developed 'dowsing' instinct, which led the healer of the tribe to the right plant and taught him or her its use ... wild animals certainly possess such an instinct ...
>
> —Ann Warren-Davies, MNIMH Medical Herbalist

> these 'dowsing' powers would explain the astonishing continuity of medicinal plant usage in the days before there were written records ... moreover how we are to account for the astonishing degree to which the same plant is employed for the same purposes in cultures so widely separated in place or time that there can have been no communication between them?
>
> —Barbara Griggs[1]

Five essential healing medicinal plants

Chamomile (Matricaria chamomilla *(L.) Rauschert)*

The universal familiarity of this plant in modern usage, in herbal teas and skin preparations could fool many of us into forgetting that chamomile packs a huge power-punch of relaxing, anti-inflammatory and nervine qualities suited to easing even the most acute symptoms of pain and distress.

Classification

German chamomile, Hungarian chamomile, Scented Mayweed, Chamomilla recutita, is currently known as *Matricaria chamomilla* (L.) Rauschert. and is a member of the Asteraceae or daisy family, once known as the Compositae family. Some older names for German chamomile are *Chamomilla chamomilla, Chamomilla recutita* and *Matricaria recutita.*

German chamomile should not be confused with another gorgeous medicinal chamomile, Roman chamomile (*Chamaemelum nobile* L.), a very similar species that previously has been called *Anthemis nobilis.* The name Matricaria gives us clues to the universal healing power of chamomile as a foremost and irreplaceable remedy in the home or the clinic. *Matrix cara*—Latin for beloved mother is one interpretation, but …

> *matrix has other meanings in biology and mathematics which refer not only to the source and the womb, but also to a ground substance which holds and moulds precious things.*
>
> —Julian Barker[2]

This speaks to another quality that chamomile has, and which Julian Barker goes on to describe—that chamomile can help to form a useful matrix, for any prescription. So that after selecting two or four herbs, chamomile can be added to bring the whole together into a rounded prescription that has the potential to have a benefit to any physiological system or tissue.

Basic botany

German chamomile, *Matricaria chamomilla* (L.) Rauschert is an aromatic, short to medium hairless annual.

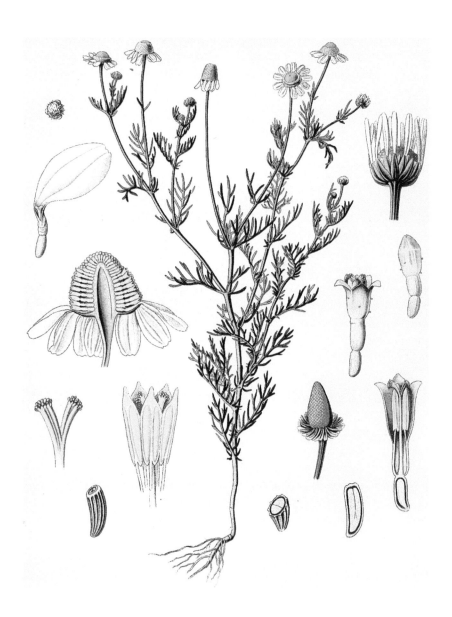

- **Stems** ascending to erect, branched.
- **Flower heads** white with a yellow conical hollow disc, 10–25 millimeters, solitary on long stalks; rays downturned soon after the flowers open. Note that the hollow conical disc floret (flower head) of chamomile is an identifying characteristic helping you ensure you have the correct plant, many authors refer to this. Flowers July–August.
- **Leaves alternate** feathery, 2–3 pinnately divided, with bristle-tipped divisions.
- **Habitat** cultivated land especially arable fields, waste and disturbed ground, saline steppes, on sandy or loamy soils, generally found at low altitudes. Found throughout Europe except for Ireland, Faroes, Spitzbergen and Iceland.[3]
- **Parts used** flowers, fresh or dried.
- **Harvesting** harvest whilst flowering.

Chamomile is grown on a large scale in Eastern Europe, Spain, Turkey, Egypt and Argentina.[4]

Main constituents

Chamomile is rich in essential oil. Two types of essential oil are recognised: one rich in bisabolol and the other rich in bisabolol oxides. Both types are rich in terpenoid compounds including matricin. The characteristic dark blue azulenes (e.g. chamazulene) can be produced by steam distillation to produce an essential oil. Flavonoids (bioflavonoids), especially apigenin, apigenin-7-O-glucoside, caffeic acid, chlorogenic acid, luteolin and luteolin-7-O-glucoside, farnesene, quercetin, patuletin and coumarin, are all essential for the pharmacological effects of this plant.[5]

Main therapeutic actions confirmed by research

Carminative and antispasmodic effects

One of the reasons that many people may not like the taste initially of chamomile tea, is due to the bitterness present. The taste of bitter acts therapeutically and pharmacologically to stimulate the digestive cascade, and to nudge the normal sequence of events into their correct order along the digestive tract. The combination of mild bitters and highly aromatic compounds with well-recognised spasmolytic and anti-inflammatory effects means that chamomile can act to soothe but also correct digestive function. It corrects tone of the membranes lining the gut and encourages good function of the cells, tissues and organs. A regular dose therefore can gradually improve function over time, as well as providing instant and reliable soothing relief.

Anxiolytic and antidepressant effects

As part of a randomised, double-blind, placebo-controlled study, researchers examined the antidepressant action of oral chamomile extract in subjects with co-morbid anxiety and depression symptoms. It was demonstrated that chamomile may have a clinically meaningful antidepressant activity that occurs in addition to its previously observed anxiolytic activity.[7]

Anti-inflammatory

Chamomile is well known as a useful external preparation for conjunctivitis (applied as a tisane over the closed eye), and has also been similarly used externally in mastitis, ulcers, wounds, haemorrhoids, anal fissure, sore gums and dental infection.[2]

The effects of chamomile (in particular the azulenes and bisabolol) have also been shown to inhibit the contractions provoked by histamine, acetylcholine and bradykinin. This confirms the traditional use of chamomile as providing relief from the histamine-induced reactions of hay fever, allergic asthma and eczema. Chamomile can form part of a hayfever-season tea for drinking, but also can be applied to sore itchy eyelids, or used as a fantastic bathing herb for the skin. A chamomile bath is a wonderful experience in any case!

To conclude, a systematic review on the efficacy of *Matricaria chamomilla* (L.) Rauschert was carried out by a team of researchers in Iran, where chamomile grows freely and is prized as a medicine. The authors concluded that

> *The findings of this study indicated that this plant is commonly used for its antioxidant, antimicrobial, antidepression, anti-inflammatory,*

antidiarrheal and angiogenesis activity, anticarcinogenic, hepatopro-
tective, and antidiabetic effects. Besides, it is beneficial for knee osteo-
arthritis, ulcerative colitis, pre-menstrual syndrome, and gastrointestinal
disorders. Antimicrobial activity (antiparasitic, antibacterial, antiviral
properties) was reported. Many studies confirmed the antioxidative effects
of this plant; finally, more complementary studies in different thera-
peutic effects of this herb in clinical trial studies may be appropriate for
future studies.

—S. Miraj and S. Alesaeidi[6]

Historical use of chamomile

Receipt books, traditionally handed down through families, comprised
of recipes handwritten in the 17th–19th century by the householder.
Many examples survive in museums and records offices. They serve as
an interesting record of healing foods and herbal medicines available to
the family in the home. Often there is a mixture of food and medicine,
utilising commonly found items in the service of a home remedy. One
of these remedies thought to date to 1791 simply says:

For deafness in the ears. Take Camelmild (chamomile) and seeth it and
putt into the eares and wash the eares with it and in a few days itt
Heales.

—A. Revell[8]

Similarly, Maria Treben (1995) records a village woman known as the
'chamomile witch' helping five people with deafness by gently frying
green field onion in chamomile oil and dropping the cooled oil into
the ear.[9]

Onions and garlic have long been effectively utilised for ear infection
as well as for a cough. In the same receipt book from 1791 is recorded a
recipe rather similar to Maria Treben's story:

Take a faire sound onien cut of the Red of the out part then cut of the top
where make a Convenient hole wherein put a meete quantity of venice
treacle, oyle of bitter almonds, a little sivet, let these bubble all night on the
embers in the morning Straine and put 2 or 3 drops in the eare keeping the
eare warm with wool.

—M. Treben[9]

Nicholas Culpeper (1616–1654) stated of onions:

> *The juice … dropped into the ears eases the pains and noises in them.*
>   —Nicholas Culpeper[10]

In Russian folk medicine we find:

> *for an abscess in the ear treat with flax seed and onion oil. Prepare by making small cracks in the onion skin, pouring in the flax seed oil and baking. Then squeeze a few drops into the ear two or three times a day.*
>   —P. M. Kourenoff and G. St George[11]

Potters New Cyclopaedia of Botanical Drugs and Preparations says:

> *who has not heard of roasted onion as a poultice for suppurating tumours or ear ache?*
>   —R. C. Wren[12]

The allium family has an ancient and venerable history of use as an antiseptic agent. The British government encouraged the growth of garlic and bought thousands of tonnes in order to utilise the antiseptic properties and apply this to the wounded of World War I using sphagnum moss as the dressing.[13,14]

In Martindale's British Pharmacopaea of 1972 Garlic was reported as having:

> *expectorant, diaphoretic, disinfectant and diuretic properties and has been used as a syrup in the treatment of chronic bronchitis and other pulmonary conditions. The juice has been given by mouth or has been used as a gargle or throat spray.*
>   —W. Martindale[15]

And so, it was not so long ago that the properties of medicinal plants like garlic were seen as being effective and available for use by doctors and pharmacists. Chamomile and garlic do make good dancing partners. Garlic (or onions) are strongly antibacterial, whilst gentle, anti-inflammatory chamomile soothes any pungency and potential irritation which may be caused by the inflammation, the infection, or even the garlic.

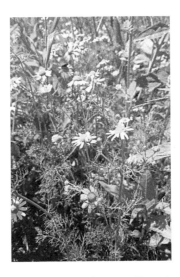

Chamomile (*Matricaria chamomilla* (L.) Rauschert)

Case history

A 4-month-old baby boy had been diagnosed with eczema that had persisted from 2 days after the birth, and he was not responding to any of the usual external treatments given by the doctor. Even steroid cream did not appear to be effective. His eczema seemed very red and deep into the skin with very well-defined patches located on his shoulders and chest. This in itself was rather unusual in presentation as childhood eczema will often appear in the creases of the body, elbows, knees, neck, wrists and so on …

The birth had been quite distressing for mother and baby and conducted in a rush and in panic after many hours of contractions. The little lad was breastfed entirely by his mother—so there was no possibility he was reacting to formula milk. Was it possible that mother and baby were 'in shock'? As a result, a series of herb baths was suggested for the little boy, and a tea for his mother to drink so that the medicinal effects would benefit them both—passing through her milk to him. The aim of the herbal mixture was to be nervine and vulnerary.

The tea was 50% *Chamomilla recutita* (L.) Rauschert, flowers with 50% *Calendula officinalis* L. flowers. A bath was made by making an infusion of 1 tablespoon of herb to 1 pint of boiling water, covered and left for at least 10 minutes. Each day this cooled tea was added to his bathwater (after sieving out the herb material). In addition, his mother drank

1 cup or more if possible, each day, made with 1 teaspoon of dried herbs. After 3 weeks the little boy was much improved and 6 weeks later his skin was 80% better.

Interestingly, this young family returned 12 weeks later as the little boy's skin had stopped improving and even slipped back a little. His mother was quite run-down, she had a head cold coming, and she was exhausted. The little boy also had hard swollen lymph glands in his neck and although his skin overall was much better, it was not completely clear. His father had noticed that the little boy no longer cried with colic and slept much more peacefully since he had received the chamomile baths.

Once again, a strong feeling of them both still recovering from shock was apparent, and so the mother was given a much more 'tonic' and immune-boosting mixture to take. The little boy could now be given teaspoonfuls of the same original herb tea rather than just bathing in the herbs. He was of course 3 months older now, and still happily breast-feeding. The prescription for his mother included *Matricaria chamomilla* (L.) Rauchert., *Melissa officinalis* L., *Sambucus nigra* L. (flowers), *Echinacea purpurea* (L.) Moench (root), and *Glycyrrhiza glabra* L. (root). Mother and baby are still doing well, and within 14 days of starting this herbal treatment plan the eczema had cleared.

Safety

The acute oral LD_{50} tests (a sadly acceptable method for defining drug safety), performed in the 1980s showed that no irritating effect could be found for chamomile, nor sensitisation or phototoxic effects. Similar safety was demonstrated for oral administration and in pregnancy. Although the Asteraceae family to which chamomile belongs has a reputation as being potentially able to cause allergic effects, in chamomile this potential is so low as to be negligible, and in fact thought to only have occurred with contamination with well-known irritants of this family, for example non-medicinal plants such as *Anthemis cotula* L. *Therefore all safety issues surround the correct identification of this plant.*

Definition—LD_{50}: LD_{50} is an abbreviation for 'Lethal Dose, 50%'. It refers to the amount of the substance required (usually per body weight) to kill 50% of the test population.

Pharmacy

Chamomile eye bath, or full-body bath

We would like to encourage you to now experience a wonderful bath in flowers! If you do not have a bath at home, you may like to try a foot bath, or perhaps experience an eye compress. All of these are made using an infusion method.

Pour boiling water over 1 tablespoon (2 or 3 tablespoons if you have a big bath!) of dried chamomile flowers in a heat-proof vessel such as a 1-pint jug or bowl. Instantly cover your herb tea with a plate or something to seal in all the precious volatile compounds including the essential oils. Leave to stand for at least 10 minutes, but preferably 30 minutes or more (it can even be left overnight).

It is worthwhile giving thought to and planning your preferred bathing method. Imagine you are in an old-fashioned hospital and this treatment is part of a very serious protocol that includes care and wellbeing for the patient (you!). We are told that in ancient Arabic hospitals patients were given baths in flower waters, sang to and had poetry recited to them at their bedsides, with gardens and water fountains available to them as part of healing and convalescence!

> *Can we imagine a modern society where herbal medicine in all its myriad forms can be as standard **alongside** conventional medical treatment and surgery for those people in hospital or recovering from major illness?*

If you are drawing a full bath, you may need to consider the water temperature (not too hot) especially as you will be adding your infusion (which may now be cold). If you are making a foot bath, consider what bowl will be comfortable to keep your feet in and will fit your feet comfortably.

Note: A quick reminder about using anything as an eye compress!

- Make sure all utensils are clean and perhaps even sterile where possible, including clean hands!
- Use clean cotton wool (organic) pads or boiled flannel type cloth, do not use kitchen roll or toilet paper as both of these harbour a huge amount of bacteria!
- Only dip a cotton pad once into the strained/sieved tea, never re-dip it.

- Only put one pad to one eye—do not then put it on the other eye (risk of transferring infection).
- Use a clean pad each time to dip into your infusion ... Sorry that's a lot of information—but hopefully you have understood the key point here.

Eyes are our only external organ, and are kept sterile by our body. Therefore only use herbs over the closed lid of your eye. *The medicinal compounds found in these herbs will pass through the membranes of the skin and reach their target.*

If you are making an eye compress, you may like to consider a comfortable seat or propped up in a bed, but you will need easy access to your herb infusion, and some cotton wool pads, somewhere to put used pads, and maybe a nice blanket to help you relax back and enjoy the experience.

Summary

Albert and Lilian Priest, writing in 1982 for the National Institute of Medical Herbalists and reflecting a herbal tradition still embedded within physiomedicalism, describe chamomile as a stimulating nervine. They suggest it is indicated for those experiencing neural irritability or a 'sthenic' background to their problem. In their recommendations for individuals, *Matricaria chamomilla* (L.) Rauschert is suited to easing flatulence, colic, abdominal distention and spasm. Also pre-menstrual irritability and spasmodic dysmenorrhoea, infantile convulsions from colic, teething, or earache.[16]

In practice, the use of strong infusions or tinctures of this seemingly delicate little plant can have significant and profound therapeutic effects on patients experiencing exactly these symptoms and in these situations. Even when very strong conventional painkillers have not given complete relief, something as straightforward as chamomile can give similar levels of relief but without any negative adverse effect. In fact due to the complete lack of liver or kidney damage when using chamomile, it is possible to use it alongside conventional medicine in almost every case. (It is always best to consult a medical herbalist if a person is using numerous conventional medications).

Definition—Sthenic: of or having a high or excessive level of strength and energy.

Fennel *(*Foeniculum vulgare *Mill.)*

Who has not experienced fennel in their lives, as a culinary herb and seed, along with many other familiar herbs of this family; parsley, coriander, aniseed and dill. And yet they all improve our experience of food, bringing flavour, delight, nutrition and digestive support. Just nibble a few seeds after a meal to aid digestion and ease flatulence. The simplicity of this act obscures the miracle going on internally and the probably thousands of little correcting reactions that spark from that one fennel seed.

> *Fennel was important enough to be mentioned in The Nine Herbs Charm as one of the plants of the 'wise lord' made while he was hanging in the heavens, and later in mediaeval times it was hung over doorways on Midsummer's Eve to ward off fire and witchcraft.*
>
> —Stephen Pollington[17]

Classification

Fennel is a member of the Apiaceae family, once known as the Umbelliferae family. It originated in the Mediterranean. Florence fennel (*Foeniculum vulgare* var. azoricum) is the source of the delicious fat bulb of fennel used in cooking, and *Foeniculum vulgare* var. dulce is an annual with a sweet taste.

Basic botany

A tall, elegant, greyish-green, hairless, pungent perennial with hollow stems.

- **Flowers** umbels of yellow flowers. Each number has between 30–50 yellow flowers on short pedicels.
- **Leaves** feathery with finely dissected terminal leaves.
- **Seeds** small, ridged and oval-shaped.
- **Parts used** the seed of bitter fennel in medicine (*Foeniculum vulgare* Mill.), sweet fennel bulb and leaves in cooking (*Foeniculum vulgare var. dulce*). Hybridisation occurs between these two cultivated varieties, and with dill (*Anethum graveolens* L.).
- **Harvesting** harvest leaves any time before seeds form. Harvest seeds between September and Oct. Harvest sweet or Florence fennel bulb

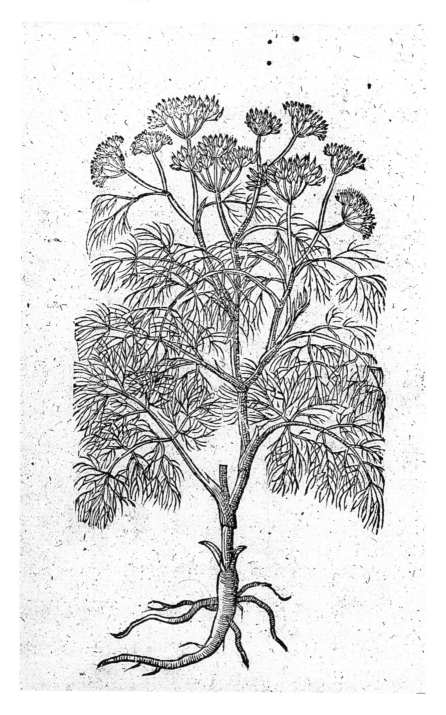

mid-summer/autumn after mounding up the earth around the bulb to help it swell.

Main constituents

- *Essential oils*: Trans-anethole, fenchone, estragole. The ratio between these oils varies between sweet fennel and bitter fennel.[4]
- *Other constituents*: Fixed oil, flavonoids, organic acids, stilbene trimmers and plant sterols including beta-sitosterol. There are only low levels of furano-coumarins in fennel fruits (seeds).[18]

Pharmacodynamics — researched plant compounds

Anethole—a compound found in fennel and some other plants like dill for example, has a similar resemblance chemically to the catecholamines—naturally occurring neurotransmitters found in the brain and nervous system such as adrenaline, noradrenaline and dopamine. Neurotransmitters allow smooth functioning of motor control (movement of our body), cognition (thinking), emotion, memory processing and endocrine modulation (hormone homeostasis). The similarity of structure between the catecholamines and anethole is likely to explain the various sympathomimetic effects seen with modern herbal medicine practice and traditional use of fennel and aniseed (*Pimpinella anisum* L.). Fennel and aniseed have well-known bronchodilation (opening the airways of the lung) effects (like adrenaline) for example.[18]

Main therapeutic actions confirmed by modern research

Effects on smooth muscle

Research has also suggested that fennel has smooth muscle effects that are spasmolytic.[18] Muscle spasm reducing effects have been noted for the uterus also. Dill (*Anethum graveolens* L.), a plant closely related to fennel, is a traditional preparation for childbirth and helps to reduce labour pains in Iran. Research has confirmed this empirical evidence.[19,20]

Definition—*Smooth muscle*: Smooth muscle refers to a special type of involuntary muscle found throughout the body, for example in the digestive system. It can contract spontaneously, and is influenced by hormones, drugs and neurotransmitters, especially the parasympathetic nervous system.

Definition—*Spasmolytic*: This word is made up of two words— spasm, and lysis meaning to destroy or break down. In other words, spasmolytic is a technical word meaning to break down or destroy muscle spasm.

Digestive effects

These include increased gastric secretion, enhanced amylase (digestive enzyme) activity in the small intestine and pancreas, and improvements in bile production and food-transit time in the gut.[18]

Oestrogenic and related effects

Improved fat content and quantity of breast milk has long been acknowledged traditionally. Research also has demonstrated this for goats given fennel oil.[18] Fennel use has been employed traditionally for enhancing fertility, for easing menstrual pain, aiding breastfeeding, and can be most helpful at menopause because of its digestive effects and aiding the nourishment and integrity of the vulval tissues. There are various studies confirming the usefulness of fennel for dysmenorrhoea (period pain).[21,22]

Respiratory effects

Mild cough suppressant effects have been observed with the use of fennel, as have improvements in the volume and thickness of respiratory tract fluid. Fennel tea has been demonstrated to increase muco-ciliary escalator transport, and opening of the respiratory airways (bronchodilation).[18]

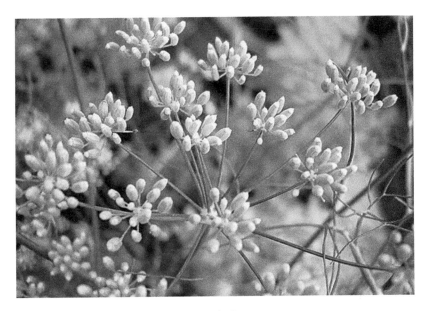

Fennel seeds forming.

Safety

Do you remember in Chapter 1 we stated that adverse drug reactions (ARDs) are defined as occurring when a person has taken a drug at normal dosage? Overdose can occur with extremely enthusiastic use, and this does happen sometimes with plants like fennel. Taking excessive quantities of anything may provoke an unwanted reaction—but this is not an adverse reaction—its just excess.

But back to fennel—fennel has been categorised as a spice allergen (for those people recognised as having a syndrome of sensitivity to celery, carrot and mugwort). This syndrome is related to occupational exposure to umbellifer (Apiaceae) family plants' sap on the skin, which can then increase susceptibility to further reactions. However allergic reactions to fennel as a medicine are known to be rare.[18]

We have never seen this in practice with fennel itself, and in this family only with hogweed (*Heracleum sphondylium* L.) and giant hogweed (*Heracleum mantegazzianum* Sommier & Levier), and very occasionally with the sap of angelica (*Angelica archangelica* L.). Remember that the Apiaceae (Umbelliferae) family include deadly hemlock, fool's parsely and water dropwort, so be careful of any cow parsley type plant (Apiaceae family) that you have not 100% identified.

Very high doses of fennel essential oil should be avoided in persons with liver problems (hepatic disorders). As we discussed in Chapter 1, the essential oil of a plant forms only up to 1% of the total constituents, and therefore represents an exaggerated dose of certain constituents. In other words, use essential oils with care. Adverse events are negative symptoms reported *at the normal dose*.

Use in pregnancy and breastfeeding

No evidence of harm in pregnancy has been found. Reduced fertility has been observed in mice, but many herbalists will confirm that fennel does not pose any significant risk to conception in humans. Fennel has a long successful tradition of use in breastfeeding mothers and is considered by regulatory authorities to be compatible with breastfeeding. A close relative of fennel, dill (*Anethum graveolens* L.) has been the main ingredient of gripe water for babies with colic for many, many years.

Fennel Elecutuary

Electuary of fennel and linseed. Electuaries are a very old traditional way of administering herbs, by powdering them and mixing them with honey to make a sweet, medicinal herbal paste, that can be held in the mouth.

Have a go at making your own electuary using the mixture of foods and medicinal herbs in the recipe below. Fennel seed ground into a powder will serve as a fine example of the method of preparing an electuary, and is an appropriate herb to make into an electuary, having been used historically to do so. Fennel seed and electuaries themselves have often been used to relieve a cough, but also to bring a feeling of wellbeing to the digestive system.

Ingredients
Fennel seeds 50 g
Linseeds (flax) 100 g
Raisins 50 g
Honey 50–100 ml

Method
Grind the linseeds (flax seeds) in a clean dry coffee grinder (or similar) or buy them freshly cold-milled. Keep them to one side. Do the same with fennel seeds, as fine as you can. Keep them with the linseed. Now using a food

processor (or a very strong arm and pestle and mortar...) pulp the raisins into a smooth paste. Add the ground linseeds and fennel to the paste and use the food processor to blend together. Finally, add the honey (or, for a vegan version—birch syrup, molasses or date syrup) and blend again.

Using a spatula or palette knife, draw your electuary out of the food processor and pack into a clean sterile jar. Press the electuary to the edges of the jar and try to press out any air pockets. This will help the electuary keep fresh for longer. This electuary will keep for a very long time preserved in the honey and raisins. The oils in the seeds seem to be more stable and do not go rancid as easily as they would be if they had been stored simply as a packet of milled linseeds.

Use the electuary in small teaspoonsful two, three or four times daily to aid digestion or to ease a tickly cough. The texture is perfect to hold in your mouth and slowly dissolve. This would be ideal for someone who needs a little nourishment at the same time! You can vary the recipe to be more complicated or to use a different powdered herb, or a different dried fruit.[23]

Summary

- Fennel has antispasmodic and carminative effects in the digestive system, clearing wind and discomfort.
- Fennel has the capacity to nourish and balance hormone levels aiding breastfeeding and also relieving common symptoms associated with pre-menstrual syndrome (PMS) and menopause.
- Fennel is nourishing and clarifying in character and clears stagnation and inflammation.
- Fennel is safe to use during pregnancy and in children's medicine.
- Fennel is an ideal companion to chamomile as a medicine.

We have found a mixture of chamomile and fennel to be ideal for relieving even extreme cramping brought on by gastro-enteritis. Also a mixture of the two is ideal for breastfeeding mothers to calm and aid breast milk formation, whilst relieving colic for the baby. It can be given in teaspoonful doses, building up to a few ounces at a time for helping with weaning babies and soothing toddlers tummy ache. A tea of chamomile and fennel can be placed over a closed eye to relieve sore dry eyes or as part of a complete treatment strategy for treating conjunctivitis. Ask your herbalist for an internal medicine to complement this.

Elder (Sambucus nigra L.)

The elder tree, such a magical and symbolic healing gift it thrives and helps us do so too. From its feminine early summer blossoms and their joyful but clarifying zingy exuberance, right through to their masculine beetrooty resilience-enhancing berries. Elder is a year-round herbal ally.

> *The elder tree grows everywhere, and you will rarely find it in a place where any other tree or shrub grows, which is a most enviable characteristic.*
>
> —M. Blochwich[24]

Classification

The elder tree is a member of the Adoxaceae or Caprifoliaceae family.

Basic botany

This deciduous shrub or small tree, native to Europe (except the far north), North Africa and Asia grows up to 10 metres in height. The bark is corky, grey-brown with a white pith, often with yellow lichen, and in maturity may harbour the edible jelly ear fungus. Branches are arching and rather brittle, from which vigorous, smooth, green new growth stems emerge.

- **Flowers** open in June–July in broad, flat-topped clusters or panicles that are 10–24 centimetres across. Every single flower is creamy–white; about 0.6 centimetre diameter, and has five equal petals, and five stamens. They have a distinctive perfume which can either seem to be lemony, or sometimes is described as 'rotting' or unpleasant.
- **Leaves** are made up of five or seven serrated leaflets, oval to eliptical. They also have a distinctive smell.
- **Berries** turn from green to red then black, globose. On reddish-purple branched stems.
- **Habitat** grows in the wild in woods, hedges and near old walls, farm buildings, disturbed land or riverbanks. Usually found on nitrogen-rich or calcareous soils up to 1600 metres. A similar variety of Sambucus is found in North America.

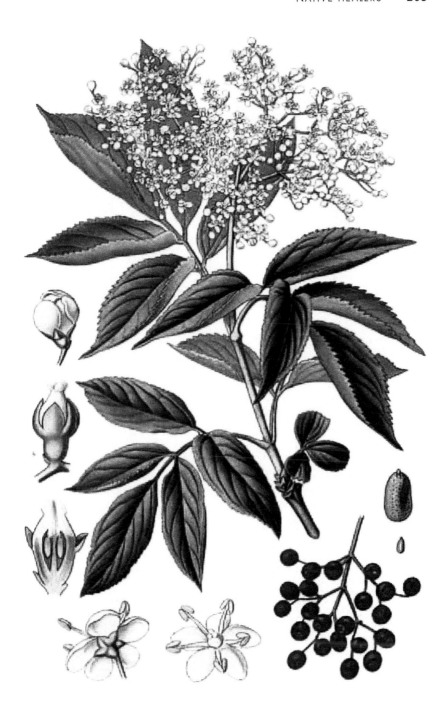

- **Parts used** mainly the flowers, and fruits, but also young leaves (externally), and the jelly ear fungus that grows on its bark. Avoid internal use of the leaves, stems or bark.
- **Harvesting** harvest flowers in early stages of flowering (June in the Northern Hemisphere), on a dry sunny day. If you are harvesting to dry them, place the whole umbels on paper to dry. Leave flowers spread out on a paper for a while to allow small creatures to escape You can use a fork to remove the flowers from the stems. Harvest berries between August and September, when they are ripe, black and shiny. You can use a fork to strip them from the stalks, thus avoiding staining your hands black with the juice. Harvest leaves in June or July for use in ointment for bruises, sprains and chilblains.

Main constituents

The main compounds and known therapeutic constituents found within *Sambucus* are:

- triterpenes including ursolic and oleanolic acid derivatives.
- flavonoids (rutin, quercitin nicotoflorin, hyperoside).
- phenolic acids such as chlorogenic acid. The flowers also contain an essential oil.[4]
- Studies have shown that elderberry wine contains quercetin, kaempferol, phenolic acids and anthocyanins.[25]

Note: The flowers and berries are best used cooked or at least heated by infusion or steam before consumption. Lectins found in them can cause mild gastro-intestinal disturbances, but lectins are easily destroyed by heat.[4]

Main therapeutic actions confirmed by research

Colds and flu

Elderflowers are part of an old classic cold and influenza (flu) tisane that also contained yarrow and peppermint. By inducing perspiration (diaphoresis) it is still thought to aid a speedy conclusion to viral infections. This recipe is one still used by many herbalists today—sometimes with the addition of boneset herb (*Eupatorium perfoliatum* L.) to help with the bone ache symptoms of flu.

Note: Diaphoresis. The concept of diaphoresis is considered crucial in activating the immune response and is a fundamental concept found in Western herbal medicine. Sweating as a health activity has been observed in various cultural traditions such as First Nations, and from Europe. Evidence of sweat houses in Ireland, called tigh 'n alluis, as well as a Neolithic building excavated at Marden Henge in Wiltshire are just two of many examples from ancient history.

The blending of ideas from the early American herbal medical schools with European naturopathic traditions meant the concept of elimination has remained important within natural medicine traditions like herbal medicine.

Sweating and properly-managed fever are, despite being uncomfortable and inconvenient, useful elements of our natural immune response. Overly suppressing a therapeutic fever is thought to elongate the duration of infections, and potentially prevent full resolution. (For more information on dealing with fever, please see chapter nine, where we talk in more detail about the treatment of colds and flu).

Antiviral effects

Recent studies show an in vitro activity against several strains of influenza virus. At least one clinical study of the berries has demonstrated a reduction in the duration of flu symptoms.[26,27] Elderberry has been shown to contain high levels of anthocyananins, especially quercetin and kaempferol and to have the antioxidative potential of red wine. These precious phenolic compounds diminish with age.[25] Fresh is best! So freeze the berries or make your elderberry products and aim to replace with fresh every 2 years.

A project called Ethnomedica or 'Remembered Remedies' at Kew is collecting information about the everyday and practical use of herbal remedies used by people up and down the country. Collaborating with the National Institute of Medical Herbalists, Chelsea Physic Garden, Neal's Yard, the Eden Project and the Natural History Museum the aim is to collect and preserve the wealth of knowledge about local uses of plants as medicines in the UK. Collection of data began in 2003 and so far about 5000 remedies have been gathered and entered into a database, preserving knowledge that may have otherwise been lost. Among the 'Top 10' remedies emerging from the project is the use of elder for treating coughs and colds.

Anti-catarrhal effects

Although the mechanism is poorly understood there are a range of herbs used to good practical effect as anti-catarrhals. Some work has suggested there is a change in the *shape* of the mucous cells lining the mucous membranes that is corrected by the use of these medicinal herbs.

The normal shape of a goblet cell could be compared to a champagne glass, but in chronic catarrh the shape becomes more brandy glass shaped and can take time and effort to restore to a normal champagne flute!

Sambucus nigra L. (flowers) is one of many mucous membrane functional restoratives. Others include eyebright (*Euphrasia officinalis* L.) and ribwort plantain (*Plantago lanceolata* L. and *P. major* L.).

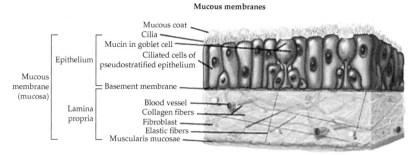

Mucous membranes

Mucous coat
Cilia
Mucin in goblet cell
Ciliated cells of pseudostratified epithelium
Epithelium
Mucous membrane (mucosa)
Basement membrane
Blood vessel
Collagen fibers
Lamina propria
Fibroblast
Elastic fibers
Muscularis mucosae

- Consists of epithelium, lamina propria & muscularis mucosae
- Lines passageways that open to the exterior: digestive, respiratory, urinary and reproductive
- Mucous coating & movement of cilia trap & remove foreign particles & bacteria from internal surfaces of body

Anti-inflammatory and allergy modulating

Elderflowers have a long traditional use for easing symptoms of inflammation of the mucous membranes especially for rhinitis and hayfever. Research has shown that elderberries ex-vivo can stimulate anti-inflammatory cytokines in human monocytes.[28] A study looking at the potential to reduce inflammatory mediators in periodontitis showed that elderflower extract was found to potently inhibit all pro-inflammatory activities tested.[29] Elderflowers are non-toxic and no side effects have been reported.[4] Elderflower is considered to have no contra-indications nor are there any official warnings or precautions based on current evidence in the UK, US, Australia and in Germany.[18]

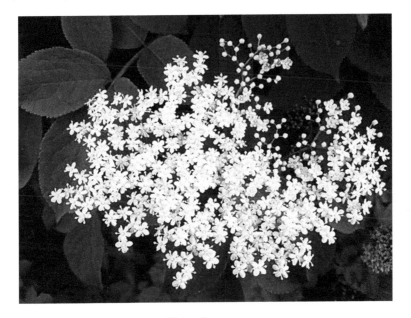

Elder flowers.

Case history

The mother of a young baby (6 months) boy came to see the herbalist concerned that the child could not breathe easily through the nose. She said he had been congested almost since he was born, and he regularly had green or yellow mucous crusting at the edges of his nostrils. This often led to noisy, laboured breathing and this was understandably worrying for his mother. He was otherwise a very healthy baby, feeding and sleeping well and growing satisfactorily. When asked, the mother was not sure if he had had lots of colds, because 'he seems to have one all the time'. Because he was so young but no longer being breastfed, a herbal tea of simply elderflowers was given, with instructions to make the tea with boiling water.

Infuse for 10 minutes in a covered vessel before straining the liquid free of flowers. One teaspoon was to be added to each of his bottles every day, whether it was milk, or another drink. In practice this meanthe would have up to 6–8 teaspoons of the prepared herbal tea per day. More teaspoonfuls could be added if necessary as the child adapted to the new flavour. In addition—some advice about his fluid intake was given—to continue to give him milk, but also sometimes water with the tea as well. The child had been previously given a sugar-free squash.

The mother returned in 3 weeks time saying that his crusty nose had cleared within 48 hours, and over the 3 weeks he had been less and less mucousy in general. His breathing was no longer laboured. This lady has used the elderflower tea for each of her children whenever they have a cold, and has found not only that it was effective, but that all four children like to drink it! As well as being anti-inflammatory, elderflowers are a classic remedy in terms of fever management, acting as an effective diaphoretic. We will be discussing fever management in more detail in chapter nine.

In children's medicine *Sambucus* can be useful for, and included in herbal treatments for an array of childhood complaints not yet mentioned including: bronchitis, allergies, chickenpox, hand foot and mouth disease, hay fever, laryngitis, measles, mumps, roseola, scarlet fever, sinusitis and teething.[26]

Due to the non-toxic nature of elderflowers and briefly cooked elderberries—it can also safely run alongside conventional treatment if necessary, but as always, if in doubt consult your qualified medical herbalist.

Elderberry

We shall briefly look at the fruit of *Sambucus nigra* L.

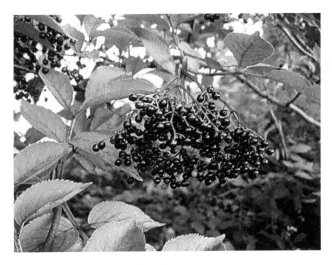

Elder berries.

Effects and uses confirmed by research

A randomized study in 2004 of the *Efficacy and Safety of Oral Elderberry Extract in the Treatment of Influenza A and B Virus Infections* demonstrated elderberry as a safe, effective and cost-effective way of treating influenza.[30]

Another study in 2002, came to the following conclusion:

> We conclude from this study that, in addition to its antiviral properties, Sambucol Elderberry Extract and its formulations activate the healthy immune system by increasing inflammatory cytokine production. Sambucol might therefore be beneficial to the immune system activation and in the inflammatory process in healthy individuals or in patients with various diseases. Sambucol could also have an immunoprotective or immunostimulatory effect when administered to cancer or AIDS patients, in conjunction with chemotherapeutic or other treatments.
>
> —V. Barak et al.[28]

Pharmacy preparations (berries and flowers)

Elderberries are also enjoyed across Europe as a spiced syrup or 'rob'. Blochwich[24] describes many interesting and more obscure ways of preparing every part of the elder into useful medicinal preparations, including: elderberry rob, tincture and wine, spiritus waters, syrups and tragea, even oil from the seeds! For the flowers he lists preserves, syrups and honeys, waters and spirits, vinegars and oxymels, wine and an infused oil. He even includes a recipe for the jelly ear fungus that grows commonly on old elder trees.

Elderberry Rob

A rob is a traditional name for a thickened juice. You can find many recipes for robs or syrups, and elderberry rob is a really worthwhile remedy to have in your store cupboard in preparation for winter, as well as being a pleasure to make and take. This is just one of them.

- Remove elderberries from stalks. (You can use a fork to do this, which may save your hands from becoming stained.
- Place elderberries in a saucepan with half their volume of water, and simmer, stirring occasionally for around 20 minutes.
- Once cooled, strain the berries through a fine sieve/muslin bag.
- Measure your juice, then add half the quantity of sugar (muscovado works well). Therefore, if you have 200ml juice you will be adding 100g sugar. You could, alternatively, use honey in a 50:50 ratio.
- Add warming spices to the mix. We recommend star anise, cinnamon, cloves, ginger.
- Simmer again for approximately 20 minutes, then strain and, while the syrup is still hot, pour into sterilized jars.

You will find a similar recipe to this one, called Elderberry and Ginger syrup, in chapter nine, where we take an in depth look at the treatment of respiratory tract infections. There are many different versions of this basic recipe, and it has proved to be an absolutely key remedy for treating viral infections.

NB: Always label your home pharmacy projects—what is in it and the date you made it!

Usually a 50:50 honey to elderberry juice ratio is used to allow preserving to take place, but cooking for longer, or storing in the fridge, will reduce the need for sugar/honey. Remember the darker the sugar the more vitamins are left in it—and honey has its own healing properties.

We have made this without sugar by cooking on a gentle heat for 2 hours, and then storing in the fridge where it has kept for several months. Occasionally a plug of white mould forms at the top of the bottle where maybe some skins of the elderberry managed to bypass the sieve, but the elderberry rob underneath the removed plug has been perfectly good to use.

A good way to sterilise bottles is to pop them in a low oven (as low as you can) for 20–30 minutes then turn off the oven and leave to cool—this helps dry them thoroughly too. Lids can melt in the oven (as can the rubber seals on kilner jars), but boiling in water for 10 minutes works well. Apparently a microwave is very effective at sterilising glassware too.

For a pharmacy preparation of the flowers we will look at an infused oil because this can be a very practical preparation for an external remedy. The oil can be used directly to the skin, or can be further prepared into an ointment (see later in this book for full details!). Please make and keep your infused oil, we will use it later on in this course to make another pharmacy preparation.

Summary

Once again, the wonderful medical herbalists Priest and Priest tell us that elderflowers are mild with diffusing and relaxing and diaphoretic properties.[16] They also say the elder has mild alterative properties—we shall discuss alteratives later in this book.

The use of *Sambucus* in children's medicine is affirmed by Priest and Priest especially for children prone to fevers. They additionally say it is relaxing to the eliminative organs—which is a wonderful concept—that we can be relaxed into improving the elimination of normal waste products of metabolism and waste products of infection! They use *Sambucus* therefore for fevers, catarrh, night sweats, skin eruptions.

This wide range of applications comes from the understanding of the effect that *Sambucus* has on the body—one which can be experienced by taking it, to open up all the many small processes in the body that allow movement of blood, lymph, serum, catarrh and sweat. It seems to us that Priest and Priest really know their herbs and have much clinical experience because they seem to speak with such clarity about complex ideas. Their experience seems to match our experience of the use of elder.

Lemon balm (Melissa officinalis L.)

Also known as bee balm, and honey plant, it is interesting to consider what properties a bee would think Melissa contributes to honey making. Lemon balm's capacity for perennial survival, popping up all around the nooks and crannies of the garden and returning each year speaks of its hardy resilience. Its slightly sour and dry taste albeit wrapped in a relaxing lemony exterior, speaks of increasing our resilience and perhaps the retention of our own inner sparkle.

Classification

Lemon balm is a member of the mint or *Lamiaceae* family.

Basic botany

Melissa is a medium to tall, sometimes hairy, lemon-scented perennial, with flowering stems, ascending to erect.

- **Flowers** whitish or pale yellow, often becoming pinkish, 8–15 millimetres long, in leafy whorled, interrupted spikes, the upper lip erect, the lower three-lobed.
- **Leaves** paired. Oval to diamond-shaped, deeply toothed, stalked.
- **Habitat** widely naturalised in northern Europe as a culinary and medicinal herb[31] native to Eastern and Central Europe, from the Caucasus to Iran.[23]
- **Parts used** leaves and stems especially just before full flowering.
- **Harvesting** harvest leaves/flowering tops just before or right at the start of flowering.

Main constituents

- Volatile oils (including monoterpenes, citral, citronellal, geraniol), tannins, bitters.

Main therapeutic actions confirmed by research

Nervine, sedative, antispasmodic

Many of the monoterpenes have central nervous system calming activities, and appreciable antiseptic properties. Antispasmodic action has been demonstrated in low concentrations. In Germany, it is the main

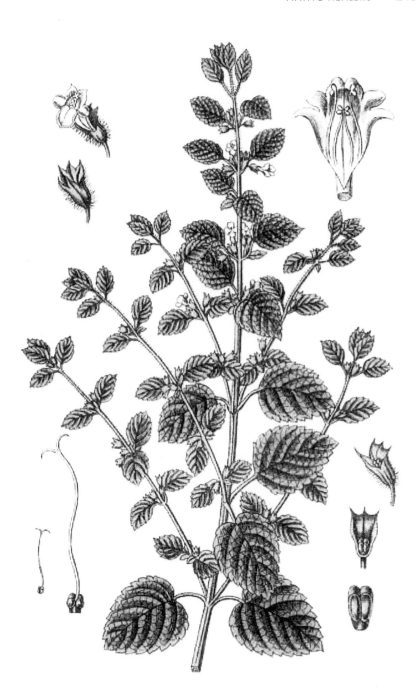

ingredient of a popular medicine called Melissengeist helping symptoms such as restlessness, excitability, headaches and palpitations, a combination of symptoms the Germans call 'psychological-autonomic'. *Melissa* has demonstrated efficacy for these problems in double-blind clinical trials.

Anti-cholinergic effects have been shown in human cerebral cortical cell membrane studies which could explain interactions between the nervous system and hormone production.[32] Effects on GABAergic synapses have also been reported from research (GABAergic synapses are a major form of synapse located in the central nervous system).[33]

Cognitive performance and mood enhancement

Using dried leaf of *Melissa officinalis* has been shown to enhance both mood and cognitive performance, leading it to be considered as a possible adjunct herb in the treatment of Alzheimer's disease.[34]

Antiseptic/antiviral

Melissa extracts have performed well topically for *Herpes simplex labialis* (cold-sore) resulting from HSV-1 infection.[34] Dioscorides (who was a physician to the Roman army) noted its capacity to prevent putrefaction and gangrene on the battlefield.

Endocrine effects

Inhaled volatile compounds have been found accumulating in the limbic system. This has suggested the calming effect and possible hypnotic potential of lemon balm. *Melissa officinalis* L. has been investigated and shown to help reduce the severity of symptoms of PMS.[35] Animal studies showing that in large quantities *Melissa* may reduce excessive thyroid hormones has led to a suggestion that it should not be used to excess in people with low thyroid function.

Note: Thyroid function. It should be remembered that low thyroid function is often brought about by excessive or prolonged stress resulting in excessive cortisol secretions. These block the protein transport mechanism for thyroid hormones causing a relative lack of thyroxine. Feedback mechanisms aimed at correcting this result in stimulating the already over-worked thyroid gland leading to its eventual exhaustion. Sufficiently early intervention, calming and reducing those stressors may then—theoretically and in practice—reduce cortisol levels and allow the thyroid gland to rejuvenate. Treatment with a herbal practitioner will include support for the whole endocrine system, nervous system and will include rejuvenating adaptogens.

Lemon balm can be made into an infused oil by placing the fresh leaves into warm oil and then repeating the process. The word 'balm' means a soothing oil or unguent.

Melissa infused oil

Method

Measure out three times the amount of oil you wish to end up with (you will lose some in the straining off process). Harvest a few handfuls of fresh lemon balm stems and leaves. You will need the same weight as you have millilitres of oil. So, if you have 300 ml of oil, you will need 300 g of the fresh herb.

Strip the leaves of the fresh lemon balm into the oil and warm the oil slowly for up to 3 hours taking care to keep it covered. You can do this in an airing cupboard, on a warm radiator or stove, or by placing a heat-proof container in a water bath and heating gently.

Remove the lid carefully and pass the oil and leaves through a sieve lined with butter muslin. Collect the warm infused oil in another clean dry vessel trying to avoid any dark droplets of oil at the bottom of your pan (these will be water from the fresh plant and will spoil the oil).

Collect another batch of fresh lemon balm, equal to the amount you had before, and repeat the process using your collected first infusion. Repeat again and again, until you are happy that you have a good scent of Melissa now in your oil. Use the oil as part of any cosmetic product that requires oil, or use directly on the skin, it can be applied directly to cold sores for example.

You can make an infused oil from a dried herb too. Elderflowers, lavender or rosemary would be great as infused oils for therapeutic use. Later we will describe how you can make this infused oil into a solid ointment or lip balm.

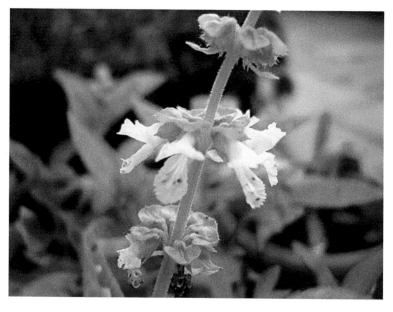

Lemon balm flowers.

Summary

Lemon balm (*Melissa officinalis* L.) is a gentle but effective mood-lifting yet anxiety quelling tonic or nervine for the nervous system. Regular use illustrates how the properties of herbs with nervine actions may have immediate observable effects but also tend to encourage a calmer happier state of being over the long term with no side effects.

Having a mild bitter effect, *Melissa* can also heal and strengthen the functionality of the digestive system and also illustrates the interconnectedness of the nervous system and the gut.

> **Definition—*The enteric nervous system*:** *Medical* herbalists are very interested in the enteric nervous system (ENS), which can be seen as the third part of the autonomic nervous system (ANS). A vast network of neurons are dispersed throughout the gut acting as a dominant neural regulator of the function of the gut.

The ENS regulates the secretion of digestive acids, mucus, and enzymes. It regulates motility and peristalsis, including sphincter function. Importantly the ENS has a broader role in immunity and defence of the mucosal wall (the complex border between the inside and outside of 'us'). When the ENS does not regulate digestive functions correctly it has been suggested as the root of conditions such as inflammatory bowel disease, disruption to gall bladder function, gastric reflux and irritable bowel syndrome (IBS).

The interior 'ecosystem' of the gut flora or 'microbiome' is influenced by the environment created by the ENS and its good function (as well as dietary factors).

The enteric nervous system is connected directly with the brain but also with the immune system, and with the endocrine (hormone) system.

In practice this means that stress and emotions create neural activity that may trigger immune responses and/or hormone (endocrine) responses from within the gut.

The enteric nervous system is not only an afferent nerve pathway (it is not only triggering activity), but it is also an efferent (sensory) pathway, and is constantly relaying positive or negative messages to the brain about the state of things within the gut. Therefore a chronic digestive problem can result in feelings of anxiety or nervousness because the brain is constantly being told 'something is wrong'. And of course, the opposite is true.[36] An exploration of the significance of the microbiome will follow in Chapter 5, 'Food, nutrition and wellness.'

As a popular and easily spreading garden plant, *Melissa* can be utilised when fresh—which is ideal—and demonstrates the usefulness of having 'garden plants' as a home pharmacy. The essential oils of lemon balm are sited in the little glands along the leaf surfaces and are easily lost by drying. Capture the scent of lemon balm in an infused oil, or perhaps just by freezing the whole leaf stems in your home freezer to use as a 'fresh' tea through the winter.

Melissa is an important ingredient in Chartreuse, Benedictine and L'eau de Melisse des Carmes and formed the main treatment for hysteria and nervous exhaustion of women, by the nuns of the Santa Maria Novella convent in Florence. Their spiritus water uses alcohol, one method of trapping more of the volatile compounds. We will look at the preparation of tinctures later in this book.

Melissa is ideal for nervous and depressive states. It has also shown activity against the herpes family of viruses, and so can be applied to the management of cold sores for example. Once again, the link here between the nervous system and how such viruses can lodge themselves within nerves is evident in conditions like cold sores and shingles. Safe in pregnancy and for children, it is an ideal ingredient in digestive, nervous and restless complaints and is usually well-tolerated due to the pleasant aroma.

Tending to be slightly drying in its nature, it is helpful where there is over-activity in the bowel, and heals the membranes of the mouth and digestive system. We have found it to be helpful when used for several weeks' before and after immunisation. We have a sense that it may help build resilience beforehand, whilst pacifying and soothing the experience afterwards.

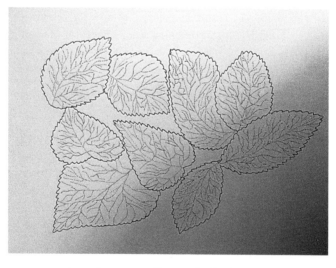

Line drawing of lemon balm leaves.

Meadowsweet *(Filipendula ulmaria L.)*

Meadowsweet, beloved of wet water-meadows, shares with us its capacity to transform the energy of water into solidity and uprightness; its ultimate expression in the uplifting scented flowers with their flash of intense pungency, lifting our spirits. Queen of the meadow, mead-sweet, eases our pains and fevers, and helps us overcome infections, and heals the membranes that deal with our own water balance and are vulnerable to infection and inflammation there.

Classification

Meadowsweet is a member of the rose family, the Rosaceae.

Basic botany

Tall (60–120 centimetres) upright leafy herb, sometimes forming dense stands.

- **Flowers** numerous small, creamy, sweetly scented flowers in dense clusters. Five petals and five sepals. Flowers in summer.
- **Leaves** dark green pinnate, silvery green on the underside. 2–5 pairs of larger toothed leaflets are interspersed with smaller ones.
- **Seeds** small, etched fruits become spirally twisted and fused together.
- **Habitat** common throughout northwestern Europe. Found in ditches, damp meadows and woods, riversides, wet rocky places, marshes and fens but not on acid peat.
- **Parts used** leaves, stems and flowers.
- **Harvesting** harvest flowering tops in summer on a dry sunny day. Leave flowers spread out on paper for a while to allow small creatures to escape.

Although meadowsweet does grow in meadows, the name is thought to come from its former use to flavour mead,[2] beer, and in France—wine. It was 1 of 50 ingredients in a drink called 'Save' recounted in *A Knight's Tale,* by Chaucer.[37] Meadowsweet seeds are spiral-shaped giving it its old name *spirea* and informing the naming of the pharmaceutical drug aspirin. The compound salicylic acid was originally discovered in meadowsweet before being extracted eventually from willow bark (*Salix* species).

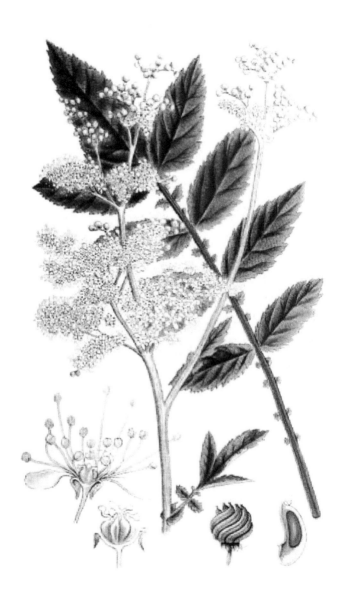

Aspirin and meadowsweet provide a useful contrast says Barker,[2] since both are effective for fever and pain relief, but aspirin (with its acetyl group attached to the salicylate) irritates the mucosal linings of the gut, whereas meadowsweet heals and soothes them. Meadowsweet is a traditional remedy for gastric ulcer. See picture (colour stained electron micrograph) of Aspirin below.

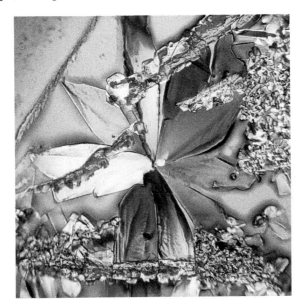

Main constituents

- Flavonoids, phenolic glycosides, such as spiraein, monotropitin and isosalicin. Essential oils (0.2%) containing volatile constituents including methylsalicylate.
- Tannins (10–15%) such as Rugosin-D.
- Salicylic acid (0.6 to 0.8%) and its methyl ester.
- Vanillin, vitamin C and mineral salts.

Main therapeutic actions confirmed by research

Meadowsweet is considered to be a valuable phytomedicine traditionally used in Europe and further afield for atonic dyspepsia with heartburn and hyperacidity, diarrhoea, acute cystitis, rheumatic pain and in the prophylaxis and treatment of gastric ulcer. One uncontrolled research trial showed evidence of benefit to women with cervical dysplasia.[38]

Back in 1691, John Aubrey wrote to John Ray about a woman in Bedfordshire who was achieving 'great cures' with meadowsweet, for agues and fevers.[39]

Meadowsweet is often useful where fever is present, it has diaphoretic effects, and can help restore normal temperature. In particular, meadowsweet should be considered where there is urinary tract infection or gastrointestinal infection.

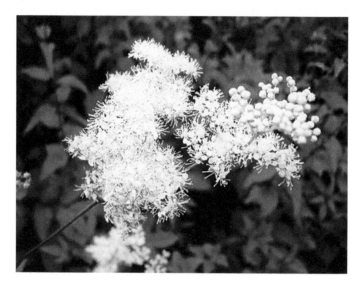

Meadowsweet flowers.

Case history

A woman in her mid-50s experiencing a period of acute personal stress and menopausal symptoms consulted the medical herbalist. She was having lots of distressing vasomotor symptoms (hot flushes), but also recurrent urinary tract infections, general viral infections, lethargy, anxiety, insomnia and also had acute flare-ups of acne rosacea.

In among other helpful plant medicinals, she enjoyed drinking a tea blend that included meadowsweet, *and* a tincture of *Filipendula ulmaria* L. was often included in one of two herbal tincture blends that were made for her. Each time the meadowsweet was used in her medicine, her skin improved and she experienced more comfort and less urinary tract infections.

The recipe for this particular patients' medicine was changed regularly and in response to symptoms and life situations that were changing rapidly. As well as demonstrating how the herbalists' approach is uniquely tailored to each individual, it allowed analysis of the therapeutic effects of the herbal medicine over a relatively long period of consistent treatment (over 2 years).

Phytotherapists consider it to be important, if not essential, to treat the digestive system, particularly the gastric and duodenal parts of the digestive mucosa when treating patients with acne rosacea. It has been our experience that the use of herbs like meadowsweet, even in the absence of digestive symptoms, can have a beneficial effect on the skin.

Other herbs with observable digestive benefits, often employed in the treatment of this patient with acne rosacea included *Berberis aquifolium* Pursh, *Glycyrrhiza glabra* L. and *Centella asiatica* (L.) Urb.

Potential interactions

None known.

Meadowsweet has relatively high levels of therapeutic tannins. There is therefore a theoretical concern that mineral absorption may be reduced (iron in particular), based on evidence from studies on other foods including regular *tea* (*Camellia sinensis* (L.) Kuntze) drinking and chewing. Once again, this is an example of over-enthusiastic use of a single plant, and is not really an adverse event.

A recommendation nevertheless could be that meadowsweet is taken 2 hours away from medication or food. In practice, it is preferable that the meadowsweet has an opportunity to be in contact with the membranes of the digestive system so that it can have maximum vulnerary and anti-inflammatory effects, so this fits in nicely with that recommendation.

Chronic inflammation of the digestive tract may also lead to mineral depletion as a result of mal-absorption. One chronically anaemic patient seen recently, has consistently increased her iron levels (confirmed by regular blood tests), despite the fact she has been taking a medicine with *Filipendula ulmaria* L. as a significant ingredient for more than 6 months.

Lets quickly revisit what we know about tannins! Hydrolysable tannins turn brown on exposure to air and are usually used only externally. Condensed tannins can turn a reddish colour known as tannin reds, or phlobaphenes, a characteristic found in many plant tissues and medicinal plant tinctures.[40] These tannins are related to flavonoids and polyphenol compounds all of which show no hepatotoxicity and have a variety of pharmacologically useful effects. Meadowsweet contains a polyphenol called Rugosin-D a hydrolysable tannin that is safe to take internally, and is found in other rose family members such as the petals of *Rosa rugosa* L.

Rugosin-D is closely related to arbutin—a polyphenol found in bearberry (*Arctostaphylos uva-ursi* (L.) Spreng), that is highly antiseptic to the urinary tract. It is also related to the nattily named sanguine H-6 found in Rosaceae family members such as raspberry leaves (*Rubus ideaus* L.), agrimony (*Agrimonia eupatoria* L.), great burnet (*Sanguisorba officinalis* L.), in strawberries (*Fragaria × ananassa*) and cloudberries (*Rubus chamaemorus* L.).

> **Definition—Berries:** The berries of this family, such as raspberry (*Rubus idaeus* L.), blackberry (*Rubus fructicosus* L.), and cloudberry (*Rubus chamaemorus* L.), are known to contain alpha-linolenic acid, an essential fatty acid that cannot be made by the body.

These therapeutic compounds exhibit effects against pathogenic bacteria. This links neatly with their similar taste and action—meadowsweet and bearberry both can be helpful in urinary tract infections, red raspberry leaf, agrimony and meadowsweet care both helpful in checking diarrhoea and they all ease acid indigestion. Raspberry leaf and great burnet are traditional herbal medicines from Traditional Chinese and Western herbal medicine used for bleeding wounds and excessive uterine bleeding.

Meadowsweet is not recommended for use with *warfarin* or other anticoagulant drugs. This is based on theoretical concerns based on animal studies demonstrating the anti-coagulant activity of meadowsweet.

> **Note: Anti-coagulant drugs.** Warfarin and its modern equivalents such as rivaroxaban, are drugs with an extremely narrow therapeutic range. This means that there is a very small difference between a therapeutic dose and a lethal dose. Using herbal medicines alongside these incredibly problematic drugs is not recommended outside of a strong therapeutic relationship/professional herbal setting. In practice, patients often experience wild fluctuations in symptoms and adverse effects *in any case* as a result of, and whilst taking, these medications and they often do not respond as expected to other conventional medicines prescribed alongside such anti-coagulant drugs.

Pregnancy

There have been one or two animal studies that have raised the possibility of foetal toxicity, but it has been acknowledged that the doses administered in the studies were (ridiculous) considerably higher than would be considered therapeutically and so are unlikely to be relevant. Women in pregnancy are more likely to become iron deficient—so we should think about that when considering meadowsweet as a therapeutic choice during pregnancy. Meadowsweet is compatible with breast-feeding, but use with care—as salicylates (not from meadowsweet) have occasionally been blamed for macular rashes in breast-fed babies.

Practical pharmacy

You can use beautiful meadowsweet as a tea, an underrated intervention! Or if you are feeling more creative—externally as a soothing anti-inflammatory muscle rub. The following recipe comes from Julie Bruton-Seal and Mathew Seals marvellous book, Hedgerow Medicine.[41]

Meadowsweet ghee

Ingredients
- one packet of butter
- five or six heads of meadowsweet flowers
- a clean jar

Method
Make the ghee: Take the butter, melt in a small saucepan and simmer for approx. 20 minutes. Skim off and discard the foam, and pour the clear, golden liquid into a clean saucepan, leaving any white residue behind.

Place the meadowsweet flowers into the ghee and gently heat for around 10 minutes. Strain and pour into jars to set.

Use this external rub for sciatica, muscle aches and pains, arthritis, painful joints and backache.

One of the questions we are often asked as herbalists is—how do you know what herbs can be combined together? One of the reasons that these five herbs have been chosen for this chapter is because each one of them can be combined with any of the others. Now the only thing to work out is what effect do you want to have and what is the person like who will be using this medicine?

And so—we have seen that you can make a medicinal bath or external application of a tea for chamomile, fennel, elderflower, lemon balm and now also for meadowsweet. You could drink meadowsweet tea with any one of the other herbs for achieving a greater or lesser effect in a particular area.

Summary

- Meadowsweet, along with many other fellow members of the rose family, contains therapeutic tannins that lend a healing, styptic, anti-inflammatory effect with very few potential adverse effects.
- Meadowsweet, like elderflower, can help control a fever without suppressing the healing response, and can ease aches and stiffness arising from 'stagnation' in the tissues.
- Meadowsweet has a particular affinity for the digestive mucosa especially the mouth, throat, stomach and small intestine, and also the urinary membranes of the bladder and urethra.

We hope that you have enjoyed meeting each of the plants discussed here, reading around a small selection of their huge histories and then making them into a kitchen pharmacy product. You should feel much more confident to use these five herbs in your home medicine chest—whether it is to treat a cold, to soothe sore or inflamed membranes or to aid sleep or relaxation.

You will have explored some central themes of Western herbal medicine and phytotherapy—including the management of fever and therefore the treatment of viral infections, the significance of the mucous membranes and the raft of herbal strategies that can be used to restore their function, and the significance of the nervous system to everything. Calming the excitation of nerves, reducing anxiety and depression, aiding healing sleep, allowing the digestive system to rest—all these things are important aspects of how a modern medical herbalist makes an assessment of a person's situation.

We look forward to revisiting with you, some of these principles and many others in further chapters and expanding your herbal knowledge and confidence.

References

1. Griggs, B., *New Green Pharmacy; The Story of Western Herbal Medicine*. 1997: Vermillion.
2. Barker, J., *The Medicinal Flora of Britain and Northwestern Europe*. 2001: Winter Press.
3. Grey-Wilson, D. C. and M. Blamey, *Cassell's Wild Flowers of Britain and Northern Europe*. 2003.
4. Heinrich, M. et al., *Fundamentals of Pharmacognosy and Phytotherapy*. 2012: Churchill Livingstone.
5. Edwards, S., E. and M. Inês da Costa Rocha Heinrich.
6. Miraj, S. and S. Alesaeidi, *A systematic review study of therapeutic effects of Matricaria recuitta chamomile (chamomile)*. Electron Physician, 2016. 8(9): pp. 3024–3031.
7. Amsterdam, J. D. et al., *Chamomile (Matricaria recutita) may provide antidepressant activity in anxious, depressed humans: an exploratory study*. Altern Ther Health Med, 2012. 18(5): pp. 44–49.
8. Revell, A., *A Kentish Herbal*. 1984, Maidstone: Kent County Council.
9. Treben, M., *Health Through God's Pharmacy: Advice and Experiences With Medicinal Herbs*. 1995: Ennsthaler.
10. Culpeper, N., *Culpeper's Complete Herbal*. 1995: Wordsworth Press.
11. Kourenoff, P. M. and G. St George, *Russian Folk Medicine*. 1976: Pan Books.
12. Wren, R. C., *Potters New Cyclopaedia of Botanical Drugs and Preparations*. 1956.
13. Ayres, P., *Wound Dressing in World War One—The Kindly Sphagnum Moss*. Field Biology, 2013. 110: pp. 27–33.
14. Petrovska, B. B. and S. Cekovska, *Extracts from the history and medical properties of garlic*. Pharmacogn Rev, 2010. 4(7): pp. 106–110.
15. Martindale, W., *Extra Pharmacopoeia*. 1972.
16. Priest, A., *Herbal Medication: A Clinical and Dispensary Handbook*. 1982: C W Daniel.
17. Pollington, S., *Leechcraft: Early English Charms, Plantlore and Healing*. 2008: Anglo-Saxon Press.
18. Mills, S., *The Principles and Practice of Modern Phytotherapy*, K. Bone, Editor., Churchill Livingstone.
19. Heidarifar, R. et al., *Effect of Dill (Anethum graveolens) on the severity of primary dysmenorrhea in compared with mefenamic acid: A randomized, double-blind trial*. J Res Med Sci, 2014. 19(4): pp. 326–330.
20. Mirmolaeea, S. T. et al., *Evaluating the effects of Dill (Anethum graveolens) seed on the duration of active phase and intensity of labour pain*. Journal of Herbal Medicine., 2014. 5 (1): pp. 26–29.

21. Namavar Jahromi, B., A. Tartifizadeh and S. Khabnadideh, *Comparison of fennel and mefenamic acid for the treatment of primary dysmenorrhea.* Int J Gynaecol Obstet, 2003. 80(2): pp. 153–157.

22. Modaress Nejad, V. and M. Asadipour, *Comparison of the effectiveness of fennel and mefenamic acid on pain intensity in dysmenorrhoea.* East Mediterr Health J, 2006. 12(3–4): pp. 423–427.

23. Mills, S., *Out Of The Earth: The Essential Book of Herbal Medicine.* 1991: Penguin Books.

24. Blochwich, M., *Anatomia Sambuci: The Anatomy of the Elder.* 1677 (original). Re-edited 2010: Berrypharma AG.

25. Schmitzer, V., A. Robert, S. Veberic and F. Stampar, *Elderberry (Sambucus nigra L.) Wine: a product rich in health promoting compounds.* J Agri Food Chem, 2010. 58: pp. 10143–10146.

26. Zakay-Rones, Z. et al., *Inhibition of several strains of influenza virus in vitro and reduction of symptoms by an elderberry extract (Sambucus nigra L.) during an outbreak of influenza B Panama.* J Altern Complement Med., 1995 Winter. 1(4): pp. 361–369.

27. Vlachojannis, J., M. Cameron and S. Chrubasik, *A systematic review on the sambuci fructus effect and efficacy profiles.* Phytotherapy Research., 2010. 24(1): pp. 1–8.

28. Barak, V. et al., *The effect of herbal medicines on the production of human inflammatory and anti-inflammatory cytokines.* Isr Med Assoc J., 2002. 4: pp. 919–921.

29. Harokopakis, E. et al., *Inhibition of proinflammatory activities of major periodontal pathogens by aqueous extracts from elder flower (Sambucus nigra).* Journal of Periodontology, 2006. 77(2): pp. 271–279.

30. Zakay-Rones, Z. et al., *Inhibition of several strains of influenza virus in vitro and reduction of symptoms by an elderberry extract (Sambucus nigra L.) during an outbreak of influenza B Panama.* J Altern Complement Med., 1995 Winter. 1(4): pp. 361–369.

31. Blamey, M. and C. Grey-Wilson, *Wild Flowers of Britain and Northern Europe.* 2003: Cassell.

32. Wake, G. et al., *CNS acetylcholine receptor activity in European medicinal plants traditionally used to improve failing memory.* J Ethnopharmacol, 2000. 69(2): pp. 105–114.

33. Fermino, B., N. Khalil et al., *Anxiolytic properties of Melissa officinalis and associated mechanisms of action: A review of the Literature.* African Journal of Pharmacy and Pharmacology, 2015. 9: pp. 53–59 doi: 10.5897/AJPP2014.4180.

34. Astani, A., M. H. Navid and P. Schnitzler, *Attachment and penetration of acyclovir-resistant herpes simplex virus are inhibited by Melissa officinalis extract.* Phytother Res, 2014. 28(10): pp. 1547–1552.

35. Mirghafourvand, M. et al., *The efficacy of Lemon Balm (Melissa officinalis L.) alone and combined with lemon balm (Nepeta mentoides) on premenstrual syndrome and quality of life among students: A randomized controlled trial.* Journal of Herbal Medicine, 2016. 6: pp. 142–148.

36. Blomhoff, S. et al., *Emotional responses' impact on intestinal reactivity.* Journal of Digestive Diseases and Sciences, 2000. 45: pp. 1153–1165.

37. Grieve, M., *A Modern Herbal.* Reprinted from 1931 edition. ed. 1988: Penguin Handbooks.

38. Peresun'ko, A. P. et al., *[Clinico-experimental study of using plant preparations from the flowers of Filipendula ulmaria (L.) Maxim for the treatment of precancerous changes and prevention of uterine cervical cancer].* Vopr Onkol, 1993. 39(7–12): pp. 291–295.

39. Allen, D. and G. Hatfield, *Medicinal Plants in Folk Tradition: An ethnobotany of Britain and Ireland.* 2004: Timber Press.

40. Pengelly, A., *The Constituents of Medicinal Plants: an introduction to the chemistry and therapeutics of herbal medicine.* 2nd ed. 2004: CABI Publishing.

41. Bruton-Seal, J. and M. Seal, *Hedgerow Medicine Harvest and Make Your Own Herbal Remedies* 2009: Merlin Unwin Books.

CHAPTER FIVE

Food, nutrition and wellness

Y*ou may wish to read this section on nutrition in conjunction with the section on the anatomy and physiology of the digestive tract, which you will find in Chapter 3.*

Introduction

As practitioners of herbal medicine we inevitably live in what often feels like a grey area between food and medicine. This is in part brought about by the obvious overlaps between what we are using as medicines and what many people use to bring colour, flavour and excitement to their food.

We herbalists also have an ingrained preference for the use of whole plants as opposed to a substance reduced and refined to its so-called active constituents. This means that our bodies will often recognise the medicines that we give them as much more akin to food, and processes them accordingly, with much less potential for problems to occur.

But let's take a step backwards for a moment, and ask a much more simple question: why do we eat?

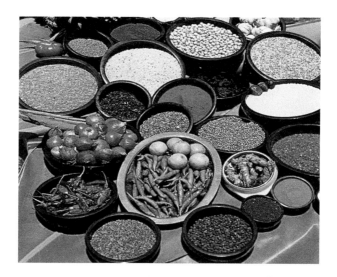

Although this list is by no means comprehensive we can see that there are many reasons beyond the practices that shape your decision to eat. How often do we eat because it's the right time (i.e., tea time) rather than because we are actually hungry? Eating at certain times out of expediency or habit is very familiar to us all, but can interfere with the body's own internal rhythms.

The reality for most of us, of course, is that food and meals tend to be made to fit around other (more important?) activities, or eaten at a time when it is most convenient for everyone in the family to be in one place together. Practicalities constantly assert themselves over ideal-world behaviour. Going back to our list for a moment, how many of these reasons are psychological in nature?

We mentioned the notorious *placebo effect* in Chapter 1. The power of the mind, and the meaning responses we have to our food do of course play a significant role also in how our bodies respond to the things that we eat.

Think of a lovely ice cream sundae, or perhaps a slice of your favourite cake. If you eat the treat with joy in your heart your hypothalamus will communicate this to the parasympathetic nervous system, which will, in turn, activate the secretion of all the lovely digestive juices necessary for you to get the best out of your sugary delicacy. You will

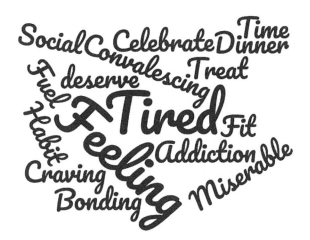

have an efficient breakdown of calories and optimise the intake of all available nutrients. All will be well. But maybe you are feeling guilty about the pudding. Maybe you are, in your own mind, committing a dietary sin, and judging yourself accordingly. Now those negative feelings may be transmitted down sympathetic nervous system pathways, rather than parasympathetic ones. Digestion will be inhibited rather than aided. The sugary treat may not be metabolised as effectively, and may stay in your gut for longer, causing you to feel a bit sick maybe, and altering the balance of your gut flora. Toxins may find their way into your system. In this emotionally stressful state, more cortisol is released into the system, which ultimately drives glucose levels up, which then drives insulin levels up. Insulin increases fat storage. Ergo: if you are eating because you are stressed, you will tend to put on weight. Our emotional state definitely affects how our bodies process our foods. The thoughts you think about the food you eat can indeed become a reality.

The act of eating is undertaken for a whole array of reasons. Further to that, *what* we are eating can be dictated by culture, mood, expediency, financial constraints, health and illness, religious beliefs, ethical and moral concerns and much more. Clearly there are many issues tied up in our food. We would like to take this opportunity to explore a few of them that may be familiar to you, and to look specifically at the area of food as medicine.

But first—let's have a nice cool soothing glass of water ...

Water

Water is Life's matter and matrix.
Mother and medium.
There is no life without water.

—Albert Szent-Györgyi

We would like to take a moment here to just talk about the health benefits of the water that we drink. Let's start with a few really simple water facts:

- There is the same amount of water on Earth as there was when the Earth was formed.
- The water from your tap could contain molecules that were once drunk by dinosaurs.
- Nearly 97% of the world's water is salty or otherwise undrinkable. Another 2% is locked in icecaps and glaciers. That leaves just 1% for all of humanity's needs—all its agricultural, residential, manufacturing, community and personal needs.

Consumption of good quantities of water every day has also been linked to weight loss over a period of time. One randomised trial showed how simply increased water consumption reduced weight in obese children, although most children in the study did not even manage the required 8 cups per day.[1] Never work with animals or children!

In the big picture, the concepts of flow, complexity and connectivity tend to recur when talking about biology and the natural world. Water embodies this both symbolically and in an actual way. Here are a few short excerpts taken from the excellent book *Energy Medicine East and West; A Natural History of Qi*, concerning muscle fascia.

> *Another perspective comes from considering the vital role of water in the body. Each collagen molecule has a helical shell of water molecules immediately associated with it ...*

The highly regular and nearly crystalline arrays of collagen molecules organise equally regular arrays of water molecules, which tend to have a particular orientation with respect to the collagen because of interactions between repeating charges on the collagen and the electrically polar water molecules …

I suspect that this "water system" in the body acts as an antenna, which is very sensitive to resonant interactions with chemicals or signals in the environment. This sensitivity arises because water forms a coherent phase-correlated system …

This property can explain the way vibrational frequencies from therapeutic devices, herbal remedies, essential oils and homoeopathic remedies can all interact so sensitively with the living system.

—James L. Oschman[2]

Water may thus take on the role of interacting directly with the foods and medicines that we ingest, and transmitting some of those energy signatures to our body's internal milieu.

Speaking of our bodies internal milieu, up to 60% of the human body is, in fact, water. We have a vast array of different mechanisms to make sure that our water output matches input and we do not go into water deficit. Maintaining the flow of lymph, blood, mucous, sweat etc. is vital for a healthy system, and it is not hard to see how stagnation can lead to all sorts of problems relating to a build-up of toxins and waste products etc. Keep the water flowing! Now let's have a look at some of the components that make up the other 40%.

Nutrient food groups—biomolecules and macronutrients

Let's start with the basics.

Food can be classified according to food groups. A food group consists of foods with similar nutritional properties. The major food groups in terms of the body's needs are the biomolecules: carbohydrates, proteins, fats, plus macronutrients such as vitamins and minerals. Micro and phytonutrients are yet other distinct groups to be found in vegetables and medicinal plants.

The five basic categories of nutrients (biomolecules and macronutrients) are needed by the body to provide energy, to provide the raw materials required for growth and repair of tissues, and to act as important co-factors in many biochemical processes in the body. One food item can contain a number of different biomolecules and macronutrients. For example, walnuts contain fat, protein, carbohydrates and the minerals manganese and copper. (They are also delicious!)

And, medicinally, from their *phytonutrients*, walnuts (*Juglans regia* L.) have been shown to contain at least six antimicrobial bioactive compounds including glansreginin A, azelaic acid, quercetin, and eriodictyol-7-*O*-glucoside,[3,4] ten antioxidant compounds[4] (especially the leaves), and the nuts contain up to 60% linoleic acid[5] as well as measurable antioxidant and antimicrobial effects.

> **Note:** The World Health Organization (WHO) state that 'Good nutrition—an adequate, well-balanced diet combined with regular physical activity—is a cornerstone of good health'.

But what exactly is a balanced diet? To achieve the optimal amount of the many different nutrients which the body needs to function, we need to eat a good cross-section of different food groups, in appropriate proportions.

Let's take a look at the first three food groups in a bit more detail.

Carbohydrates, lipids, proteins and nucleic acids

These large molecules are composed of basic building blocks called monomers.

Carbohydrate = monosaccharides
Lipids = fatty acids and glycerol
Proteins = amino acids
Nucleic acids = nucleotides

Carbohydrates

Carbohydrates are made up of carbon, hydrogen and oxygen. The smallest structural units of carbohydrates are called monosaccharides. These then join together to form other, larger carbohydrates.

$$
\begin{array}{c}
\mathrm{H} \diagdown \overset{1}{\mathrm{C}} \diagup \mathrm{O} \\
\mathrm{H} - \overset{2}{\mathrm{C}} - \mathrm{OH} \\
\mathrm{HO} - \overset{3}{\mathrm{C}} - \mathrm{H} \\
\mathrm{H} - \overset{4}{\mathrm{C}} - \mathrm{OH} \\
\mathrm{H} - \overset{5}{\mathrm{C}} - \mathrm{OH} \\
\overset{6}{\mathrm{CH_2OH}}
\end{array}
$$

Glucose

- *Monosaccharides* (*mono means one*) include glucose itself, also Fructose and Galactose.
- *Disaccharides* (*di means two*) when two or more of the monosaccharides are joined.
- *Oligosaccharides* (*oligo means 'few' or 'less than 10'*) when a few, or less than ten glucose, or fructose molecules are joined e.g., fructo-oligosaccharide.
- *Polysaccharides* (poly mean 'many' or 'more than 10') starches, or long chains of monosaccharides joined to form useful molecules like glycogen, cellulose and inulin.

Why we need glucose

- The primary use of glucose (a monosaccharide) is for energy. Red blood cells (erythrocytes) and nerve cells (neurons) rely entirely on glucose, which is crucial for their function, hence our body maintains blood glucose levels via homeostasis.
- As a 'fuel' for energy, glucose metabolism creates *heat* as a by-product, warming our body.
- Glucose is converted into glycogen by our body for energy storage.
- Glucose forms part of the structure of DNA and RNA.
- Glucose is required to make cell receptors on cell membranes (receptor sites). For example—oligosaccharides are responsible for our cell-to-cell recognition such as in the blood types A, B, O, AB: oligosaccharides form the structure of these four different receptor sites.

A small amount of carbohydrate absorption occurs in the mouth (via amylase contained in saliva), but most of it occurs once food we have swallowed has been through the stomach and enters the duodenum. It is now subject to enzyme breakdown in the small intestine. The pancreas secretes amy*lase* (enzyme) and the long polysaccharide chains of our carbohydrate meal are broken down to disaccharides.

Disaccharides can now be absorbed into the cells of the microvilli (villi and microvilli line the walls of the small intestine) and taken into the enterocytes. Here the *disaccharides* are subject to more enzymatic action from enzymes such as maltase, lactase, and villase so that the *monosaccharides* can be absorbed into the (portal) bloodstream.

Once glucose (and other monosaccharides) are in the bloodstream any of the following can occur:

a) glucose stays in the blood to be ready for use
b) glucose is converted into glycogen and stored
c) glucose is oxidised into energy as adenosine triphosphate (ATP)
d) excess glucose is converted into fat (triglycerides)
e) some glucose goes into the pentose phosphate pathway, making the
   building blocks of our DNA and RNA
f) liver uses glucose to regenerate glutathione. Glutathione is used by the
   body to mop up free radicals that result from metabolism (oxidisation).

Definition—*Glycogen*: Glycogen is a special structure of polysaccharides produced in the liver, which allows the body to store glucose. Conversion occurs in the cell cytosol (the fluid inside each cell that surrounds the cell organelles). Glycogen arranges the polysaccharides in a highly branched molecule allowing multiple 'free ends' to be exposed and available for breakdown back into glucose for energy use.

Note the beautiful spiralling flower-like arrangement of this structure! Glycogen breakdown is affected by/managed by:

Glucagon (a hormone) made by the *pancreas*, allows for an increase in blood glucose levels when needed.
Adrenaline (a hormone) made by the *adrenal medulla*, increases blood glucose levels because glucose will be needed in 'fight or flight' mode.
Thyroxine (a hormone) made by the *thyroid gland* controls metabolic rate and metabolism of glucose.

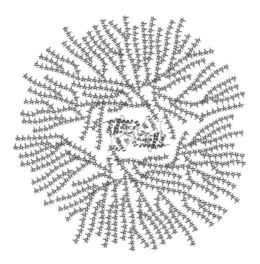

Glycogen molecule

Glucose and energy release (catabolism)

Glucose + Carbon dioxide (CO_2) + Water (H_2O) = Energy

Catabolism occurs inside cell organelles known as mitochondria, in little steps, releasing energy at each step.

One glucose molecule = 38 molecules of ATP (adenosine triphosphate)

NB: *When we exercise and breathe sufficient O_2 this is an aerobic process. If we exercise beyond the immediate supply of O_2 the process becomes anaerobic. Anaerobic exercise is less efficient and leads to waste product accumulation such as lactic acid (which causes cramp).*

Glucose catabolism results from the breakdown of glucose (glycolysis), a complex process involving the krebs cycle (aka the citric acid cycle or TCA cycle) resulting in ATP molecules being produced. Cyanide poisoning and carbon monoxide poisoning affect the flow of the electron transport chain in our mitochondria and results in blockage of ATP production and energy starvation.

Gluconeogenesis

This describes the ability within the body to make glucose from other sources. Certain amino acids can be converted into glucose. The glycerol from triglycerides can also be broken down into glucose.

Definition—*Cellulose (A polysaccharide)*: In living organisms, cellulose is used for structure (plant cell walls resulting in plant leaves, stems, branches) or storage. It is the most abundant organic compound on Earth. Plants also make other polysaccharides for energy storage—glycogen and starch. Plant cellulose is a major provider of essential dietary fibre and fructooligosaccharides. Oligosaccharides from many edible plants are known to have many beneficial effects including improved mineral absorption and other prebiotic effects.[6]

Definition—*Inulins*: Inulins are polysaccharides and oligosaccharides made by many plants in the Asteraceae family (Jerusalem artichoke, elecampane, chicory, dandelion) and Amaryllidaceae (onion) family. Inulin can be made commercially as a source of fructose and forms a sweet white crystalline powder. It is not absorbed in the small intestine and so, like cellulose, contributes to the microflora in the large intestine resulting in functional and nutritional benefits.[6]

Lipids

Lipids are all insoluble in water (hydrophobic). They include: triglyceride (a true fat), cholesterol, phospholipids and waxes.

Triglycerides (also known as fats).

- Are stored as adipose tissue
- Are composed of a glycerol and fatty acids (see in the picture below how one glycerol binds to three fatty acids)
- Can be manufactured in the body from carbohydrate (see how the structure of carbohydrate is similar to a triglyceride)

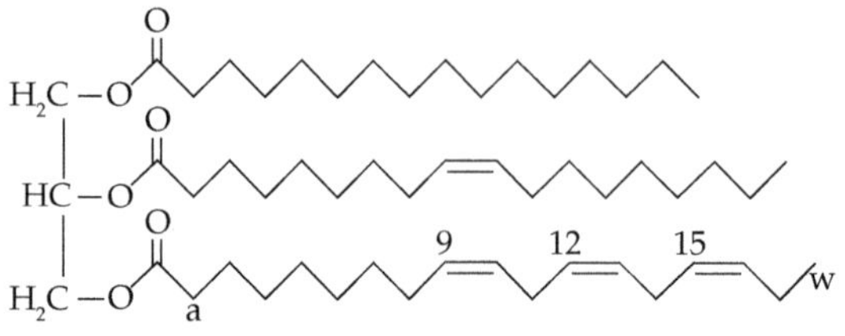

Triglyceride molecule

The structure of a triglyceride is three fatty acids attached to one glycerol. The long arms of the fatty acid chains have a backbone composed of carbon molecules. These carbon molecules possess four binding sites, where they can bind with other molecules. They use two of them to bind with the two carbon molecules either side of them. This leaves two free binding sites.

Saturated, unsaturated and polyunsaturated fats

In the past we have all seen advertisements and articles telling us how polyunsaturated fats are good for our health, and saturated fats are not (although opinions on this are now changing again). Well, this is what that is all about! The details of the structure of triglycerides have led to them being called saturated, unsaturated or polyunsaturated, and it is all to do with the carbon atoms that make up the fatty acid side chains of triglycerides.

With *saturated fats* all four arms of their carbon molecules are occupied (hydrogen often binds to spare binding sites). Because the binding sites of saturated fats are all used, this affects melting, and so saturated fats are often solid at room temperature.

With *unsaturated fats* some of the four arms of their carbon atoms are not occupied (unsaturated). They therefore form 'double bonds' with nearby carbons instead. Unsaturated fats are often liquid at room temperature. They are usually found from vegetable sources because plants make them as energy storage e.g., sunflower oil.

Mono-saturated and polyunsaturated! This depends on how many (one or more than one) carbon to carbon bonds there are ... C = C.

Polyunsaturated oils are more likely to spoil, or go off. This is because they are more 'reactive' due to these double carbon bonds that are able to interact with other atoms more easily. Trans-fatty acids are found in processed food as hydrogenated oils. Extra hydrogen atoms are introduced in the manufacture of hydrogenated oils, and these hydrogen atoms sit either side of the carbon atoms joined to each other—hence the word *trans*. This increases shelf life but is now considered to be associated with cardiovascular disease, and so hydrogenated fats are used less often in the food industry. Linoleic acid is derived from walnuts (among other foods) and is a polyunsaturated fat. Linoleic acid has an important role in inflammation within the body, and therefore with certain anti-inflammatory prostaglandins. Linoleic acid is an essential fatty acid, which means that our body cannot make it and it has to be found from our diet. Prostaglandins are made from polyunsaturated lipid compounds and can be pro-inflammatory or anti-inflammatory.

Why we need triglycerides:

- To provide us with energy (e.g., migratory birds use stored triglycerides).
- To provide us with protection such as fat pads around kidneys and adrenal glands.
- To provide us with insulation.
- To enable absorption of fat-soluble vitamins (e.g., vitamins A, D, E, K).

Sources of triglycerides: plant oils, meat, dairy, baked goods. Alcohol can be converted into triglycerides very easily.

Cholesterol

The structure of cholesterol looks very different from triglyceride. It is more of a ring structure with a tail of carbon and hydrogen atoms.

Cholesterol is similar in structure to steroid compounds and is involved in hormone production, cell membrane construction, bile production (essential for emulsification of dietary fats), myelin sheath construction and thus the optimal function of the nervous system. Compare the pictures of cholesterol and testosterone; see how similar they are.

Cholesterol structure   Testosterone structure

You can see how easy it might be for the body to make testosterone from cholesterol. Sources of cholesterol include full-fat dairy products. We also manufacture about 20% in our body.

Phospholipids

Phospholipids are vital for formation of the cell membrane. They possess a non-water repelling (hydrophilic) head with two water-repelling (hydrophobic) fatty acid tails.

If you look back at the picture of the structure of triglycerides, you can see how we can potentially make phospholipids from triglycerides due to their similar structure. Phospholipids also have a phosphate group on top. Phospholipids tend to group together with all of their hydrophilic heads facing outwards, and their hydrophobic fatty acid legs dangling inwards. This then naturally forms the basic structure of a cell membrane.

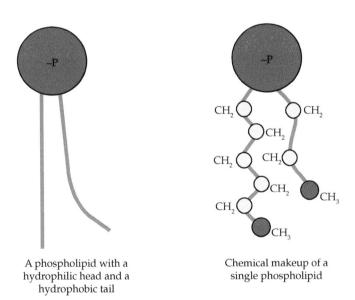

A phospholipid with a
hydrophilic head and a
hydrophobic tail

Chemical makeup of a
single phospholipid

All animals can make phospholipids. Phospholipids can be derived from egg yolk, soya bean and lecithin.

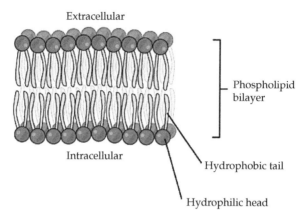

Phospholipid structure of a cell membrane.

Waxes

Waxes, like all lipids, are hydrophobic, but waxes also actively repel water. They are found on the surfaces of many plant structures such as leaves and the outside of fruits. Waxes can also be found in the outer coating of many animals to protect and repel water. Human ears have wax to protect the eardrum. Bees use plant waxes to make the comb for their honey storage.

Now we have seen how essential lipids are in the body, how do we get them into our body tissues?

Note: Our bodies absorb fat via a different route to carbohydrates or proteins. The pancreas secretes an enzyme called lipase. Triglycerides are broken down by lipase into monoglycerides and fatty acids. These form micelles, little balls of fatty acids, which are taken up by the brush border of the epithelium of the small intestine and enter via enterocytes. Cholesterol has in addition a carrier protein that encourages its uptake from the small intestine. Carbohydrate absorption from the gut enters the bloodstream, but lipid absorption from the gut (via enterocytes) enters mainly via the lymphatic system. This causes lymph in the digestive region to appear milky, due to the fat present.

Fats (triglycerides) are stored by our body as adipose tissue. There is also something called brown adipose tissue (BAT). BAT is found in hibernating bears and newborn babies. BAT generates heat and helps regulate body temperature (useful when hibernating!). This is also useful in the first few weeks of a baby's life. A newborn baby has a greater surface area of skin compared to body size, so is vulnerable to heat loss and poor temperature regulation. Heat generation is possible in adults via shivering but this is not yet possible in newborns as the muscles have not developed this capacity. Higher levels of BAT therefore help newborn babies stay warm.

Proteins

Proteins are comprised of varying combinations of 20 main amino acids. You may remember that lipids and carbohydrates are formed from carbon, oxygen and hydrogen atoms. Amino acids have an extra nitrogen molecule (and sometimes a sulphur molecule). We are made mainly of protein, and some of the amino acids (nine of them) required for our body's protein cannot be made (synthesised) by our body, and so they are essential to our diet.

An amino acid (glycine)

The picture above is of the structure of an amino acid called glycine. Note the nitrogen molecule left of centre. Glycine has the simplest structure of the 20 amino acids. It is found extensively in collagen where it is involved in the formation of the helical structure of that substance. We break down proteins from the food we eat, mainly in the stomach itself. Because we are comprised mainly of proteins, we make and secrete proteolytic (protein digesting) enzymes initially in an inactive form. This avoids undesirable (!) auto-digestion (autolysis). We certainly don't want to start to break down our own proteins! Once the enzyme is safely secreted into the stomach however, our own proteins are protected by a nice layer of mucous. One of these enzyme precursors, pepsinogen is made by chief cells lining our stomach, and other cells (parietal cells) produce hydrochloric acid (HCL). Hydrogen ions from the HCL act on the pepsinogen to form the active proteolytic (protein digesting) enzyme pepsin.

Ingested proteins (long chains of amino acids) are broken down in this way into either individual amino acids or into peptides (two or more short-chain amino acids).

Now it is the turn of the pancreas! Inactive precursors of proteolytic enzymes—trypsinogen and chymotrypsinogen, are secreted by the pancreas in response to the acidic chyme released into the duodenum. Meanwhilst the enterocytes within microvilli lining the small intestine secrete enterokinase which activates the proteolytic enzymes, and proteins are further broken down into amino acids. Amino acids can be absorbed across the gut wall passively by diffusion, and also with the expenditure of energy, in an active transport mechanism. They are absorbed into the capillaries of the microvilli into the portal circulation, where they are transported to the liver.

Why we need protein; the role of the liver in protein metabolism:

- Amino acids can be de-aminated in the liver by removal of the nitrogen (N) atom. The nitrogen forms urea, which is excreted by the kidney.
- Gluconeogenesis can take place from amino acids that have lost their N, and thus make new glucose for energy, or be converted and stored as fat (triglyceride).
- The nitrogen might be removed from some amino acids to be used in the making of other amino acids.
- Amino acids can be used to make transport proteins (i.e., albumin) to transport useful things around the body. Albumins are made in the liver, and used to transport hormones and some drugs for example, and are also used in the production of clotting factors.
- Some hormones are made from amino acids (e.g., insulin). You will remember that some hormones are also made from cholesterol.
- Antibodies are made from amino acids and are a vital part of our immune system.
- Amino acids can be used as an energy source—although this is as a last resort after glucose, and then triglyceride (fat).
- Amino acids are vital for the growth and repair of all body cells. Much of this repair takes place while we are asleep—a possible

reason for children and teens (who are growing and making lots of extra hormones) to need extra sleep!

As you can see, the main molecule of our body is protein. There is a constant synthesis and breakdown of protein, and amino acids are not especially 'stored'. There is a small 'pool' in the bloodstream, and a surplus is converted to glucose to be used as fuel, or converted to triglyceride to be stored as fat. So we need to eat and replace our protein on a regular basis. Traditionally protein was thought to come mainly from eating meat. However, it is found in dairy products, eggs and a variety of vegetable sources. Eating excess animal proteins (eating meat) is now recognised as a major associated factor in the development of many cancers, and this is particularly notable with consumption of processed or mechanised meat. Vegetable sources of proteins can be combined to access all required amino acids including the essential amino acids. For example combining whole grains and pulses is an especially successful method and forms the basis of traditional diets across the globe. All nine essential amino acids are found in quinoa, buckwheat, hemp seeds, chia seeds and spirulina (an edible algae).

Note: The nitrogen removed from the amino acid monomers in the process of de-amination forms ammonia. Ammonia is one of the most toxic substances produced by the body, and excess can lead to brain damage and death. The body therefore very efficiently removes nitrogen in the form of urea and excretes this via the kidneys.

And finally—nucleic acid

Our final biochemical, and the one responsible for encoding our genetic information, nucleic acid, is constructed from long chains of nucleotides. Nucleotides are organic molecules forming the nucleic acid polymers deoxyribonucleic acid (DNA) and ribonucleic acid (RNA), both of which are essential biomolecules within all life-forms on Earth.

- Nucleic acid is synthesised in living organisms from nucleotides.
- Nucleotides are structurally comprised of phosphate, glucose, and nitrogen.

- Nucleic acids hold our genetic information and direct the process of protein synthesis from amino acids.

> **Note:** Remember—DNA cannot function unless it is given instructions from the environment in which it exists. It also depends upon that environment for its existence. It does not act in isolation. We can change our internal environment. Thus we can modulate how our DNA functions.

Vitamins

What do you think about when you think of vitamins? We have become very used to the concept of vitamin supplementation, and many manufacturers of these products use bright colours in their advertising to try and emphasise the natural nature of the potential health benefits to be had from them. But what exactly are vitamins?

As a result of a series of animal feeding experiments at the turn of the last century, the British scientist Frederick Hopkins postulated the existence in normal diets of tiny quantities of unidentified substances that are essential for animal growth and survival. These hypothetical substances he called accessory food factors.

We get the word vitamin from the words *vital* and *amine*, and the term was first used by a Polish biochemist. In 1912 Casimir Funk discovered a complex of micronutrients, which had been previously discovered by a Japanese scientist Umitaro Suzuki in 1910. Funk called this complex a vitamin, meaning vital amine, and it was subsequently renamed vitamin B3 (niacin). (An amine is an organic compound derived from ammonia.)

It was Funk who suggested that illnesses such as rickets, pellagra, coeliac disease and scurvy could be cured by vitamins. This name soon became synonymous with Hopkins' accessory food factors, and by the time it was shown that not all vitamins are amines, the word was already in popular usage. Vitamins are compounds that the body needs in very small amounts to carry out vital processes. Because the body cannot synthesise them itself they are vital to the diet, although many are only required in very small quantities. There are many sources of information out there regarding what vitamins are needed for what actions in the body.

Recommended dietary allowance (RDA)

The intake amount of a vitamin that meets the needs of half (50%) of the population is used to set the recommended daily allowance or RDA for vitamins and minerals. Once the amount needed by 50% of the population (Estimated Average Requirement or EAR) has been established, the RDA is then calculated as a figure two standard deviations above EAR.

> **Definition—*Standard Deviation*:** Standard deviation is a statistical calculation used to express the amount of variation present in a set of variables.

Most countries have a set of RDA's that are recommended for public health and nutrition. These are updated from time to time as new research on nutrition becomes available, but they will always be a rule of thumb rather than an absolute, as they suggest minimal nutritional requirements rather than optimal ones, and individual needs should always be considered. Even seasonal variations occur which are not accounted for by RDA's. Vitamin D from UV light is in much scarcer supply in December than it is in August for those of us in the Northern Hemisphere.

Also, the presence of a number of vitamins and minerals together in a food is rarely taken into consideration. For example: Vitamin D works synergistically to aid calcium absorption; Vitamin C aids the absorption of iron. Therefore vitamins and minerals present in whole foods can act synergistically together to increase overall nutrient levels. Looking at these substances in isolation does not give us the whole picture. There is potential for over-emphasis on specific quantities of specific vitamins. The dynamic interplay of nutrients both between each other and within the complex system that is the human body, and microbiome, is often overlooked.

You may have heard of vitamin C referred to as ascorbic acid. This refers to the use of vitamin C in the treatment of a disease called scurvy. The letter A in the word ascorbic signifies *no* or *without* (i.e., asexual means without any sexual leanings), and scorbutus was the old Latin name for scurvy. Here is a picture of the chemical known as vitamin C.

Vitamin C molecule

Looking at this image, it is easy to imagine this molecule as a substance in its own right, isolated from complex interactions with other substances around it. The biochemical reality is of course very different. The actions of this molecule are dependent upon all sorts of different variables within the biological terrain in which it may find itself. Activity can only occur when all the relevant dancing partners are present, the co-factors, the enzymes, the co-enzymes, various trace metals etc. The isolated 'vitamin' in a refined supplement is a very different thing from the complex of vitamins, and trace elements found in good quality whole foods. We shall return to vitamin C throughout this chapter as an example of the complex synergy of plants as food and medicine.

Vitamin C — a short history

Scottish physician James Lind has gone down in the history of the biological sciences as being the first person to have conducted a clinical trial.

During his years as a naval surgeon, he observed that citrus fruits and lemon juice seemed to cure and indeed prevent scurvy among sailors. He wrote a treatise recommending their mandatory consumption by British sailors. By 1795, lime juice was being issued to all naval vessels, resulting in the gradual elimination of scurvy within the entire British fleet. At the time, no one, including Lind himself, knew of the existence of ascorbic acid/vitamin C.

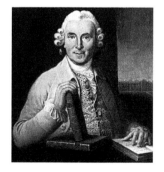

James Lind

In the 1930s Albert Szent-Györgyi discovered the chemical ascorbic acid, which enables the body to efficiently use carbohydrates, fats, and protein. His discovery was among the foundations of modern nutrition.

He enrolled at the University of Budapest, but his studies were interrupted by the outbreak of World War I. Fervently anti-war throughout his life, Szent-Györgyi deliberately wounded himself to escape combat and returned to the university to finish his studies in 1917. He was reputed to have said that he was:

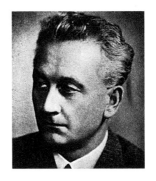

Albert Szent-Györgyi

> *Overcome with such a mad desire to return to science that one day I grabbed my revolver and in my despair put a shot through my upper arm.*
> —Albert Szent Gyorgyi

His research presented unexpected difficulties in terms of trying to purify ascorbic acid. One night, Szent-Györgyi recalled, his wife served him fresh red paprika for supper. As he wrote in his autobiography, 'I did not feel like eating it so I thought of a way out. Suddenly it occurred to me that this is the one plant I had never tested. I took it to the laboratory. By about midnight I knew that it was a treasure chest full of vitamin C'.

Linus Pauling is our last character in terms of the history of vitamin C.

He was the only person ever to be awarded two Nobel prizes in his own right (Chemistry and Peace). He was also one of only two people to have been awarded Nobel prizes in two different fields (the other being Marie Curie). You will all be familiar with one of Linus Pauling's theories—large doses of vitamin C will help cure the common cold. This is why people automatically reach for vitamin C supplements when they get a head cold. For

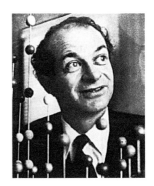

Linus Pauling

much of his working life his research centred around the nature of the chemical bond, and he is generally viewed as one of the founders of modern quantum chemistry.

Dr Pauling's grasp of the nature of chemical bonds and molecular structure was so formidable that Albert Einstein commented that he would have to 'brush up on the subject' of chemical bonds before again trying to engage the young Dr Pauling in a conversation. He was a life-long pacifist and campaigner against nuclear weapons, and in his later life became interested in the role of vitamins in healthcare, ultimately attracting a lot of criticism from orthodox medicine circles for his recommendations of the use of high levels of vitamin C in the treatment of cancer.

Note: Rosehips. It is hard to escape the image of oranges when talking about vitamin C isn't it! However, did you know that, pound for pound, rosehips contain more vitamin C than oranges? This is what made them such a valuable commodity during World War II, when school children were sent out to pick rosehips and sell them to local pharmacies for the production of rose hip syrup. This also of course makes rose hips a very valuable addition to any cold and flu medicine.

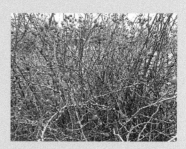

Even better is the fact that the hips of the most common native wild rose, *Rosa canina* L. or dog rose, has been shown to contain the highest quantities of vitamin C.[7] In nature, this vitamin C is found as part of an array of bioflavonoids, not ascorbic acid in isolation. Bioflavonoids have bioactive benefits far beyond the effects of vitamin C alone.

Once again we would like to make the point that organic compounds do not work in isolation, and there are an array of phyto(micro) nutrients adding to health benefits. For example—in one recent study, in comparison with a control drink, 6 weeks of daily consumption of rose hip resulted in a significant reduction of systolic blood pressure, and an improvement in cholesterol ratios.[8]

We have focussed specifically on vitamin C here to explore the fact that there is much more to vitamins than just a cause and effect supplement. This is true of all the vitamins we know about.

Minerals

Minerals have a very similar story. There are a number of minerals and elements which comprise the overall structure of the body (such as carbon, hydrogen, iron, calcium etc.) and many more that the body needs in trace amounts for a wide range of physiological functions. There is plenty of information already published concerning the many minerals that our bodies require for maintenance and good health. The following table is therefore meant as a simple, (and not comprehensive) guide to some of the more familiar ones. This is just to give you an idea as to how the body uses some of these compounds.

Minerals: Brief Notes

Mineral	What does it do?	Where can we get it from?
Calcium	• Necessary for blood clotting • Necessary for muscle contraction • Necessary for nerve conduction • Important component of bones and teeth	Green vegetables Some fish (ie sardines) Eggs Dairy
Iodine	• Necessary for formation of thyroid hormones	Sea-foods Seaweeds Vegetables grown in iodine rich soil Natural sea salt
Iron	• Formation of haemoglobin in red blood cells • Carbohydrate metabolism • Synthesis of some hormones • Synthesis of some neurotransmitters	Pulses Nuts Eggs Red meat Wholemeal bread Green leafy veg
Magnesium	• Structure of bones and teeth • Cofactor for many enzymes • Influences membrane permeability	Green vegetables Avocados Bananas Nuts Broccoli Green beans

(Continued)

Minerals: Brief Notes (continued)

Mineral	What does it do?	Where can we get it from?
Phosphate	• Essential part of DNA and RNA • Component of phospholipids (cell membranes) • Component of ATP (Energy storage in body)	Dairy products Red meat Fish Poultry Bread Rice
Potassium	• Intracellular cation (positively charged ion) • Necessary for muscle contraction • Necessary for nerve transmission	Very common in fruits and vegetables
Sodium	• Extracellular cation (see potassium) • Necessary for muscle contraction • Necessary for nerve transmission	Fish Meat Eggs Milk (Salt) High in processed foods
Zinc	• Immune system health • Cell division and growth • Wound healing • Carbohydrate catabolism • The senses of smell and taste • Structure of receptor proteins on cells	Oysters Red meat Chicken Crab Dairy Can be found in most foods
Manganese	• Connective tissue formation • Production of sex hormones • Production of blood clotting factor	Nuts Brown rice Dark chocolate Beans and legumes Leafy green veg Oatmeal
Chromium	• Metabolism of fats, (also proteins and carbohydrates) • Glucose metabolism	Broccoli Potatos Garlic Basil Wholemeal bread

(Continued)

Minerals: Brief Notes (continued)

Mineral	What does it do?	Where can we get it from?
Selenium	• Anti-oxidant actions • Thyroid hormone metabolism • Healthy hair and skin	Whole grains Dairy Fish Eggs
Copper	• Helps form haemoglobin—red blood cells production • Helps in absorption of iron from gut • Immune system health • Connective tissue maintenance	Nuts Shitake mushrooms Liver Oysters Dark chocolate

The bottom line is, assuming that your digestive tract is functioning well and you are eating a good cross-section of whole foods, there is no reason why you should not be getting the vitamins and minerals you need to function on a day-to-day basis. It has been debated whether eating frozen or organic food helps or not. Because of our interconnectedness with our microbiome, it is likely that organic agriculture enhances the plants' microbiome and therefore ours. So simply counting vitamin and mineral content does not allow for this possible benefit.

Ill health may change our capacity to absorb and utilise our macronutrients, so that anxiety for example might result in us using more nutrients whilst also affecting our digestion enough to hinder nutrient assimilation. Working with individual cases there may be a lot that can be done through dietary changes to support specific situations, through enhancement of living, dynamic, digestible foodstuffs, *alongside* herbal therapy that can help reduce the negative effects of say—anxiety.

Finally, and rather romantically, let us take heart from the fact that we really are stardust. All elements, except helium and hydrogen are created at the centre of stars.

Inflammation and diet

Just to recap: there are two types of inflammation—acute and chronic.

Acute inflammation is a normal healing response, vital for life, e.g., a wound/insect bite/burn (also oxidised foods, environmental toxins) results in inflammation essential for preventing infection/toxicity and mopping up and healing damaged tissue.

Traditionally the five cardinal signs of an inflammatory response are—redness, heat, swelling, pain and loss of function. Acute inflammation may be caused by injury or by a pathogen (virus, bacteria etc). Injured or infected cells respond chemically to the problem, releasing histamines, kinins and prostaglandins. This initially causes localised tissue damage, keeping any potential poison or foreign body from invading the body any further. The powerful chemicals released by damaged cells attract other cells to help (chemotaxis), and this, in turn, causes vasodilation, swelling and oedema which can lead to pain, but also helps inhibit pathogens and aids white blood cells in their work. Finally vascular permeability is increased (the blood vessel walls become more porous) releasing clotting factors from the blood vessels and allowing large white blood cells to move out from the bloodstream into the affected tissues. In injuries, the response to tissue damage may cause localised leakage of red blood cells from blood vessels, leading to bruising, and blockage to venous and lymphatic channels causing initial acute swelling.

Chronic inflammation involves a slightly different pattern of events, and different cellular chemotaxis occurs involving macrophages and B and T lymphocytes. Macrophages can form giant cells (granulomatous inflammation) e.g., tuberculosis, and Crohn's disease. T and B Lymphocytes activate cytokines and interleukins that can result in immune-led apoptosis (cell death). All chronic disease is a result of the stresses of chronic inflammation. Examples include cancer, cardiovascular disease, diabetes, Alzheimer's disease, arthritis, auto-immune disorders, neurological diseases.

Prostaglandins are biochemicals and key compounds in the inflammatory response. Pro-inflammatory prostaglandins promote inflammation—very useful if you are wounded or infected by a pathogen. Anti-inflammatory prostaglandins are essential in reducing inflammation once the pathogen/injury is dealt with. The optimum ratio for dietary omega 6 and omega 3 oils necessary for prostaglandin production in the body is 4:1, but modern Western diet is thought to be about 220:3—in other words, extremely out of balance in favour of inflammatory prostaglandins.

What role does diet play?

1) The balance of omega 3 to omega 6 fatty acids affects prostaglandin formation.
2) There is a broad spectrum of anti-inflammatory effects from plant-based foods containing polyphenols and flavonoids.

3) There are anti-inflammatory effects of aromatic compounds in herbs (as well as direct antiviral, antibacterial, and antiseptic effects).

4) There are indirect effects of a plant-based diet on the microbiome; growing research data links the diversity of the microbiome from a plant-based diet (especially via flavonoids in the gut) with reduction of inflammation.

5) Pro-inflammatory Insulin-like growth factor (IGF-1) is produced by our liver, but also found in all dairy products. It is possible that consuming large quantities of dairy may lead to elevated IGF-1 which is pro-inflammatory.

6) Any food that results in inflammation for that individual can potentially lead to an immune response and inflammation, e.g., coeliac disease, lactose intolerance.

Omega 3 F.A.'s from fish, Algae (spirulina/chlorella), some nuts, linseed, all generally encourage anti-inflammatory prostaglandins. Omega 6 F.A.'s are found in non-mechanised meat, and some cold-pressed vegetable oils (corn, sunflower, safflower, peanut). They promote both anti-inflammatory and pro-inflammatory prostaglandins, e.g., arachidonic acid—high in meat, is helpful for cell membrane phospholipids, but can promote pro-inflammatory cytokines. Things are rarely black and white, and usually a lot more complex than we bargain for.

We looked at the process of inflammation in Chapter 3 when we explored the immune system. Many people are of the opinion that chronic inflammation in the system is the underlying reason for a wide range of chronic disease states experienced by people, and that treating inflammation directly and vigorously will significantly improve treatment outcomes. Whether or not inflammation is responsible for disease states, or a sequelae to them, there is no doubt that chronic inflammation is a definite feature of many health issues such as arthritis and fibromyalgia, but also including less obvious conditions such as atherosclerosis and cancer.

Foods with 'bad press'

Salt

In ancient Rome, you were worth your salt if you were competent and good at your job. Historically salt was a valuable commodity, in short supply in some parts of the world. At one point there was a belief that Roman soldiers were actually paid in salt.

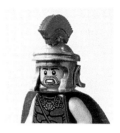

Although this is now disputed, it is true that we get our modern-day word 'salary' from the Latin 'salarium' which referred to a Roman soldier's allowance to buy salt. So, what is salt?

Starting from the good old pedant's viewpoint of the world, in chemistry a salt is an ionic compound, comprised of two groups of oppositely charged ions; a positively charged *cation* and a negatively charged *anion*. The positive ions usually come from a metal and the negatively charged ions usually come from a non-metal. We are used to talking about sodium chloride ($NaCl$), the stuff we might sprinkle over our chips with vinegar, but there are many other different types of chemical salts, such as aluminium oxide or magnesium iodide. Salt is just one of those words that we use rather casually to mean something very specific.

Now that's all cleared up, let's continue with our slightly inaccurate use of the word 'salt'.

In the body:

- Sodium represents the dominant (positive) cation in extracellular fluid and is also crucial for the maintenance of plasma volume.
- The chloride (negative) anions absorbed in sodium chloride are also used by the body to make essential hydrochloric acid (HCL) by the parietal cells of the stomach.
- Our body has an optimal internal pH, between 7.35 and 7.45, i.e., slightly on the alkaline side of neutral. Apart from their vital roles in the formation of bones and cartilage, healthy nerve function, as co-factors in enzymatic reactions and much more, minerals help to keep our internal pH on the alkaline side, which is exactly what we need.

But is that all there is to salt found on our table and in our food? Of course not! Table salt undergoes a refining process. Chemicals are usually added to remove all minerals, except sodium chloride and ultimately a number of different substances are added to the sodium chloride such as anti-caking agents. Thus much of the good stuff is removed and some 'less than good stuff' albeit in small quantities, is added. *Anti-caking agents include sodium ferro-cyanide, ammonium citrate and aluminium silicate.* This refined salt may then be processed via a very harsh method involving extremes of heat and pressure, thought by some to potentially damage the molecular structure of the salt.

Unrefined sea salts are usually processed via much gentler, slower methods, leaving the sodium chloride, but also approximately 16% of the naturally occurring minerals including: silicon, magnesium, iron, zinc and calcium, and around 60 other trace minerals.

Note: It is the action of fungal mycorrhiza in the plant's microbiome that convert minerals from rock and decomposing organic matter, into ionic mineral salts. Only in this form can they be absorbed and used by plants including sea vegetables (and then by us!).

Why is salt refined?

The refining process prolongs shelf life, and makes the product look more attractive. Looked at like this, it doesn't seem very logical does it? Confusion about the word and meaning of salt obfuscates the links between many causes of the chronic healthcare issues affecting the Western world and the overuse of refined salt.

So let's look at a few things that we can do to avoid falling into this trap:

* Replace refined salt with unrefined sea salt or mineral salt.
* Introduce seaweed and unrefined sea salt into your diet.
* Generally use more herbs and spices to flavour your food, rather than just depending on salt.

Unsurprisingly seaweed is a highly alkaline food, and we will look at its use as a lovely adjunct to our diet shortly.

Sugar

Much like the salt issue, the word sugar is actually a general term referring to sweet, soluble carbohydrates. The table sugar that we all know and love is actually sucrose, which is a disaccharide composed of glucose and fructose.

Amazingly enough, sugar produced from sugar cane was originally used in ancient Greece for medicinal purposes only.

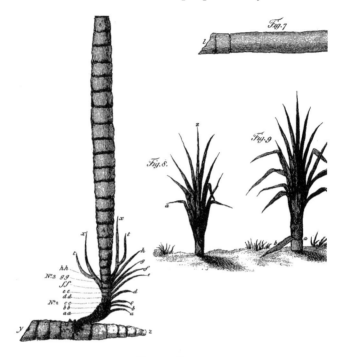

Sugar Beet

Sugar is made in Arabia as well, but Indian sugar is better. It is a kind of honey found in cane, white as gum, and it crunches between the teeth. It comes in lumps the size of a hazelnut. Sugar is used only for medical purposes.
—Pliny the Elder, *Natural History*

Honey remained the main form of sweetener in use in Europe until the 18th century. Subsequent to this demand for sugar became so great that it was, in part, responsible for the colonisation of many tropical Islands where sugar cane could be grown, and the associated rise in slavery.

Molasses is a by-product of the refining process of sugar cane. You may have heard of blackstrap molasses. This is produced by a third boiling of the sugarcane juice, and produces a thick, dark syrup which is high in vitamin B6, as well as minerals such as calcium, iron and magnesium.

A few sugary facts:

- Refined sugar undergoes 32 processes, unrefined only 6 processes.
- If you buy refined brown sugar you often get white sugar dyed brown—it has merely been mixed with cane molasses.

Natural and refined sugars

Confusion has developed over the years concerning the difference between the refined sugars that we instantly associate with the word sugar, and the natural sugars and carbohydrates found in foods. In particular, because the overconsumption of sugar as sucrose has become such a huge problem, all forms of carbohydrates are now viewed as bad by many people. This is especially the case when considering such issues as suitable diets for diabetics or patients with glucose intolerance. Carbohydrates of course, can be more or less refined.

As we have seen in our introduction to biomolecules, foods containing natural sugars (carbohydrates) play a role in providing essential nutrients for daily health. Don't forget that our red blood cells and our brain both rely on glucose as their only source of energy, so some sugars in the system are actually crucial to health.

Food manufacturers often add chemically produced sugar, typically high-fructose corn syrup, to foods and beverages, including crackers, flavoured yoghurt, tomato sauce and salad dressing. Low-fat foods are often the worst offenders, as manufacturers use refined sugar to add flavour and texture. This can be confusing to the consumer.

As can be demonstrated with salt, sugar and carbohydrates in general, if they are processed foods, they add calories and sugar with little nutritional value. By contrast, using plant-based, unrefined ingredients provides biomolecules, macro and micronutrients and fibre helping slow down sugar release. Longer lasting, slower impact glucose consumption, is less stressful for the body and keeps us feeling fuller for longer.

Metabolism matters

How the body metabolises the sugar in fruits or milk differs from how it metabolises the refined sugar added to processed foods. The body breaks down refined sugar rapidly, causing blood sugar levels to spike, and necessitating a rapid and strong response from the pancreas to produce insulin and normalise the situation.

Because refined sugar is digested quickly, you don't feel full after you're done eating, no matter how many calories you consume. Refined sugars are calorie-dense with virtually no accompanying nutrients. This leads to obesity in the first instance as the body converts the excess glucose first to glycogen, then to fat.

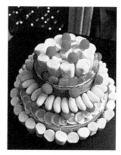

Then there is the whole sugar addiction thing. When we eat sugar an area of the brain called the nucleus accumbens becomes flooded with the neurotransmitter dopamine. This has been described as a reward circuit. This pleasurable reaction in our brains when we eat sugar has been linked with addictive behaviour and explains why some people find it incredibly difficult to kick the refined sugar habit.

The fibre in fruit, nuts and seeds, herbs and vegetables slow down metabolism. Fibre expands to make you feel full, but also has an essential role in maintaining the microbiome and therefore indirectly helping blood glucose control. Blood sugar levels rise more slowly when sourced from a plant-based diet, and do not spike as refined sugars do. The pancreas can respond over time rather than as an acute situation.

Bread — (The staff of life?)

Bread has been with us for a long time. Wheat, the cereal we primarily use in bread production today, is the result of cross-pollination of three different species of grass, which is thought to have occurred in Turkey around 10,000 BC. The earliest evidence for bread (made from cereals and plant tubers) has recently been found at a Black Desert site in Jordan, and dated to 14,000 years ago.[9] And yet, how many people can you think of who have problems eating bread? How often do people say they feel bloated or lethargic after the lunchtime sandwich? Is this a wheat problem, a bread problem, or something else? The organisation *Coeliac UK* list three defined conditions involving wheat-related intolerances:

1) *Coeliac disease*: A well-defined auto-immune disease involving the production of auto-antibodies, damage to the gut lining and reduced ability to absorb nutrients.

2) *Wheat allergy*: A more generalised reaction to wheat, triggered by the immune system and occurring within seconds or minutes of ingesting wheat. Symptoms tend to be more 'allergy-like' in general and may include rash, runny nose and asthma. Wheat allergy is thought to be rare.

3) *Non-coeliac gluten sensitivity*: Symptoms are similar to coeliac disease but no auto-antibodies are detected and there is no damage to the gut wall. Symptoms can include, diarrhoea, constipation, headaches, bloating and fatigue.

So what's going on?

Bread making using traditional methods can be time-consuming, as several cycles of kneading and resting are required in order for a yeast-based loaf to produce the desired flavour and texture.

As a result, bread making in the 20th century has undergone some radical changes, which may go some way to explaining our current issues.

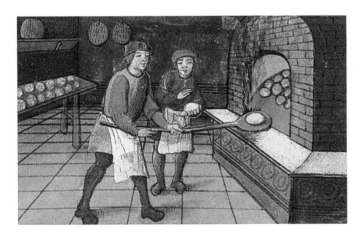

The Chorleywood method was developed in 1961 by the British Baking Industries research department and by 2009 it was used to produce over 80% of the UK's bread. As well as using a new, fast-action yeast, the method involves high energy mixing, which allows for the use of inferior grain. Both significantly reduce the fermentation time, and thus the time taken to produce a loaf. Taste and nutritional value have both been the victims of this process. This system is able to produce a loaf of bread from flour to sliced and packaged in about 3 and a half hours.

A third factor is the growing list of chemical additives used which both speed up mixing time and further reduce fermentation time. Dough not requiring fermentation because of chemical additives is called 'quick bread' by commercial bakers. Chemicals are often added to the dough in the form of a prepackaged base, which also contains most or all of the dough's non-flour ingredients. The impact of these chemical additives and their potential allergenic properties is an area of growing concern. Factory-made bread may also have extra gluten added.

One of the most informative books on how bread making on a large scale has evolved in the UK, and how it has impacted on the health of the nation is *Bread Matters*, by Andrew Whitley. He devotes over five pages to the subject of additives in bread and how they may be detrimental to health. To take a quote from his book, concerning the Chorleywood method:

> ... *you can't miss it. From the clammy sides of your chilled wedge sandwich to the flabby roll astride every franchised burger, the stuff is there, with a soft, squishy texture that lasts for many days until the preservatives can hold back the mould no longer. If bread forms a ball that sticks to the roof of your mouth as you chew, thank the Chorleywood Bread Process— but don't dwell on what it will shortly be doing to your guts.*
>
> —Andrew Whitley[10]

As a result of this the UK is now notorious for producing cheap, poor quality bread.

> *How can a nation be called great if its bread tastes like kleenex?*
> —Julia Child. (American cookery teacher and author)

It may be stretching a point to claim that the Chorleywood method is responsible for all of our bread-related woes. As with so many things in life, it's probably just another bit of the jigsaw. Finally, a quick note about sourdough bread.

This has become very popular in recent years, possibly as a part of the artisan bread making kick-back against industrially manufactured poor quality bread, but also, on a more positive note, due to perceived health benefits relating to gut flora. It is of course, the original method of developing yeast in flour to make bread. The yeasts

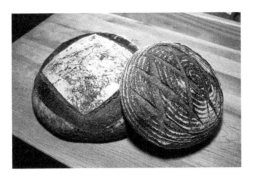

naturally present on the grain that made the flour, allow for fermentation into bread.

It seems that sourdough bread brings benefits in terms of iron absorption, compared to other methods of bread making. When sourdough, conventional yeast and Chorleywood methods were compared, the following findings were reported:

> *The iron released in solution after a simulated digestion was 8-fold higher in sourdough bread than with others but no difference in cellular iron uptake was observed. Additionally, when iron was added to the different breads digestions only sourdough bread elicited a significant ferritin response in Caco-2 cells (4.8-fold compared to the other breads) suggesting that sourdough bread could contribute towards improved iron nutrition.*
>
> —Rodriguez-Ramiro et al.[11]

Important nutrients such as iron, zinc and magnesium, antioxidants, folic acid and other B vitamins become easier for our body to absorb as a result of the long slow fermentation that produces sourdough bread. Gluten is also broken down more thoroughly and therefore becomes less of a problem. There is also a lower surge in blood sugar levels as a result of eating sourdough bread—good news for diabetics!

Gut biota and the microbiome

> *Slain, after all man's devices had failed, by the humblest things that God, in his wisdom, has put upon this earth.*
>
> —H. G. Wells

Trillions of microorganisms live in our digestive tract.

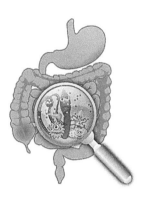

Efforts to identify and name them have as yet been overwhelmed with the complexity of the task. In recent years, scientific interest has been directed at this incredible dynamic ecosystem and what its role is in our health. Estimates suggest the microbiome forms 2 or more kg of our body weight, and it is now considered an organ system in its own right. It is difficult to imagine, but this microbiome also spills out across our body organs and tissues such as our skin, so our unique microbiome is always interacting with our external environment.

Functions of gut flora:

- Ferments undigested carbohydrates to produce short-chain fatty acids (SCFA's)
- Synthesises vitamins (B7—biotin and K)
- Improves vitamin absorption
- Metabolises bile acids
- Metabolises 'foreign' substances such as drugs
- Stimulates cell growth
- Provides defence against some disease, by contributing to gut wall integrity.
- Increases the gut's absorption of water, reduces counts of damaging bacteria, increases the growth of human gut cells and stimulates the growth of indigenous bacteria

Research is now showing that it also comprises an essential part of our immune system; performing a vital role in preventing and helping us overcome infection, but also allergy and (according to new research) playing a large role in switching on or off auto-immune disorders. The gut microbiota also interacts with and modulates the hypothalamic, pituitary, adrenal axis (HPA axis) and, further to this may be regarded as an endocrine organ in its own right.[12] Microbes co-evolved with and exert an influence on the human immune system, but communications are bidirectional—there is a cross-talk between gut microbiota and the immune system and the immune system also helps to regulate the gut flora.

Finally, we present recent evidence to support that disturbances in the bacterial microbiota result in dysregulation of adaptive immune cells, and this may underlie disorders such as inflammatory bowel disease. This raises the possibility that the mammalian immune system, which seems to be designed to control microorganisms, is in fact controlled by microorganisms.

—J. Round and S. Mazmanian[13]

Birth and early life have an influence on establishing microbiota. Children with eczema have been shown to have predictably altered microbiomes.[14] It has been demonstrated that an absence of microbiota or a depleted microbiome can account for many common digestive symptoms such as those found by sufferers of irritable bowel syndrome (IBS). Because hormones are conjugated and excreted via the gut, the microbiome and gut function play a vital role in hormone homeostasis. Links have also been made between microbiome depletion and allergy, auto-immune disorders, brain diseases such as dementia, Parkinson's disease, obesity, and also cancer development and lowered cancer survival rates.[15]

There is still much to discover about what exactly constitutes a 'healthy' microbiome, but diversity seems to be important and our diet plays a significant role. A so-called 'American diet' (high meat, high carbohydrate) has been shown to have significantly less diversity than a so-called 'Mediterranean diet'. Some Japanese islanders have demonstrated positive microbiome changes due to their complex diet and high consumption of seaweeds for example. Greater microbiome diversity and seasonal variation in microbiomes have also been demonstrated in tribal populations.[16]

Non-refined, plant-based diets with fibre, particularly soluble fibre, provide substrates for intestinal microbial metabolism and food-associated commensal microbes. One other point to consider comes from American cell biologist Bruce Lipton.

When humans digest genetically modified foods, the artificially created genes transfer into, and alter the character of the beneficial bacteria in the intestine.

—B. Lipton[17]

Our diet affects our metabolism and our microbiome. Our microbiome interacts with our metabolites, shaping a complex interacting network that relates to gut health and beyond.

Interesting Fact: Poo transplant

Strange but true! Conventional research has gone down the path of investigating microbiota 'transplantation', such as taking a faecal supplement (a capsule of poo) from a person with a 'healthy' microbiome and so 'seeding' a new colony in a person who is lacking.

A long-standing idea within many traditions of herbal medicine is that the whole body can be seen as a functioning ecosystem, interacting in a dynamic way with our body's cells, tissues and organs. Modern microbiome research appears to support that view.

One overlooked area is that the function of each and every section of the digestive system has an impact on the self-maintenance of the microbiome. This means that although diet has an important role in providing the 'soil' for our internal 'rainforest', the function of our gut is also vital in providing the correct conditions for our forest to thrive! This is where the herbalist has access to a huge choice of medicinal, digestive function enhancing plants, arising from a deep interest in them through history.

Let's now explore some of these ancient ideas with regard to our food and our health, firstly taste.

Taste

The concept of taste has a much broader meaning to the herbalist than simply bitter, salty, sweet and sour. Historically correspondences were drawn between a taste and its elemental quality (fire, water, earth and air), and between elements, organs, tissues and emotions. Using a meditative tasting method as described in Chapter 2, shows that taste in the context of plant medicines can represent dynamic functions within the body. Early scientists used taste to help identify chemical compounds, and this can still act as a guide to compounds even today. Think of the taste of bitter almonds for example and the presence of cyanide-like compounds, or the taste of the presence of mineral salts, or fruit acids.

In a deeper elemental sense tastes are 'qualities' that can inform our understanding of health.

The taste sweet has historically always been linked with the heart. The Latin for heart '*cor*' gives us clues to what depth of meaning lies behind a simple word like 'heart'. A cordial therefore was a sweetened drink, but to be cordial can mean 'friendly' or 'sincere' even 'hearty'!

Sweet things were used as medicine for the heart, and the heart was thought to contain the soul, and be responsible for the emotion of love and joy—or the lack of it (hence 'broken-hearted').

Salt refers to the minerals and mineralisation of the body, the minerals in bone for example, controlled by the organ of the kidney. Salt increases water content in the body. The taste of salt therefore can relate to water, minerals, the kidney or lymph flow in the body.

Sour—perhaps the *least* well-understood taste/function—is associated with the capacity for assimilation, and to hold on to nourishment. It is related to the Chinese organ-concept of spleen, whereby the use of sour can help 'shore up leaks of the assimilative capacity of the body'.

Bitter—the least popular taste perhaps—is associated with the liver (and gall bladder) in traditional herbal medicine. Its use stimulates and triggers the cascade of normal physiological functions from mouth to anus. The primary quality of bitter is Cool and this reduces inflammation, returning the body to normal warmth.

Tongue maps like this once suggested that we have different taste receptors in different parts of our tongue. It is nowadays considered that all tastes can be detected across the whole tongue but that certain papillae may be more pre-disposed to particular receptors.

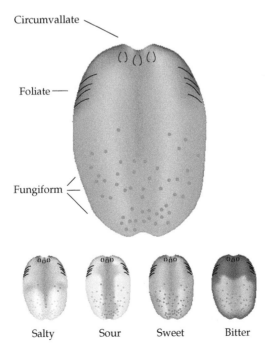

Circumvallate

Foliate

Fungiform

Salty   Sour   Sweet   Bitter

Furthermore, it is now thought that we have bitter receptors through-out our body, and these are in some way linked to the health of our immune system.[18,19]

The four temperaments of Greek and Unani medicine

The Ancient Greeks had an understanding of four basic qualities making up the natural world—of which we are part. Hot, Cold, Dry and Moist co-exist in varying degrees and quantities. This was not literal, but rather figurative and allowed for the observation of patterns in nature or the patient. Pattern recognition is still a vital component of the assessment of the patient for modern medical herbalists.

The Greeks and then subsequent translators and practitioners of these concepts such as the Arabic Unani (Tibb) physicians developed this into an empirical observation of people and their health. Galen-ism—the persistent dogmatic perusal of ideas originally expressed by Galen of Pergamon (we met him in Chapter 1) led to a stagnation and lack of evolution of the ideas of the four humours, and they are now largely discredited as inaccurate redundant concepts. A sympathetic view of the concepts behind the humours allows us to see that physicians were recording what was observed, and therefore some of what was described have modern explanations. Let's take a look at some of the fundamentals.

The primary, active polarity of Hot/Cold is the easiest to understand and refers to the relative level of energy or activity present in a system or entity. Hot denotes a high level of energy or activity. Hot activates, excites, expands, disperses, moves and circulates. Cold denotes a low level of energy or activity. Cold slows down, sedates, contracts, congeals and obstructs. Moisture is essential for life, and lubricates function, but without some dryness, there can be no retention of matter and energy, so dryness allows for the integrity of the structures of the body.

From these four qualities—it is possible to create mixtures that constitute the temperament of a thing/person. So that Cold and Dry is the temperament of melancholy, Hot and Moist is sanguine. Phlegmatic is Cool and Moist and choleric is active or Hot and Dry. Each temperament has correspondences such as seasons of the year, food, diseases etc. Let's reflect on one key concept from this tradition—the concept of how we digest (concoct) and absorb (assimilate) our food and nourishment.

Digestive fire

A persistent theme of herbal medicine traditions is the concept of digestive fire: the capacity of our digestive system to successfully digest (cook, concoct) the food we eat into the perfect balance of micro-ingredients required to manufacture and maintain our body cells and tissues (blood and flesh). Sufficient digestive vigour/fire and the correct balance of cooked/raw/types of food for our constitution are necessary so that we can produce healthy tissues.

Excess food, excessively 'Cold' food, or a lack of digestive fire in a person could mean that what is eaten is insufficiently or imperfectly 'cooked'. This creates phlegm. Phlegm itself is vital as lubrication in the body, and, for example, perfect mucous membrane function; but excess could lead directly to phlegm (excess moisture and cold) building up in the tissues of the body. This concept is thought to lead to the production of excess catarrh, flesh, rheumatic aches or benign growths and lumps.

In contrast, over-cooked food, or excessive digestive 'fire' or choleric behaviour could lead to 'burnt' food. This over-burning eventually increases the qualities of cold and dry—in other words melancholy. Excessive Cold and Dry leads to lack of flow, stagnation, inflammation, morbidity and even cancer in a traditional view. Small amounts of melancholy were important to form the structures of the body, but in excess could lead to disease of the mind or body. Today, we are aware of the causes of oxidative stress and free radical formation from fried foods, especially burnt barbequed meat, and how it is linked to inflammatory processes. We might also agree that a lack of exercise, and allowing 'stagnation' in the sense of physical activity might lead to the melancholy of the mind, as well as chronic inflammatory diseases.

Modern Western medical herbalists use some level of constitutional assessment—a recognition of the individual nature of a person's whole wellbeing—to go beyond the initial diagnosis of just having 'arthritis' or 'migraine'. Many modern herbalists would also use any dietary advice offered in a constitutional way, suggesting that certain foods or liquids (including herbs used) could be warm, cool, moist or dry to support the transition of a persons' health back to a more balanced position.

This concept also suggests that it might be better to eat more salads in the summer, and warm cooked food in winter. Grating or fermenting raw vegetables can be helpful for winter vegetable consumption.

Vegetables available seasonally often seem appropriate to our needs emotionally and physiologically. We have also observed this in prescribing for our patients. We might choose different herbs in summer to those for use during the winter.

Introducing a winter slaw (inspired by Anna Jones, *A Cook's Year*, 2017, 4th estate).

Shred half of a light green cabbage.
 Grate one large raw beetroot.
 Grate one unpeeled apple.
 Finely slice two large spring onions or one small red onion.
 Finely slice one red pepper.
 Mix all of the prepared vegetables with 1–2 tablespoons of cold-pressed nut/seed/olive oil, the zest and juice of one organic unwaxed lemon, a teaspoon of quality sea salt (or rock salt), a pinch of pepper, several whole mint leaves and 3 tablespoons of toasted pumpkin or sesame seeds. Leave at room temperature before serving.

Seasonal eating and foraging

We are living through a time of a popular revival of foraged food. Richard Mabey's book *Food for Free*, published in 1972, helped start a reconnection with food from our wild spaces and a need to care for our diminishing countryside. Many traditional herbal medicines were essentially foraged foods, known to all country dwellers. Educated and wealthy people were often remembered for their scientific advances, but the ordinary, and (often hugely knowledgable) people used foraged herbs and foods as nutrition and medicine. Their voices have occasionally been (thankfully) recorded in books[20] and via the Ethnomedica— Remembered Remedies Project at Kew Gardens for example. See http://www1.kew.org/science/directory/projects/MedicUsesBrit Plants.html.

Take a moment to think about what benefits you perceive are to be gained from going out there and harvesting food from the wild. They could be practical, emotional, spiritual, intellectual or nourishing to name but a few.

Going back to the gut biome for a moment, it is interesting to consider the potential impact of introducing seasonal wild foods into the diet on our gut flora. Natural yeasts, unrefined sugars, a broad cross-section of phytochemical constituents from plants which have had to survive in an uncontrolled environment; the type of food in fact that we have co-evolved with. One study of the Hazda people of Tanzania concluded with the following statement:

> We show that the Hadza have higher levels of microbial richness and bio-diversity than Italian urban controls. Further comparisons with two rural farming African groups illustrate other features unique to Hadza that can be linked to a foraging lifestyle.
>
> —S. L. Schnorr et al.[16]

In terms of gut flora populations, it is not only the type/species of microflora that are important to our health, but also the diversity of different species. Greater diversity in terms of gut microbiota helps us to deal effectively with a wider range of potential challenges. The Hazda have a distinct advantage here it would seem.

Seaweeds—a foraged food

Wild seaweed and coastal plants have been harvested for food, and used in traditional herbal medicine for centuries. Seaweed is well documented as important in the human diet across the globe. An ancient Korean tradition is to serve brown seaweed soup called miyeokguk to postpartum mothers. Wake is the key ingredient in a Korean birthday soup, which symbolises rejuvenation. It also serves as a reminder that seaweed was the first food eaten by the mother and through her breastmilk, her newborn.

Have you ever eaten nori?? Well, we would like to take this opportunity to introduce you to Kathleen Mary Drew-Baker, Mother of the Sea. Kathleen Mary Drew-Baker was born on the 6th November 1901. She graduated from the University of Manchester in 1923, with a degree in botany, subsequently becoming a lecturer in botany for the university. Her marriage in 1928 to a fellow academic resulted in her being dismissed from the university faculty as they had a policy of not employing married women. She was demoted to an unpaid research assistant.

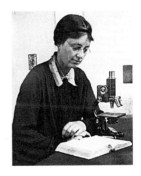

Kathleen Mary
Drew-Baker

Kathleen studied the red algae *Porphyra umbilicus* (Kutzing), subsequently publishing its life cycle in the academic journal *Nature* in 1949. Japanese researcher Segawa Sokichi then developed artificial seeding techniques based on her work, which ultimately led to a significant increase in production in the Japanese seaweed industry. In honour of her contributions to Japanese aquaculture and her role in rescuing the commercial production of nori, she was named Mother of the Sea in Japan, and since 1953, an annual 'Drew festival' is celebrated in the city of Kumamoto in Japan, where a shrine to her was also erected. She was a co-founder of the British Phycological Society in 1952 and its first elected president.

For those of us who are fortunate enough to live by the sea, the opportunity for a spot of seashore based wild foraging is a fine thing. Edible seaweeds are packed full of vitamins and minerals, partly because the sea is not farmed as the land is, and is therefore not depleted of its mineral content. As we discussed in the section on salt, the minerals are present in seaweed in a highly bioavailable form.

Researchers have found benefits from key compounds such as mucilages can lead to strengthening the protective layer of membranes lining the gut (remember goblet cells?), and a general slowing down of digestive processes, allowing food to release its energy more slowly.

Medicinally through phytonutrients, they bring many benefits, and certainly Bladderwrack, (*Fucus vesiculosus* L.) and Carrageen moss (*Chondrus crispus* L.) are both often to be found in the herbalists' dispensary. If plants thrive due to their own microbiome, and we ingest plants, or animals that have eaten those plants, then the health of the ecosystem within which that plant lives is likely to impact the plant's own microbiome and ours too. We are of the Earth ...

Fermented foods

Another type of food our ancestors will have surely experimented with, and sometimes relied upon, is fermented food. Storage of food in an age before refrigeration would have been key for survival—and many traditional techniques survive even where they are no longer a required storage method. Fermented foods have also been gaining recognition for their healthful effects in recent times. Popularity and awareness of sauerkraut, kimchi, kefir, kombucha and apple cider vinegar, for example, has increased.

This area of nutrition has a natural affinity for medical herbalists because of our focus on gut function and the inevitable improvements to the microbiome. Foods that can be fermented such as cabbages, beetroots or apples are traditionally associated with encouraging a reduction in inflammation; fermentation just adds another layer of benefits. A broad-based gut flora equips us with the ability to effectively deal with a much broader array of digestive challenges from the foods that we ingest, resulting in fewer potential problems arising to disrupt or dampen our digestive fire. It also reduces inflammation throughout the body tissues.

Self medication with culinary herbs

If you are looking for an area where food and medicine definitely do overlap, look no further than the wonderful world of culinary herbs and spices. Exotic herbs and spices have been imported into Europe for many centuries, cumin, the second most popular spice in the world today (after black pepper), was once used as payment for rent in mediaeval England.[21] A little knowledge concerning the medicinal uses of culinary herbs is a fantastic way to develop a working domestic medicine chest, and of course the good news is that many of these herbs are easy to grow, and some remain available even in the winter months. Let's look at a few of the well-known favourites:

Parsley

Petroselinum crispum (Mill.) Fuss

Parsley is a low-calorie, highly concentrated source of vitamins, minerals, fibre and antioxidant compounds. It is specifically high in potassium and is one of the foods listed by the World Health Organization as being high in potassium and therefore beneficial in the treatment of high blood pressure. Any time you are contemplating how to acquire a good quality vitamin and mineral supplement, consider parsley. This, along with nettle and watercress, is an excellent source of trace minerals and vitamins.

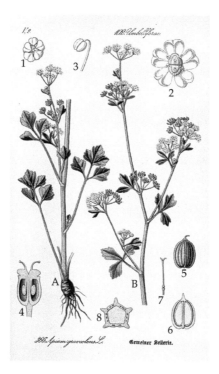

Health benefits of parsley's phytonutrients (including the flavone apigenin) include acting to boost the immune system, acting as a cleansing diuretic, soothing indigestion, helping with gas and constipation and improving bone health. Parsley has been investigated for its antioxidant effects in humans.[22] Don't leave the parsley garnish on the side of the plate at restaurants—eat the lot. Eat a small handful of parsley every day. Grow it in your garden. Enjoy.

Sage

Salvia officinalis L.

Why should a man grow ill when sage grows in his garden?

The above quote is sage advice about sage, going back many centuries; some people attribute it to Hippocrates. Easy to grow and delicious in cooking, sage gets its name from the Latin form 'to save' giving us perhaps a hint at its high historical value as a medicinal plant. The aromatic qualities of sage make it a great herb for the digestive tract, acting as a carminative to ease indigestion and helping to digest fatty foods.

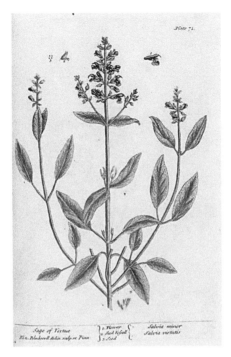

Sage is antiseptic and astringent and has a long history of use as a cold tea to treat hot flushes during menopause. It is also specific for problems with gums and mucous membranes of the mouth, and the cooled infusion can be used as an excellent antiseptic mouthwash, particularly when combined with cloves.

A recipe for a poultice to ease the pain of sprains:

Sage poultice

- Bruise whole, fresh sage leaves by flattening them with a rolling pin. Try not to break or tear them.
- Put the sage leaves in a pan and just cover them with vinegar. Simmer gently for 5 minutes over a very low heat. The vinegar should not boil, but it should steam so that the sage leaves soften and blanch.
- After 5 minutes take out the leaves and lay them on a clean cloth (i.e., muslin). Working very quickly and carefully as the leaves will be very hot, fold the cloth into a package to cover the affected area.
- Apply as hot as can be tolerated and cover with a towel to retain the heat. Leave on for an hour or so until the swelling has subsided.[23]

Rosemary

Salvia rosmarinus Spenn.

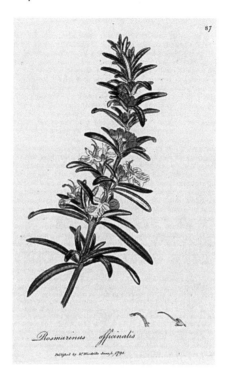

There's rosemary, that's for remembrance. Pray you, love, remember.
—Shakespeare, Hamlet. Act 4, Scene 5

Rosemary is the ideal infusion to drink if you are feeling fuzzy-headed, perhaps from too much study (surely not!). It has been the subject of much research in terms of its ability to improve blood flow to the head and brain, and one interesting piece of research finished with this sentence:

> *The positive effect of the dose nearest normal culinary consumption points to the value of further work on effects of low doses over the longer term.*
> —A. Pengelly et al.[24]

This speaks to the potential value of using healing herbs regularly in your food. A warming digestive tonic, and circulatory stimulant, with an underlying reputation as a heart tonic, this lovely aromatic herb graces any garden and the infusion makes a great addition to the bathwater to relieve aches and pains. In addition rosemary herb has been shown to contain antimicrobial compounds,[25] that could complement foods for those recovering from viral and bacterial infections. Rosemary and garlic infused oil used regularly with soups, stews, drizzled over pizzas and pasta, and used to roast vegetables and potatoes is very delicious.

Dill

Anethum graveolens L.

Antioxidant, antibacterial and containing high levels of calcium, dill is possibly best known for its antispasmodic effects on the gut. Although recipes vary for gripe water for colic in infants in different countries, one of the core herbs in its preparation has always been dill.

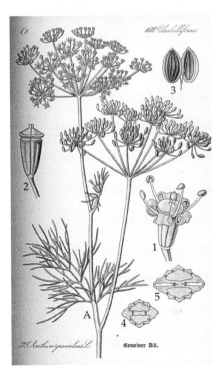

Other valuable uses for this remarkable plant are still being investigated however today. One study at an Iranian hospital found that ingestion of dill seed extract (traditionally used in Iranian folk medicine) leads to contraction of uterine tissue, and a decrease in duration and intensity of labour pain.[26] More research work done in Iran in 2014 on *Anethum graveolens* L., concluded that it was as effective as mefenamic acid in the treatment of painful periods.[27] If you know someone who suffers from painful periods, it is important to establish the underlying cause where possible, but getting them to include dill in their diet as a regular feature may well be of benefit. Use in pickles, salad dressings, salads etc.

Well, there we have it—a very brief foray into the uses of some culinary plants as medicines. Domestic medicine can be flexible, effective and fragrant all at once. Developing and using your favourite remedies from your kitchen cupboard or garden is a hugely resourceful and empowering thing to do, and it also reminds us of some of the benefits we are getting simply from ingesting these plants on a regular basis as part of our diets.

Antioxidants, free radicals and phytonutrients

We began this chapter by introducing biomolecules, vitamins and minerals. Phytonutrients, including antioxidants in all their forms, are another class of essential nutrient now gaining attention within the scientific community. Phytonutrients are not classical nutrients, nor are they vitamins; they are a group of compounds, found in many medicinal and food plants that are more than just antioxidants, they are also involved in other key anti-inflammatory pathways, mopping up free radicals, and acting to help repair DNA. But first, let's define antioxidants and free radicals and their associated terms.

Antioxidants and free radicals

Any stable atom is made up of a nucleus with electrons orbiting around it. Unstable atoms do not have enough electrons orbiting the nucleus to be stable, and will therefore try to become more stable by stealing electrons from other atoms with electrons to spare. These unstable atoms are known as free radicals and are formed as a result of oxidation—a normal process occurring as a result of cooking food and metabolic processes within every cell in our body. Because free radicals are unstable they can interact with living tissues causing damage. An antioxidant is an atom with electrons to spare. Antioxidants can give away electrons to free radicals and yet remain stable themselves. Because of this heroic capacity they are known as non-radical species.

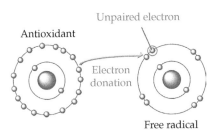

Sometimes there can be so many free radicals and not enough non-radical species that a domino chain reaction of electron stealing takes place. The instability of this chain reaction can lead to oxidative stress causing dysfunction, inflammation, and sometimes death of living cells. Oxidative stress has now been identified as the underlying pathogenesis of many degenerative disorders.

The electron transport chain, which is involved with energy production in cells, is part of all normal cellular processes, but the by-product is the creation of free radicals. Other causes of free radical production include physical or psychological stress, smoking and environmental pollutants, and radioactive exposure. Our body manufactures some antioxidants to help deal with this, and we can absorb antioxidants from our diet to try to mitigate our cellular and environmental free radicals.

Reactive *oxygen* species (ROS), reactive *nitrogen* species (RNS), reactive *hydrogen* species (RHS), and others are all examples of free radicals that are formed. Curiously there are also benefits to free radicals. Macrophages and neutrophils (white blood cells) use and generate free radicals to kill bacteria during phagocytosis. Thyroxine synthesis in the thyroid gland uses the free radical hydrogen peroxide. Nitric oxide is vital in the vasodilation pathway (dilating blood vessels), and during childbirth free radicals are used in the positive feedback process of labour.

Our body synthesises antioxidants to help protect our cells from damage and from excess free radicals that could lead to oxidative stress.

Occasionally the body becomes overwhelmed by oxidative stress and this leads to cell damage. For example:

- Cellular damage can occur to cell membranes, or to proteins or nucleic acids leading to chronic conditions and cell ageing or death.
- Lipids are also easily damaged especially polyunsaturated fats (you'll remember their double bonds make them highly reactive). Oxidisation leads to inflammation.
- Phospholipids of the cell membrane (remember them from our brief look at fats) are vulnerable to oxidative stress.
- Amino acids used in every cell are also vulnerable, and ultimately can lead to nucleic acid and DNA damage.

Endogenous antioxidants (made by the body) donate their electrons, stabilise free radicals and stop the domino effect of oxidative stress; they behave like scavengers of tissue damage. Examples include superoxide dismutase (SOD) an enzyme found in green vegetables, especially cruciferous vegetables, and omega fatty acids of flax oil. Catalase and peroxidase are other enzymes that have antioxidant effects. Glutathione peroxidase is another powerful endogenous antioxidant (manufactured by the liver). It requires the mineral selenium as a co-factor.

Exogenous antioxidants include vitamin C, which is a highly effective electron donor, and is recycled by glutathione. It does not act in isolation however, often working with vitamin E. These antioxidants from nutrients in our diet have an affinity for and stabilising effect on cell membranes.

Other familiar antioxidants from micronutrients in our diet are beta-carotene and lycopene—which are absorbed in the small intestine and distributed to adrenals, liver, prostate and testes. The largest groups of antioxidants are the phenols and polyphenols and these scavenge lipid peroxyl radicals. They are found particularly in red and purple fruits and vegetables and are often cited as accounting for the strong taste of herbal medicines. They are highly anti-inflammatory as well as antioxidant. Others to mention include flavonoids and flavonols, proanthocyanidins and gallo tannins (found in many herbal medicines including green tea). Flavonoids, which are among the largest group of polyphenols, enhance SOD production thus enhancing vascular integrity.

So, in summary: free radicals are an inevitable consequence of living, breathing and energy production within cell mitochondria. Free radicals are used in many body processes, but in excess they can cause oxidative stress, inflammation and cell damage.

Our body manufactures antioxidants, and also absorbs antioxidants from our diet, to manage and reduce oxidative stress, inflammation and cell damage. Macro and micronutrients found in foods and medicinal plants offer our body a rich source of these antioxidants.

Plants also produce free radicals as an inevitable consequence of energy production; they also use free radicals in normal growth processes such as producing lignans to form plant tissues such as bark. It is now considered likely that many crucial cellular pathways in humans have evolved requiring phytonutrient co-factors for optimal function. There are multiple lines of evidence supporting their critical role in establishing and maintaining health.

Some examples of phytonutrients include:

Sirtuins: a class of protein molecules which have been shown to activate calorie restriction in human cells. This reduces the production of reactive oxygen species (ROS), free radicals associated with the ageing processes, *and aids* apoptosis. Apoptosis is the capacity for our body to recognise and kill off rogue or cancer cells. Sirtuins therefore have a number of potential therapeutic applications. Sirtuin genes were discovered in yeast and function as so-called anti-ageing genes.[28]

Nrf2: a basic leucine protein that regulates the expression of antioxidant proteins, (produced by our bodies), which protect against oxidative damage triggered by injury and inflammation. Glutathione is an example of one of these endogenous antioxidant proteins, made by our liver (and also found in many medicinal mushrooms). Reactive oxygen species and other endogenous reactive molecules are constantly generated from normal aerobic metabolism, and increased under 'stress'. The body tries to maintain homeostasis and keep open normal enzyme pathways to protect healthy cells from damage, and this is enabled by Nrf2.[29]

So it is becoming clearer that there is an array of dietary micro-nutrient phytochemicals that are important for optimal health and ageing, and which act as homeostasis and wellbeing enhancers.[30] It is interesting to consider just how many plants from antiquity were prized as agents to increase longevity. We hope to make the case throughout this book that it is in fact the complexity of constituents working synergistically which provide the most benefits.

Recap of phytonutrients of interest to science (you may have heard of some of these!).

- Berry anthocyanins.
- Polyphenolics from green tea, cocoa and pomegranate juice.
- Curcumin from turmeric.
- Resveratrol from grapes, and Japanese knotweed.
- Flavonoids from spices, fruits and vegetables.
- Carotenoids from spices, fruits and vegetables.
- Nitrate from beetroot and spinach.
- Nrf2 primers, especially broccoli sprouts.
- Bitter phytochemicals used by the medical herbalist.

> **Definition—*Luteins:*** Luteins are found in the plant world in the form of yellow plant colourings. Lutein and zeaxanthin are xanthophyll carotenoids found particularly in yellow-orange and dark green leafy vegetables (and in egg yolks, and marigold flowers). They are widely distributed in tissues and are the principal carotenoids required by the eye lens and macular region of the retina.

Modern starchy diets lacking plant secondary metabolites (phytonutrients) are associated with multi-morbidity, or 'lifestyle diseases' including obesity, type 2 diabetes and cardiovascular disease. There is ample reason to believe that diets rich in phytochemicals provide protection from vascular diseases and many cancers, and direct antioxidant activity as well as modulation of enzyme expression or hormone activity, contribute to this effect.[31] Phytochemicals derived from diverse living foods can interact additively and synergistically; thus, the total dietary load of phytochemicals may have ever—greater important implications for health.

A dietary phytochemical index (DPI) has been proposed as a means of roughly quantifying the ultimate 'load' on the body and health.[32] Calories derived from fruits, vegetables (excluding potatoes), legumes, whole grains, nuts, seeds, fruit/vegetable juices, soy products, wine, beer and cider—and foods compounded therefrom—would be counted in the DPI index. Calories from other added oils, refined sugars, refined grains, potato products, hard liquors, and animal products—(regrettably, the chief sources of calories in typical Western diets)—would be excluded from the DPI. It is hoped the DPI index could aid epidemiologists in exploring the health consequences of diets high in phytochemical-rich plant foods, and also help health practitioners giving advice to patients. DPI has been inversely linked to hypertension and insulin resistance in epidemiological studies.

Eventually, there may be set reference values for the intake of key phytonutrients—for example—lutein and flavonoids, just as we have reference values for vitamins and minerals.[33]

To elaborate on the interconnectivity of everything a little further—another phytochemical—epigallocatechin gallate (do you remember gallic tannins from Chapter 2?), a major component of green tea polyphenols, protects against the oxidation of fat-soluble antioxidants including lutein. Many nuts and berries also contain these types of compound. So, ultimately this means there is a synergistic effect between phytochemicals that allow each individual phytochemical to do its work!

The 'Microcirculation Phytonutrient Diet' suggested by Professor Kerry Bone[34] includes the following advice:

1) Boost dietary nitrate via beetroot and spinach
2) Increase cocoa intake via 90% chocolate
3) Increase berry anthocyanin intake via berries
4) Raw crushed garlic: up to one clove/day
5) Increase herbs and spices: especially green herbs, turmeric and ginger.

Conclusion

We would like to state here that we are first and foremost herbalists. Our strong interest in food, springs from two main sources:

a) The deep understanding that we ultimately gain from the practice of herbal medicine concerning how the bodies of living plants interact with the living human body.
b) The magnificent liminal space that the practice of herbal medicine inhabits between modern-day perceptions of food and medicine as being separate entities.

Recommendations on diet in terms of health and wellbeing were incorporated into the practice of medicine from ancient times. The School of Salernum, mentioned as being Ancient in 846 CE, placed a strong emphasis on food, and the importance of healthy eating (the majority of

Hippoctaric corpus is from the last decades of the 5th century BCE and the first half of the 4th-century BCE).

> *It is not sufficient to learn simply that cheese is a bad food, as it gives a pain to one who eats a surfeit of it. We must know what the pain is, the reasons for it, and which constituent of man is harmfully affected.*
>
> —Hippocrates

So, a healthy diet is not just about the optimal concentration of carbohydrate, fat and protein, nor simply about vitamins, minerals etc. There is a lot more to think about. Recommendations for foods suited or optimal for specific conditions can always be tailored to fit the individual, and after all, that is what the practice of medicine is all about. It is often the case, however, that just observing some good, basic healthy eating practices can have a significant impact on many situations. It may seem that attaining a diet that is ethically sourced, organic, optimal for gut bacteria, and one that is suitable for your constitution, is just too confusing. One of the big things to take away from this is that food is a joy and a blessing. Ensuring that it remains so, and that we do not get too bogged down in the nitty-gritty of food science, of in-depth research and of biochemistry, can seem like a bit of a mammoth exercise. We would like to offer you these few simple pointers to keep you on track.

How to eat well

- Stay away from refined and processed foods and additives that 'preserve'. (Ask yourself, how many processes has a food been through to reach your plate?)
- Eat organic where you can.
- Consider harvesting something from the wild to eat.
- Eat a wide variety of seasonal fruits and vegetables.
- Consider how you can expand the range of foods in your diet, rather than restrict.
- Incorporate more beans, nuts and seeds into your diet. Consider sources of prebiotic foods.
- Find sources of probiotic foods.

- Consider what types of protein, fat or carbohydrate will also have the broadest array of phytonutrients?
- Use herbs and spices generously.
- Find inspiration in other traditions and cultures ways with food.
- Treat yourself. When you do this, make it as good quality as possible and eat without guilt.
- Make a food menu and shopping plan for the week if that helps.
- Never go shopping when you are hungry!

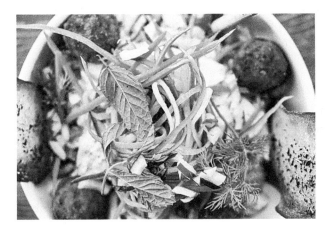

We all have to be realistic about what we can achieve. It would be lovely to make your own bread, make lots of homemade fermented foods, drink eight glasses of water every day, etc. etc. The reality is that we may be able to incorporate one or two things into life, but we cannot do it all. Pick your battles, do what works for you, and enjoy the lush richness that is good, good food. Good food does not need to be expensive. Good food does not need to be complicated. Good food *does* need to be enjoyed. Knowledge of the phenomenal and wonderful healing complexity that phytonutrients offer us is a thing to be savoured when you bite into a crunchy apple or smell a luscious homemade soup.

You may ultimately want to start your own receipt book, in the tradition of historical receipt books full of favourite recipes and simple home remedies, that you can refer back to regularly and ultimately pass on to the next generation (what a lovely heirloom).

Food engages all of our senses. It will nourish and heal us on many levels if we allow it to. It provides a gateway whereby the wild can enter into us, and it connects us to both the world and each other. To finish with some wise words from a lovely wee cookbook:

> We all have to eat, so it is empowering to realize that every time we fulfil that fundamental need we have choices which may seem small in themselves, but which cumulatively can quite simply transform our lives.
> —Ann Bowen-Jones and Phillippa Lee[35]

Bibliography

Barker, Julian, *History, Philosophy and Medicine; Phytotherapy in Context.* 2007: Winter Press

Bird, Fiona, *Seaweed in the Kitchen.* 2015: Prospect Books.

Ghayour, Sabrina, *Persiana.* 2014: Octopus Books.

Hemsley and Hemsley, *A Guide to Eating Well.* 2014: Ebury Press.

Katz, Sandor E., *Wild Fermentation. Flavour, Nutrition and Craft of Live Culture Foods.* 2003.

Ottolenghi, Yotam, *Plenty.* 2010: Ebury Press.

Raven, Sarah, *Good, Good Food.* 2016: Bloomsbury Publishing.

Rhattigan, Prannie, *The Irish Seaweed Kitchen.* 2009: Booklink.

References

1. Wong, J. M. W. et al., *Effects of advice to drink 8 cups of water per day in adolescents with overweight or obesity: a randomized clinical trial.* JAMA Pediatr, 2017. 171(5): p. e170012.
2. Mayor, D. and M. S. Micozzi, *Energy Medicine East and West; A natural history of Qi.* 2011: Churchill Livingstone.
3. Ho, K. V. et al., *Identifying antibacterial compounds in black walnuts* metabolites, 2018. 8(4).
4. Pereira, J. A. et al., *Walnut (Juglans regia L.) leaves: phenolic compounds, antibacterial activity and antioxidant potential of different cultivars.* Food Chem Toxicol, 2007. 45(11): pp. 2287–2295.
5. Pereira, J. A. et al., *Bioactive properties and chemical composition of six walnuts (Juglans regia L.) cultivars.* Food Chem Toxicol, 2008. 46(6): pp. 2103–2111.
6. Sabater-Molina, M. et al., *Dietary fructooligosaccharides and potential benefits on health.* J Physiol Biochem, 2009. 65(3): pp. 315–328.
7. Jiménez, S. et al., *Chemical composition of rosehips from different Rosa species: an alternative source of antioxidants for the food industry.* Food Addit Contam Part A Chem Anal Control Expo Risk Assess, 2017. 34(7): pp. 1121–1130.
8. Andersson, U. et al., *Effects of rose hip intake on risk markers of type 2 diabetes and cardiovascular disease: a randomized, double-blind, cross-over investigation in obese persons.* Eur J Clin Nutr, 2012. 66(5): pp. 585–590.
9. Arranz-Otaegui, A. et al., *Archaeobotanical evidence reveals the origins of bread 14,400 years ago in northeastern Jordan.* Proceedings of The National Academy of Sciences of the United States of America., 2018. 115(31): pp. 7925–7930.
10. Whitley, A., *Bread Matters: The State of Modern Bread.* 2009: Harper Collins.
11. Rodriguez-Ramiro, et al., *Assessment of iron bioavailability from different bread making processes using an in vitro intestinal cell model.* Food Chemistry, 2017. 1(228): pp. 91–98.
12. Clarke, G. et al., *Minireview: Gut microbiota: the neglected endocrine organ.* Mol Endocrinol, 2014. 28(8): pp. 1221–1238.
13. Round, J. and S. Mazmanian, *The gut microbiota shapes intestinal immune responses during health and disease.* Nature Reviews Immunology, 2009. 9(May): pp. 313–323.
14. Abrahamsson, T. R. et al., *Low diversity of the gut microbiota in infants with atopic eczema.* Journal of Allergy and Clinical Immunology, 2012. 129(2): pp. 434–440.
15. Blaser, M. J., *Missing Microbes. How the Overuse of Antibiotics is Fuelling Our Modern Plagues.* 2014: Picador Books.

16. Schnorr, S. L. et al., *Gut microbiome of the Hadza hunter-gatherers.* Nat Commun, 2014. 5: p. 3654.
17. Lipton, B., *The Biology of Belief.* 2004: Netherwood et al.
18. Lee, R. J. and N. A. Cohen, *Bitter and sweet taste receptors in the respiratory epithelium in health and disease.* J Mol Med (Berl), 2014. 92(12): pp. 1235–1244.
19. Cohen, N. A., *The genetics of the bitter taste receptor T2R38 in upper airway innate immunity and implications for chronic rhinosinusitis.* Laryngoscope, 2017. 127(1): pp. 44–51.
20. Allen, D. and G. Hatfield, *Medicinal Plants in Folk Tradition: An Ethnobotany of Britain and Ireland.* 2004: Timber Press.
21. Francia, S. and A. Stobart, *Critical Approaches to the History of Western Herbal Medicine: From Classical Antiquity to the Early Modern Period.* 2014: Bloomsbury Press.
22. Nielsen, S. et al., *Effect of parsley (Petroselinum crispum) intake on urinary apigenin excretion, blood antioxidant enzymes and biomarkers for oxidative stress in human subjects.* British Journal of Nutrition, 1999. 81(6): pp. 447–455.
23. Hedley, C. and N. Shaw, *Herbal Remedies: A Practical Beginner's Guide to Making Effective Remedies in the Kitchen.* 1999: Parragon.
24. Pengelly, A. et al., *Short-term study on the effects of rosemary on cognitive function in an elderly population.* J Med Food, 2012. 15(1): pp. 10–17.
25. Celiktas, O. Y. et al., *Antimicrobial activities of methanol extracts and essential oils of Rosmarinus officinalis, depending on location and seasonal variations.* Food Chemistry, 2007. 100(2).
26. Mirmolaeea, S. T. et al., *Evaluating the effects of Dill (Anethum graveolens) seed on the duration of active phase and intensity of labour pain.* Journal of Herbal Medicine., 2014. 5(1): pp. 26–29.
27. Heidarifar, R. et al., *Effect of Dill (Anethum graveolens) on the severity of primary dysmenorrhea in compared with mefenamic acid: A randomized, double-blind trial.* J Res Med Sci, 2014. 19(4): pp. 326–330.
28. Dali-Youcef, N. et al., *Sirtuins: the 'magnificent seven', function, metabolism and longevity.* Ann Med, 2007. 39(5): pp. 335–345.
29. Nguyen, T., P. Nioi and C. B. Pickett, *The Nrf2-antioxidant response element signaling pathway and its activation by oxidative stress.* J Biol Chem, 2009. 284(20): pp. 13291–13295.
30. Gertsch, J., *The metabolic plant feedback hypothesis: How plant secondary metabolites nonspecifically impact human health.* Planta Med, 2016. 82(11–12): pp. 920–929.

31. Bahadoran, Z. et al., *Dietary total antioxidant capacity and the occurrence of metabolic syndrome and its components after a 3-year follow-up in adults: Tehran Lipid and Glucose Study.* Nutr Metab (Lond), 2012. 9(1): p. 70.

32. McCarty, M. F., *Proposal for a dietary 'phytochemical index'.* Med Hypotheses, 2004. 63(5): pp. 813–817.

33. Wallace, T. C. et al., *Dietary bioactives: establishing a scientific framework for recommended intakes.* Adv Nutr, 2015. 6(1): pp. 1–4.

34. Bone, K. and S. Mills, *Principles and Practice of Phytotherapy: Modern Herbal Medicine.* 2nd ed. 2013: Churchill Livingstone.

35. Bowen-Jones, A. and P. Lee, *Kitchen Alchemy. Transform Yourself Through Food.* 2010: Spirituality & Health.

CHAPTER SIX

Native healers: five more key plants from the Western herbal tradition

Introduction

In this chapter we will consider and contemplate five essential and magnificent plant tonics from Western herbal medicine practice.

We will learn about their identifying botanical features, the parts of the plant used for medicine and their uses in both home and clinical settings. We will provide you with some core information about each plant and we will also look at some of the scientific research available for the safety and efficacy of each of these medicinal plants. Finally we will supply some real case examples to help illustrate how each medicinal plant has been and can be used in modern phytotherapeutic practice.

In exploring these five plants in more detail we shall also be able to consider some central concepts within Western herbal medicine, such as cordials, tonics and the role of adaptogenic herbs. This allows us to consider in more detail the effect of herbal medicines upon the heart and circulation, the skin, wound healing and allergy.

Following on from the theory, join us in making some straightforward, but effective, medicinal preparations that you can create and use at home. Some of them incorporate herbal medicines in a food-like way; others are slightly more 'pharmaceutical' in their preparation and application. And so we shall look at transforming our homemade infused oil from Chapter 4 into an ointment. This secondary process can be adapted to the production not only of ointments but also for lip balms or even suppositories.

It was once common practice to put these infused oil ointments onto bandages and create a 'plaister'—a medicated plaster that could hold the medicament close to the skin for many hours in a kind of oily compress. You can still purchase a hot chilli pepper plaster from some oriental supermarkets. This demonstrates that the application of a hot plaster in this very traditional pharmacy preparation is made for production and use today. In addition, we shall look at the methods of preserving herbs as tinctures; how this is done using a tincturing simple method, and how tinctures are categorised according to the strength of herb material and strength of alcohol. We offer some sage advice for safe use of tinctures in your own home, and when it may be better to avoid them.

> Look at lavender, or at nettles or at mint. They are modest-looking plants. One could take them as the very symbols of humility. And yet these three plants alone can deal with as many troubles as can a family medicine-chest full to bursting.
>
> —Maurice Mességué

At this point You may wish to read the section on the cardiovascular system in Chapter 3 as we will now take a look at a few herbs which interact with it.

Five magnificent plant tonics

Hawthorn (Crataegus species)

Hawthorn, mayflower, hedgethorn, this small tree is right at the centre of things, practical, metaphorical and magical. Its ubiquitous use in hedging means it is supremely abundant, and her rosy blossoms are part of the herald of summer, just as much as her haws are of autumn. If nothing else, hawthorn's capacity to live to a great age, should be a clue to us all.

Classification

Hawthorn is a member of the rose family, the Rosaceae. It is a large and important family for a whole range of ethnobotanical reasons, and can be divided into and considered as three groups: The roses, the apples and pears and the stone-fruit group (which includes apricots and almonds). The rose group includes the important medicinal herbs of meadowsweet, raspberry, blackberry, agrimony, lady's mantle and parsley piert, not forgetting of course rose itself! Every single one of these plants is to be found on our dispensary shelves.

In Europe we have two indigenous species of hawthorn, the Midland hawthorn, Crataegus laevigata (Poiret) DC, and hawthorn, Crataegus monogyna Jacq. These two species are very similar and Linnaeus did

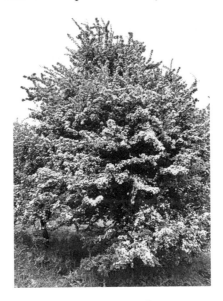

Hawthorn Tree in flower.

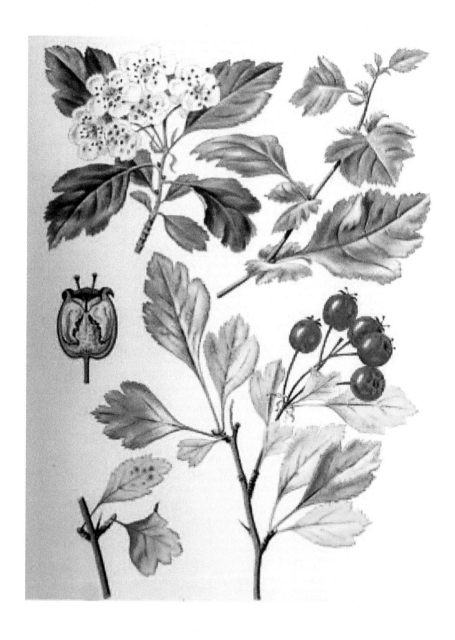

not originally distinguish between them, using the name Crataegus oxyacantha L. for them both. They are used medicinally interchangeably, and this name is still in common use today. You will also often see *Crataegus sp.* used where the species have not been differentiated.

Basic botany

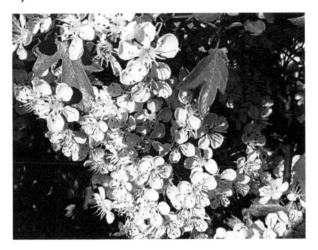

Hawthorn

The rose family shares features such as alternate leaves with serrated edges and stipules that often (especially in woody species), adhere to the leaf stalk, or fall off early (especially herbaceous species) and so appear to be absent.

- **Bark** light grey bark, sometimes with a reddish tinge. Thorny twigs.
- **Flowers** flowers are regular with sepals and petals usually five, but in some herbs reduced to four. The petals are free and in cultivars (like many roses) are doubled-up. Stamens are usually numerous.
- **Fruits** the number and arrangement of carpels give this family its distinctive complexity of fruit types including:
    A single carpel formed into a 'drupe' fruit—the stone fruit (plums, cherry, apricot, almond and of course hawthorn!).
    Multiple tiny drupes (blackberry and raspberry).
    Swollen 'receptacles' with a core (technically the fruit), and (seeds inside) as in apples.
    But in all these diverse forms, the carpels are usually five or multiples of five (or less).

- **Leaves** deeply lobed, usually 3–5 lobes, serrate at front.
- **Habitat** thickets, hedgerows, shallow stony soil, scrub. Common throughout Britain and Northwestern Europe (except Northern Scotland).
- **Harvesting** gather flowers whilst blossom is fresh and some flowers are still at bud stage. Gather young leaves between May and July. Berries are usually ready to harvest between September and October. Like apple, the hawthorn can produce many diverse hybrid forms so that you will notice the flower-colour and berry-colour often varies from tree to tree.
- **Parts used** flowers in bud or in early flowering (late April–May). 'Berries' (false fruits are known as 'haws') harvested in early September—late October depending on geographical location.[1] Fresh young leaves may also be used.

Main constituents

- Oligomeric procyanidins (OPC's) especially the leaves. The leaves also contain rutin, among many other identified compounds. Other well-investigated plants with high OPC content include pine bark (*Pinus pinaster* Alton. cortex), and grape seed (*Vitis vinifera* L. semen).[2]
- Flavonoids, including quercetin glycosides (especially the flowers), and hyperoside, which is often used as a marker compound to check if a sample of the plant is fresh and identifiably Crataegus.
- Amines, catechols, carboxylic and triterpene acids (especially the berries). It is thought that a mixture of these active constituents is required for its therapeutic effect.

Note: Flavonoids. You may have noticed how often similar constituents appear in completely different plants. This is one of the wonderful aspects to herbal medicine—that since many medicinal plants contain flavonoids, it makes most medicinal plants strongly antioxidant. Flavonoids give a brilliant blue or yellow flower-colour, and the red of red wine, but there are also colourless flavonoids that are visible to insects.

Antioxidants are compounds that have the ability to 'scavenge' and 'mop-up' free radicals (damaging compounds known to exacerbate disease states). It is these antioxidant-rich foods that give rise to the so-called 'superfoods', or 'functional foods' that crop up as being very beneficial in studies into cancer and heart disease for example.

Other well-known beneficial flavonoid-related compounds include resveratrol and combretastatin. We like to think of compounds like flavonoids as being an extremely positive and beneficial side-benefit of using medicinal plants internally.

Main therapeutic actions confirmed by research

Increases coronary artery circulation

Dilation of coronary arteries and relaxation of tone in the peripheral circulation.

Research confirms that hawthorn has the capacity to increase blood flow to the heart muscle itself via the coronary arteries.[3] It exerts a positive inotropic effect, meaning that it increases the efficiency and quality of the muscular contraction of the heart muscle.

Improves peripheral circulation and can lower blood pressure

Improved blood flow to the extremities has also been demonstrated, as has a beneficial effect on blood pressure and heart rate.[4-8] Benefits to the microcirculation and increase in the flow of erythrocytes in all vascular vessels has been shown.[2]

Note: Circulation. A Western herbal medicine perspective of the circulation is brilliantly explained by Priest and Priest.[9] They remind us of the interconnectivity and dynamism present within the enclosed circulatory system. To summarise their explanation:

1) The heart requires tonicity, trophicity (nourishment for growth) and vasomotor function. This reminds us that medical herbalists can utilise herbs to address each of these three factors.

2) The arteries are in a state of relaxation or constriction and this can occur locally or generally. There is a recognition here of the importance of adequate circulation to all parts of the body, and that blood vessels need to have the right amount of 'tone', not too relaxed, not too constricted.

3) The capillary bed has the capacity to 'bounce' back the blood from the periphery due to the contractility of the capillaries, and terminal arterioles and venules. This 'bounce' is addressed using capillary agents and diaphoretics to address *over-dryness* and *irritability* of the capillaries (requiring diffusive stimulation and relaxation)—or its opposite—clamminess, coldness and flaccidity (requiring astringing herbal stimulants).

4) The veins require general tonicity, and great importance is placed on the portal circulation and its relationship to the return flow of the blood to the heart.

These concepts are important to the practitioner of Western herbal medicine. For our purposes, it is simply important to note that:

a) different herbal medicines may act on blood vessel tone.

b) blood vessel trophic nourishment is possible with herbs.

c) herbs can influence blood vessel contraction and relaxation .

d) The effects of diaphoresis are brought about by effects to the terminal blood vessels and can relieve pressure in the system.

e) The portal circulation is significant and involves the return flow of blood to the heart. It is usually impaired in conditions afflicting areas of the body below the liver, and the liver is the 'governor' of the portal circulation.

Reduces oversensitivity of the heart

Hawthorn reduces the sensitivity of the myocardium and improves its oxygen utilisation. It has demonstrated benefits to the heart muscle also by regulating Akt and HIF-1 signalling pathways. AKt (a protein kinase enzyme) and HIF-1 (Hypoxia-inducible factor) are both substances produced by the body in response to hypoxia/low oxygen levels.[10]

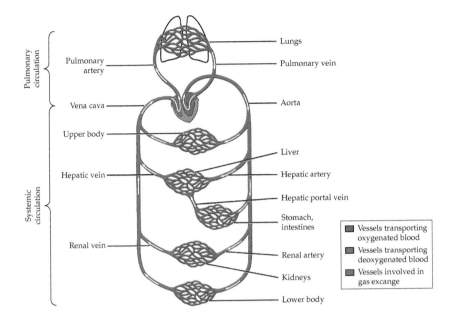

Lungs

Pulmonary artery

Pulmonary vein

Pulmonary circulation

Vena cava

Aorta

Upper body

Liver

Hepatic vein

Hepatic artery

Hepatic portal vein

Systemic circulation

Stomach, intestines

Renal vein

Renal artery

Kidneys

Lower body

| | Vessels transporting oxygenated blood |
| Vessels transporting deoxygenated blood |
| Vessels involved in gas excange |

Anti-arrhythmic

Hawthorn has an anti-arrhythmic effect via relaxation of the coronary arteries. This means it has the potential to re-establish heart rhythm without using stronger alkaloidal compounds such as those found in digitalis (giving rise to the pharmaceutical drug digoxin).[3,6–8]

Anti-sclerotic

Hawthorn demonstrates a capacity to improve the microcirculation and reduce sclerosis and 'furring-up' of the blood vessels.[11] This can have benefits to people with varicose veins, haemorrhoids (anal varicosity), and diseases of the vasculature of the eye and brain. Often this effect is attributed to the presence of antioxidant anthocyanidins, or the anti-inflammatory action of saponins. Other examples of plants with very good research data in this area include bilberry (Vaccinium myrtillus L.), horse chestnut (Aesculus hippocastanum L.), and garlic (Allium sativa L.). By improving the *integrity* of the blood vessel wall, hawthorn has the potential to reduce thrombus (clot) formation, also demonstrated in various studies.[2]

Hypocholesterolaemic

In addition Hawthorn has shown hypo-cholesterolaemic activity.[6-8,12]

Cardiotonic

It has been directly established that hawthorn reduces oxidative stress.[7,8,13,14]

This is an effect explored in Chapter 5, whereby antioxidants, and other beneficial compounds cause helpful seleque such as improved ability to reduce oxidative stress which otherwise damages cellular contents, or improve cellular apoptosis. The concept of a cardiotonic is more poetically imagined in the ancient concept of a 'cordial'.

> **Note: Cordials.** From the Latin *cor* meaning heart, cordial means to be warm and friendly. It refers to the world-view of ancient times that all our organs have a number of associations, such as emotions and astrological significances, as well as elements and temperaments. The heart in ancient Europe referred to the seat of the soul and related to the emotion of joy and where love struck its arrow. We can also be broken-hearted or say something heartfelt; and even today we use the image of the heart to mean love or friendliness.
>
> The taste of sweet was thought to relate to the heart, and so a syrup made from herbs was known as a cordial, because it was pleasing to the heart. Excess, it was acknowledged even in ancient times, could damage the heart; *too much of a good thing!*
>
> Our idea of a cordial today is very much a sweetened citrus drink to be diluted with water, although elderflower cordials are making a comeback. Herbs of Venus, in mediaeval times were often candied or made into cordials, to further encourage the good and uplifting effect to the heart! So violets, roses and mallows were all considered cooling and soothing to the heart and so were ideal to be made into 'heart-helping' cordials.
>
> Interestingly, hawthorn is described as being under the influence of Mars by Nicholas Culpeper (1616–1654). The qualities associated

with Mars are choleric and youthful, and of summer—warming and drying. When in balance choler helps us digest our food successfully, and is outgoing, active and nimble. Does this sound like hawthorn to you?

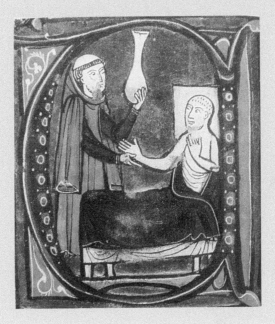

Mildly diuretic and febrifuge, mild sedative

Many herbs demonstrate mild diuretic effects. This suggests an increase in blood flow to the kidney itself. As we have demonstrated so far with hawthorn, increasing the blood to an organ has positive inotropic consequences. Increasing blood flow to the kidney may also account for some of the blood pressure corrective effects shown for hawthorn.

Note: WS1442. We would like, at this point to say a quick word about WS 1442. You will find many references to this product in clinical trials concerning hawthorn and its benefits in the treatment of cardiovascular disease. WS 1442 is a standardised extract, manufactured by

Dr W. Schwabe Pharmaceuticals©, made from *Crataegus spp.* leaves and flowers. It contains 18.75% oligomeric procyanidins (OPC) and is very popular for such things as clinical trials as it offers a standardised and therefore controlled dose of the drug under study. A growing number of clinical trials have now been undertaken using WS 1442, particularly with regard to the treatment of chronic heart failure, with very positive patient outcomes. Specifically, one trial showed a significant reduction in the rate of sudden deaths in patients taking WS 1442.[15–18]

We also suggest that a mild diuretic and diaphoretic such as hawthorn would make a useful addition to medicine for someone experiencing a viral or bacterial infection, who is weak, or has a heart problems.

Synergy

Numerous studies have suggested that the compounds in hawthorn demonstrate a highly synergistic effect. In other words for the benefits above, the whole plant should be used. Research also suggests that a mixture of leaf, flower and fruit together will provide the best combination of beneficial compounds.[19]

Methods of preparation and use

Hawthorn leaves and flowers can be eaten from the may tree (in May!) and were once picked by children who called this 'bread and cheese'. Hawthorn flowers and young leaves can be made into a fresh tisane, or dried and made by infusion into a very pleasant tea. The berries (or haws) of hawthorn should be decocted (boiled for 20 minutes in a closed vessel), as they will not release their contents easily in a tea.

A slow overnight decoction can be done by covering the berries with water, fitting an oven-proof lid, and leaving in a slow cooker or oven on the lowest heat overnight, or even for 48 hours. A tincture is often made using the flowers and young leaves in the spring and then after pressing can be mixed with the berries in the autumn giving a magnificent product in both quantity and diversity of constituents.

What is a tincture?

For our purposes we shall consider a tincture to be the liquid preparation produced by macerating prepared plant material in a mixture of alcohol and water at room temperature over a prescribed period of time. This is then pressed and filtered to yield a fluid into which active constituents of the herb have dissolved. Tinctures are one of the commonest ways a modern phytotherapist will dispense medicinal herbs, although teas, decoctions, syrups, vinegars, oxymels and glycerites are all used. Tinctures have been found in the tombs of Egyptian pharaohs and so are very ancient in origin.

Why make a tincture?

Preservation of fresh or dried herb material into a liquid that can easily be mixed in combination with other liquids is one good reason to make a tincture. It allows for preserved 'fresh' herb materials that would normally be available in the garden at different times of the year to be available for use together, and it preserves the fruits of your labours too!

Making a tincture will also extract the non-water-soluble parts of the plant and break down plant structures to further extract constituents of benefit. This is particularly necessary for herbs with oils such as thyme, lavender and rosemary, for example. Once the tincture has been pressed and filtered, it will have had removed from it the fibrous material of the plant.

Effectively any herb can be converted into a tincture, but tinctures are not appropriate to all therapeutic strategies. The main consideration here is that they contain a significant amount of alcohol, which is in itself warming and stimulating.

Tinctures are thus the preparation of choice for tonics, carminatives and circulatory stimulants and generally any situation where warming and energizing are appropriate.

—Stephen Church

An exception to a preference for tinctures might be the herbal approach to treating coughs and colds that normally involves diaphoretics—to stimulate peripheral circulation and induce sweating. This approach is best performed with a hot infusion, although if necessary a tincture can be taken in hot water.

Making a simple tincture

The herb material must be prepared optimally for tincture making. This is called comminution: The reduction of herbal material to an optimum particle size for e.g., tincture making, by chopping, grinding or shredding.

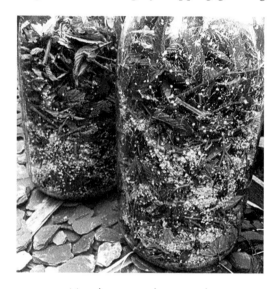

Meadowsweet harvested.

The process for making most tinctures is maceration: defined as the process of submerging and steeping herbal material in a solvent liquid (e.g. diluted alcohol) at room temperature, over a prescribed time period.

Some tinctures are prepared from decoction and percolation rather-than maceration.

Some technical terms: menstruum and marc. Once combined, the solid matter (herbal material) is referred to as the marc, and the solvent (diluted alcohol) as the menstruum. After separation (by pressing and filtering) the menstruum is now a tincture (or extract) the spent marc is usually discarded (composted).

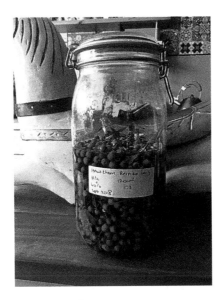

Hawthorn macerating.

Alcohol and water proportions

A liquid with less than 12% alcohol content will 'go off' very soon after being exposed to air, whilst a fortified wine such as sherry (17.5%) will survive a year or more after being un-stoppered, and spirits (34%+) may suffer from evaporation but not an infection. For the majority of tinctures, an alcohol content of 25% is the accepted standard, especially since the addition of the dried herb material will result in an effective lowering of the alcohol to approximately 20%.

Fresh herb material (not dried) will require an absolute minimum of 45% alcohol at the start of the process. It will also require some calculations to estimate the total water content in the weighed fresh herb to ensure the alcohol level does not drop below 20% by the end of the process.

The tincture 'strength' usually refers to the quantity of herb material (marc) in relation to the water/alcohol (menstruum). So that a 1:5 tincture means that 1 part herb has been macerated in 5 parts alcohol/water. The percentage of alcohol to water is then denoted by a percentage sign. If the 1:5 tincture was macerated in alcohol of 45%, then the tincture will be a 1:5 45% tincture.

Making a tincture for your own use

A method for producing half a litre of hawthorn berry tincture.

Crataegus oxycantha L. (hawthorn), fructus (berry), 1:5, 25%

Place 100 g of whole, dried hawthorn berries in a clean glass jar with a wide mouth and sealable lid.

Pour 500 ml of vodka, whisky or brandy, diluted with water to an alcohol content of 25%, over the herb. Seal the jar and shake gently to remove trapped air bubbles. Place the jar in a dark cupboard and leave for 28 days.

Remove and pour into a press* fitted with suitable filter bags. Press to full tension, running the tincture off into a jug; leave for a minute or two, after which it will be found that further pressure can be applied.

Repeat until no further significant amount of tincture can be expressed. If the result is murky you may wish to stand the tincture for a few hours to let the sediment settle before decanting into an amber glass stock bottle.

Note: the yield will be somewhat less than 500 ml, depending on the efficiency of the press, due to fluid remaining in the spent herb.

*If you do not own a small wine press or similar—the most basic method of 'pressing' is to initially strain the macerate through a boiled tea towel or strong muslin cloth in which the remains are then gathered up and wrung out by hand. This will give as good a quality as any other method but an understandably modest yield.

The finished tincture will be called *Crataegus oxycantha fructus* (berry) tincture, 1:5 25%, even though the finished product will have been diluted in the tincture making process (by adding the herb) to approximately 20%.

Using a tincture

Obviously, tinctures contain some alcohol, and this is not appropriate for all persons. However, as it may be seen above, preparation of many tinctures results in a lower alcohol product than it may at first appear.

It is worth remembering that even vinegar has some alcohol, and high quality (naturally fermented) vinegar has many health benefits. Small measured amounts of alcohol are stimulating and beneficial (to most people), and in traditional Chinese medicine, they are seen as being Qi enhancing.

Ultimately, it is all a matter of dose, as larger amounts of alcohol become depressing, and to anyone in a vulnerable state, this could prove helpful or harmful. Where a person shows (or you suspect) addiction to alcohol, then tinctures are not appropriate, however tinctures are not necessarily harmful to liver function, and many trials showing improved liver function of medicinal plants have been conducted using an ethanol (alcohol) extract of the herb. The human body produces alcohol endogenously as part of the fermentation process occurring in the gut microbiota, so our liver has pathways by which modest amounts of alcohol can be metabolised safely. So, watchful common sense should be employed when considering tincture production and use.

If you were going to use your hawthorn berry tincture as a daily 'tonic' for a general circulatory remedy over an extended period of time, you could use a much smaller dose, but simply repeat it daily. So a dose of 5 ml or less on a daily basis, could be helpful to most healthy adults.

In a therapeutic setting, it may be necessary to encourage change to achieve the desired health improvements. A more dynamic, and sometimes heroic, approach to prescribing may be called for. In these circumstances, a medical herbalist may recommend a 5 ml dose of mixed tinctures three or four times per day. In an average adult, the herbs will be processed satisfactorily by the body, and careful monitoring will allow observation that things are moving towards the desired goal. Cessation of herbal therapy is usually the aim, since a return of function and resilience in most cases will maintain the persons' health.

Note: Children and tinctures. Using smaller doses of herbal tinctures for children can be extremely useful, particularly for persistent problems such as digestive or immune system issues. However doing so requires a good relationship between the herbalist, the parent(s) and of course, the young individual themselves.

Enthusing children about the plants in their medicine, and about the ideas behind the treatment usually engages a young person to take part—even if they complain about the taste. Positive parental encouragement, and supervision is vital.

Doses should be roughly reduced by comparing the size of the child to the adult and taking a reduction in dose based on that. There are formulae available, including Clark's Rule and Youngs Rule, which involve calculations based on the weight of the child. Do take into consideration the seriousness and acute/chronic nature of the problem.

Teas can be a cheap and safe way to get herbs into a child, but dilution with fruit juices or other sweetening agents may be required.

Ideally, work with and alongside a qualified practitioner who will want to involve parent and child in the decision process but be able to add in their experience too. Be prepared to have to add herbs for flavour as well as a therapeutic effect. Be prepared to make adaptations to the medicine, and find different modes of taking herbal medicine, if tinctures will not do. Children under the age of 2–3 years should ideally not be using tinctures at all.

Tinctures for the professional

Suppliers to professional herbalists produce tinctures under very strict guidelines and methods required in the UK—Good Management Practice (GMP). They confirm via laboratory methods that the plant is identified correctly and contains a high level of marker compounds, thus assuring freshness of the original herb material and absence of undesirable chemicals such as contaminants.

Note: Marker compounds. The living plant creates its secondary metabolites gradually over the day and over the growing season. Compounds are gradually built up and most of them also begin to decay again as new ones are made.

This means that scientists can identify certain key compounds that are specific to each medicinal plant, which can act both as a measure of optimal harvesting time, and as a measure of the age of any dried herb sample (as compounds slowly degrade over time in dried plant material too). Herb suppliers who have signed up for their product to be tested and certificated in this way (GMP) can confirm authenticity and safety. This does add an extra layer of 'processing' and can make products from these companies slightly more expensive.

In the early 2000s the Medicines and Healthcare Regulatory Agency (MHRA) conducted a UK-wide assessment of herbal products for sale using these methods. They took samples from a number of medical herbalists (including ourselves), from herbalists who made their own tinctures, as well as from several health food shops and other non-practitioner outlets. Interestingly not a single product tested from medical herbalists was found to be below the guideline for marker compounds (and were in fact way above minimum requirements). Several over-the-counter (OTC) companies and health food suppliers were challenged however and GMP was made a requirement for all OTC products sold in the UK. Unfortunately these restrictions do not apply to products purchased via the internet from outside of the UK, and UK enforcement is still only done by random testing and according to MHRA budget.

Cautions and care

No adverse effects or drug-herb interactions are expected from hawthorn used in a positive clinical setting.[17,19] The World Health Organization (WHO) data and web data show a tiny number globally of mild to moderate adverse reactions including dizziness, and digestive changes. These were self limiting however, and not confirmed to be due to hawthorn.[2] There is a theoretical possibility that hawthorn could act synergistically with Digitalis glycosides or with beta-blocker drugs, but this has not been demonstrated[2,19] nor is it our experience in practice.

Summary

Hawthorn can be seen as a true 'tonic' with an affinity for the heart and circulation. You may remember in Chapter 4 we talked about chamomile as being a 'matrix' and general all-rounder for the digestive system. Hawthorn can be seen in a similar way as a regular ingredient in any herbal mixture directed at the heart and circulation. It combines well with any other combination of beneficial herbs. So we might consider combining it with motherwort(*Leonuruscardiaca*L.)

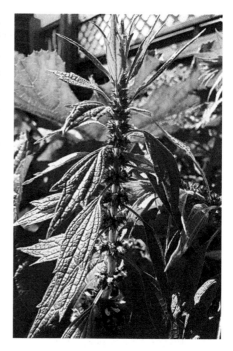

Motherwort
(*Leonurus cardiaca* L.)

in a variety of anxiety or stress situations where palpitations are a feature. Or perhaps combined with lime blossom (*Tilea europaea* L.) to relax and soothe, especially if symptoms occur at night. Hawthorn may also be a key ingredient in venous congestion supporting other venous tonics (supported by research) such as horse chestnut (*Aesculus hippocastanum* L.).

A myriad of possibilities and combinations may be crafted to individualising the prescription.

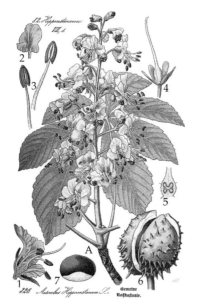

Horsechestnut
(*Aesculus hippocastanum* L.)

Marigold (Calendula officinalis *L.)*

Capturing the sun's rays, this friendly cheery plant ally has a mild and agreeable presence. Although primarily wound healing and anti-infective, it is its capacity for generosity, its tonic effect on the integrity of skin and the tissues beneath such as the lymphatics, that really make marigold irreplaceable as a reliable vulnerary tonic.

Classification

Marigold is a golden member of the Asteraceae family, a family that we looked at in more detail in Chapter 2. Other medicinal examples include daisy (*Bellis perennis* L.), feverfew (*Tanacetum parthenium* L.), yarrow (*Achillea millefolium* L.), and elecampane (*Inula helenium* L.).

Basic botany

Coarsely haired, erect (20–60 centimetres), but not rigid, tending to sprawl, branching and leafy.

- **Leaves** narrow, oblong or paddle-shaped, rather variable in outline: tending to be almost entire.
- **Flowers** large range to yellow flowerheads (4–7 centimetres across) with rays at least twice as long as involucral green bracts. Disc florets much the same colour as the rays but sometimes brownish.
- **Fruits** in this genus come in three shapes; most are boat-shaped, without a pappus of hairs to aid dispersal.
- **Habitat** naturalised in South and West Europe, often found as a weed of vineyards. A frequent casual in the British Isles where it has escaped from gardens.[1]
- **Parts used** petals, flowers and whole inflorescence.
- **Harvesting** harvest whilst plant is in full flower, preferably in the middle of the day. Repeat harvests can be made over many weeks as the plant will keep flowering. Allow some seed to form for more plants next year, as this plant is an annual.

Main constituents

- A common theme within this family of plants (Asteraceae) is the presence of polyfructanes (especially inulin), which are created by the plant as carbohydrate storage (instead of polysaccharides predominantly

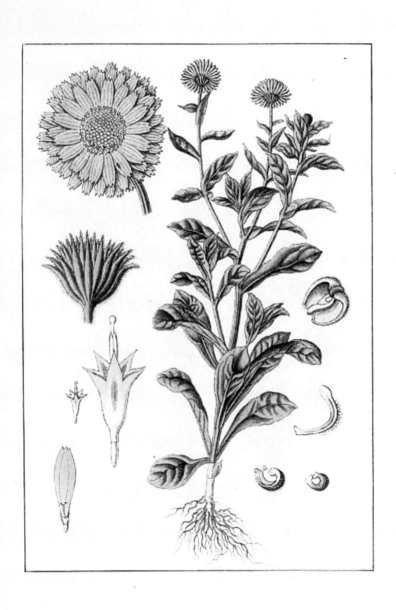

found in perennials). Inulin containing herbs are often used to create coffee substitutes such as chicory root (*Chicorum intybus* L.).

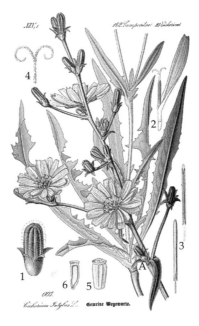

Chicory

- Some members of the Asteraceae accumulate sesquiterpene lactones, which have a significant role in the medicinal effects of feverfew (*Tanacetum parthenium* Sch.Bip.) and arnica (*Arnica Montana* L.) for example.

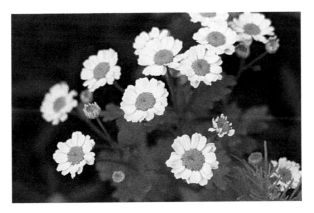

Feverfew

- Calendula flowers specifically contain saponins based on oleanolic acid and have some named after them—calendasaponins A, B, C and D. There are also triterpene pentacyclic alcohols such as faradol, arnidiol, erythrodiol, calenduladiol and heliantriols. These lipophilic (fat-loving) triterpene alcohols are known to act as powerful anti-inflammatories to the skin in particular—including after sun-damage.
- Flavonoids including hyperoside and rutin are present in Calendula.[3] You may remember these specific flavonoids are also found in hawthorn?
- Sesquiterpene and ionone glycosides such as officinosides A, B, C and D, lolioside and arvoside A.
- Glycosides are secondary metabolites found in certain plants, usually not absorbed easily from the digestive tract until the distal ileum or colon. Here they will interact with intestinal microbes to produce a significant anti-inflammatory effect and (as demonstrated in other plants with similar constituents) an array of beneficial outcomes including antioxidant, antidiabetic, anticancer, antiviral, neuroprotective and fat metabolism modulatory activity.[2]
- A volatile oil is present as are an array of polysaccharides. Polysaccharides are associated most often with immunomodulatory effects—such as those found in purple coneflower (*Echinacea purpurea* (L.) Moench).
- Resins—as with other herbs containing resins such as myrrh (*Commiphora mol mol* T Nees, Engl.), frankincense (*Boswellia serrate* Roxb.) and bayberry (*Myrica spp.*), there is a strong antiseptic and stimulating effect on the gastric mucosa which is often employed in oral health for gums and the membranes of the tongue and mouth. Traditionally they have been used for inflammation of the throat, mouth and upper digestive tract, for lymphadenopathy and recurrent infection.

Main therapeutic actions confirmed by research

Anti-inflammatory

Calendula officinalis L. has both anti-inflammatory and antiseptic properties and can help support the microflora balance on the surface of the skin which is now known to play a much more active role in skin health than previously thought. There is some empirical evidence to suggest that Calendula could play a positive role in part of a treatment strategy for patients with methicillin-resistant staphylococcus aureus (MRSA) infection related non-healing wounds.

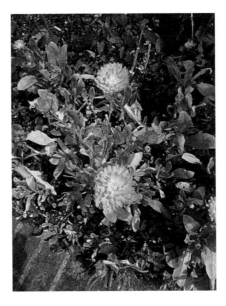

Marigold

Case history

A woman of 32 years old, working as a nurse presented with a 7 centimetres open surgical wound above her right kidney following surgery nearly 5 months previously for a kidney cyst.

She had been rather despondent as the hospital had not been able to get her surgical wound to heal, and she had now tested three times as positive for MRSA. She was otherwise relatively healthy, but had a recent history of recurrent urinary tract infections (UTIs) followed by vaginal thrush due to repeated courses of antibiotics over 3 years (approximately 3–4 infections per year). She worked usually as a registered nurse at the local hospital, and was working long shifts. She slept well except when she worked nights, and she was very worried about returning to work, as she had been off longer than expected, but could not return without a clear MRSA test.

Our strategy was to increase the vitality of her diet (more fresh and raw vegetables, and to avoid modern bread (with fast-action yeast), and sugary foods (she loved sweets). Instead she made garlic and onion soups, sweetened her porridge with prunes and cinnamon, and added linseed. She agreed to make an effort to drink more water (at room temperature or hot), to increase nourishment and restore vitality. The kidney and lung need to be warmed to be resistant to infection.

The herbal prescription was aimed at providing lots of tissue regenerators or tonics and skin wound healing effects (*Calendula officinalis* L.). It was also designed to improve general immunity (*Echinacea purpurea* (L.) Moench and *Calendula*), promote microbiome restoration (*all herbs*), kidney function (via circulation and flow—*Betula pendula* Roth., *Juniperus communis* L. and *Barosma betulina* P.J. Bergiui), prevent urinary tract infection (*Barosma* and *Juniperus*) and include what were perceived to be MRSA effective herbs (*Thuja occidentalis* L.).

Her prescription was in two parts:

A topical application of marigold flower tea which was applied twice daily and left open to the air to dry.

An internal mixture of tinctures:

Echinacea purpurea (root) 1:2	20 ml
Calendula officinalis (flower) 1:2	25 ml
Barosma betulina (leaf) 1:4	20 ml
Betula alba (leaf) 1:4	20 ml
Juniperus communis L. (berry) 1:3	10 ml
Thuja occidentalis L. (leaf) 1:4	10 ml

= 105 ml is taken as 5 ml four times daily in a little warm water.

This lovely lady found the external application to be very soothing. She said she felt it was 'doing her good' even the first time she used it. She had been a little afraid to bathe herself before, but now she felt confident using the marigold wash. She disliked the taste of the herbal mixture, but as she took it as she noticed how warm it made her feel 'that was nice'. She also noticed her urine improved in smell (an unknown symptom and unexpected outcome).

After 3 weeks the wound was nearly sealed right across and it was intact after 5 weeks. She continued with the herbs for 3 more months because she felt it was 'helpful to her whole being', and then she stopped. She returned to work and had not had another UTI throughout the herbal treatment or right up to the last time we spoke nearly a year later.

Epithelialisation and vulnerary agent

An oily extract of calendula and hypericum flower was evaluated for tissue regenerating effect on surgical wounds in 24 women following caesarean section during childbirth in Sardinia and demonstrated reduced surface perimeter of the wound against a control group.[20]

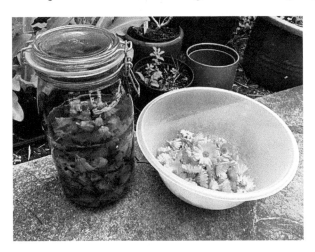

Calendula is a well-known local application for mouth ulcers used by many medical herbalists sometimes combined with other resin-containing herbs such as myrrh, or even the bee product propolis. It should be noted that Western medical herbalists recognise liver distress (usually excess heat/choler), as a causative factor in mouth ulcers and so an internal strategy addressing the liver is likely to be employed concurrently. Other common applications of Calendula flowers include as a facial wash for acne vulgaris and as a post-labour bath for mother and baby.

Anti-cancer effects

A traditional approach to people who have or are survivors of cancer begins with a general aim to support the patient with heightened nutrition via vegetable and plant means. Many plants have shown repeatedly good anti-cancer effects particularly the onion, cabbage, Apiaceae and nightshade families and edible fungi. A strong influence in traditional herbal medicine, particularly in Europe, is towards a naturopathic approach to elimination and cleansing and therefore linseed (*Linum ussittatissumum* L.), psyllium seed (*Plantago ovata* Forssk.) and slippery elm bark powder (*Ulmus fulva* Michx.) would all be indicated here.[2]

Mills and Bone state that:

> *The overwhelming instinct through history is to see cancer as an indication for cleansing … In the nature clinics of central Europe, often alpine establishments dedicated originally to the treatment of tuberculosis but switching increasingly to cancer management as the former condition diminished, the emphasis was on strict diets, invigorating hydrotherapy treatments and alternative herbal formulations. The latter might include (depending on other indications):*
>
> > *Arctium lappa (burdock)*
> > *Calendula officinalis L. (marigold)*
> > *Galium aparine L. (cleavers)*
> > *Phytolacca decandra (Syn americana L.) (poke root)*
> > *Rumex acetosella L. (sheep's sorrel)*
> > *Rumex crispus L. (yellow dock root)*
> > *Taraxacum officinale (aggr. F.H. Wigg) (dandelion)*
> > *Thuja occidentalis L. (arbor-vitae)*
> > *Trifolium pratense L. (red clover flowers)*
> > *Urtica dioica L. (nettle)*
> > *Viola odorata L. (sweet violet)*
> > *Viola tricolor L. (heartsease)*
>
> —S. Mills and K. Bone[2]

They go on to add that similar approaches are comparable in strategy within Traditional Chinese Medicine, and in the popular approaches to come out of North America (gleaned from First Nations peoples) including the Essiac formula.

Whatever doubts about efficacy, there is at least a consistency of approach here, albeit obscured by the occasional promotion of specific products for sale such as apricot kernels etc. These sit uneasily as 'alternative' culture competing directly with conventional chemotherapy.[2] It is a reminder that it is not legal to claim to treat cancer throughout the European Union. Any Western medical herbalist will in any case want to treat the person not the disease but will inevitably find themselves in a legally unsupported position when treating a patient with cancer, and will

approach the task with humility and a recognition that in most cases,
the treatment course will be set without a compass or a map.

—S. Mills and K. Bone[2]

It is often the case that herbalists can provide valuable support for patients undergoing rigorous biomedical treatments for cancer, both by helping to reduce the discomfort of the various side effects experienced as a result of treatments and by using herbs such as adaptogens to optimise physiological coping strategies. These approaches may be vastly helpful in terms of quality of life, and recovery after treatment.

Methods of preparation

As you have already seen marigold flowers are commonly prepared as an infusion and employed externally and internally, often at the same time. Marigold flowers can be preserved as a herb vinegar, and these are ideal to use in the bath for recurrent vaginitis and thrush. (See herb vinegars and oxymels in Chapter 8). Marigolds are made into two types of tincture. One, to extract more resinous compounds, is a high alcohol tincture and should be used for short-term use only if used internally, or in small doses.

More commonly, a lower strength alcohol (25%) tincture is made of fresh marigold inflorescences to extract the flavonoid and glycoside components more effectively. This is used internally as part of a prescription, often for wound healing, recurrent infection and lymphatic drainage. Marigold flowers can also be made into an infused oil. These are best done from the dried flowers or at least semi-dried. Also, ideally the oil and flowers will be warmed at the lowest possible temperature, over 3 days, then squeezed out and poured into a clean, sterile bottle, avoiding any darker brown 'blobs' resulting from any possible 'watery' component getting into the oil.

In Chapter 4 we demonstrated making an infused oil with fresh lemon balm leaves. Marigold flowers and lavender flowers lend themselves well to being made into an infused oil from dried flowers, and with a longer infusing time. This oil can then be transformed into an ointment by adding a setting agent—traditionally beeswax. An ointment is an oil-based (not water-based) external semi-solid preparation and is fairly stable with beeswax at room temperature for about 18 months. Use your ointment to make another interesting and traditional preparation, a plaister—for use in acute or 'stuck' conditions.

A plaister is a medicated bandage or dressing left in contact with the skin for many hours.

Cautions and care

Calendula is extremely well tolerated and not associated with any particular side effects or concerns.

Summary: the central role of marigold as a wound healer and skin tonic

Marigolds are a healing, antiseptic, anti-inflammatory external preparation *par excellence*, and have no irritating or negative effects. They are gentle and soft and ideal for raw open wounds including immediately after childbirth. They are safe for babies and children, and for teenage skin. Their exceptional array of well-researched phytoconstituents backs up traditional and modern practice, including their helpfulness in relieving congestive skin problems due to lymphatic insufficiency such as in breast tissue, and facial tissues.

Marigolds are ideal for softening and complementing internal healing mixtures of herbs where other more 'targeted' herbs can be used alongside. So, as we saw in the case history, marigold appears alongside more targeted herbs for the kidney and to address MRSA infection.

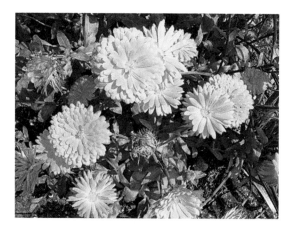

Marigolds

Lime blossom *(*Tilia x europea *L. and* Tilia cordata *Mill.)*

Linden—heady syrupy ecstasy, lie back to the hum of bees, sink into the per-
fumed embrace. Tilia has gentle power to enter via our olfactory centre straight
into our brain and help us trust our heart to relax. From softness comes
strength. With relaxation comes mental vigour. Acceptance brings healing.

Classification

Linden or lime blossom trees belong in their very own Tiliaceae, lime tree
family. The Tiliaceae is a largely tropical family which is a source of timber and fibre, Jute (*Corchorus capsularis* L.) being one example. The inner
bark, often fibrous and mucilaginous, is known as bast, which accounts
for the name given to some American trees that are a source of fibre—
Basswood. Otzi, 'the iceman' whose mummified remains were found in

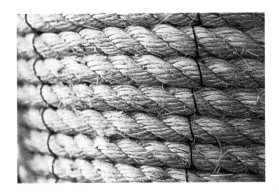

the mountains of Europe had a variety of useful tools and clothing items,
and lime bast was identified as the source of some rope he had with him.
   There is no connection whatsoever with the citrus lime fruit.

Basic botany

Large-leaved lime (*Tilia platyphyllos* Scop.) and small-leaved lime
(*Tilia cordata* Mill.) as well as common lime (*Tilia x vulgaris, Tiliea x*
europea L.)—which is thought to be a hybrid of the first two—are all
used. All three species are quite similar being large or very large deciduous trees—at their tallest Tila grow to around 46 metres, which is the
tallest non-coniferous species found in Europe.

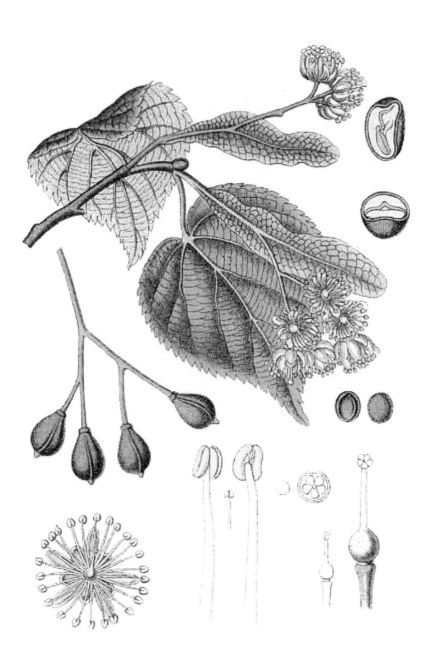

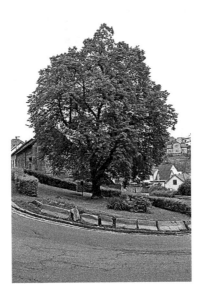

- **Leaf** a similar shade of green on both sides. More or less heart-shaped leaves with toothed margins. It can be asymmetrical at the base. Leaves appear in late April on long stalks that are alternate, sometimes in small rows.
- **Flowers** the heavily scented sweet flowers are in small clusters whose common stalk is attached to a long papery dull yellow-coloured bract. This is shed later with the flowers to aid dispersal. The flower itself, rich with nectar has sepals and petals in fives, they are pale yellow with many bunched stamens. Bees can often be found in profusion around this tree at flowering time, so much so that this tree may be found by listening.
- **Habitat** it is not native to Britain, but much planted and naturalised. Common throughout France through to some Mediterranean countries.
- **Parts used** the greeny-yellow inflorescence, including the bract.
- **Harvesting** harvest flowers early, when the first flowers in each cluster have opened, they are highly perfumed and somewhat sticky.

You will often find tea and teabags freely available as a popular beverage throughout Europe especially France, Greece and Spain where it can be known as lime flower, lime blossom, linden, Tilia and tilleulle.

Main constituents

- Volatile oils (including linalool, germacrene, geraniol, 1,8 cineole, 2-phenyl ethanol and others).
- Flavonoids (hesperidin, quercetin, astragalin, and tiliroside).
- Saponins and tannins.
- Phenolic acids such as chlorogenic, caffeic and benzoic acids.
- Mucilage of arabinose, galactose and rhamnose polysaccharides.

Main therapeutic actions confirmed by research

Diaphoretic

Lime flowers have a long traditional history of use for fevers, coughs, colds catarrh and influenza. They are used as a herbal infusion taken hot to induce diaphoresis (sweating), and as we saw from the section on hawthorn, diaphoresis induces an effect to the microcirculation in a similar way to elderflowers (*Sambucus nigra* L. flores).

As described earlier, the importance of circulation in herbal medicine cannot be underestimated. In particular, with the wide range of peripheral vasodilators available to the herbalist, Tilia included, we can see how the mechanism of diaphoresis is actually addressing the peripheral circulation and quite likely the blood flow to the kidney. Despite a general lack of research in this area, Tilia is thought to act as a mild diuretic too, thus aiding the treatment of hypertension (high blood pressure) as part of a considered approach.

Case history

A 70-year-old gentleman came along to seek help with hypertension which, despite two conventional medications (taken for approximately 10 years) perindopril (an ACE inhibitor) and a loop diuretic furosemide, remained above the ideal. His readings (on his medication) were on average 155/92 mmHg. He was mainly well, although extremely anxious in his manner. His main complaint apart from the blood pressure reading was that he was permanently dry of mouth, and felt quite low a lot of the time.

We agreed he should start using some herbal medicine alongside his conventional medication; although he was also hoping to stop his medicine he was too anxious to do so. In any case, it would be unwise to start withdrawal from a long-term conventional therapy without knowing the patient well, and before seeing how the patient responds to herbal treatment. We started with a simple prescription, a tincture of three herbs:

Rx
Passiflora incarnata L. 1:3   35 ml
Hypericum perforatum L. 1:2   35 ml
Tilia x europaea L. 1:2   35 ml
= 105 ml to be taken 5 ml three times daily.

After the first 6 weeks the patient returned, he was disappointed he said because his blood pressure readings looked much the same. He had kept meticulous records thankfully. This was most disappointing to him because he knew he felt a lot better, and he was visibly much calmer and more cheerful. He was particularly pleased with the advice that he should be kinder to himself from the first appointment, and this had for some reason resonated with him.

On checking his recorded blood pressures there was only a very slight downward trend in his blood pressure reading to an average of 148/90, but significantly his pulse rate had reduced markedly and definitively from an average of 86 beats per minute (bpm), to around 74 bpm. He was delighted at realising this, having not noticed at first, and so he happily continued his prescription for another 6 weeks. At the second follow-up, his blood pressure had also reduced to an average of 136/86 and his pulse was still in the low 70s.

He had experienced no negative effects, he was still feeling happier and well, and his mouth was much less dry. He had spoken to his doctor about stopping his conventional medication—and his doctor had (probably in a very difficult position) said, 'yes you can but I wouldn't advise it'. We aimed therefore to work together, keeping his doctor informed and slowly reducing his medications, one at a time, and under regular monitoring. His blood pressure continued to improve, and at his last appointment the average was 126/82 mmHg.

Sedative

The mucilages in *Tilia spp* adhere to the digestive tract and epithelial tissues and produce a demulcent effect. This is relaxing to the nervous system and induces a sensation via biofeedback messages to the central nervous system of calm. It has been suggested that Tilia acts on gamma-amino butyric acid (GABA) receptors in the central nervous system (the same mechanism of action as such pharmaceutical tranquil-lizing drugs as benzodiazepines). This would, in part, explain Tilia's actions in aiding relaxation and reducing anxiety. Tilia is non-toxic however and no side effects have been reported.[3]

Antispasmodic

As either a beneficial side effect of reducing anxiety or as a direct effector of muscular spasm, Tilia has a long history of use throughout Europe as a spasmolytic as well as an anxiolytic. Traditionally large doses of Tilia were consumed, and large-dose, long-term therapy is well tolerated especially as infused teas. A commonly held position is that mucilages presented to the gut will aid muscle relaxation and reduce tension by reflex. Certainly the opposite is true, as people experiencing regular or acute anxiety will often have corresponding digestive effects involving spasm of muscle—either constipating or causing urgent evacuation.

Nervine tonic and trophorestorative

Herbal medicine has had to adapt from its traditional roots, particularly in the case of mental health and perspectives on anxiety and depres-sion. Traditional concepts of neurasthenia encompassed a very wide range of disorders including nervous exhaustion, but also what we would more precisely in our language today describe as specific anxi-ety states, depression and so on. Nevertheless the idea that the nervous system itself could benefit from a 'tonic', and a 'trophorestorative' has remained strong in Western herbal medicine.

Tilia could be included in a list of nervous system trophorestoratives that would almost certainly include oat flower (*Avena sativa* L.), passion-flower (*Passiflora incarnata* L.), St John's wort (*Hypericum perforatum* L.), skullcap (*Scutellaria altissimo/lateriflora* L.), valerian root (*Valeriana offici-nalis* L.) and vervain (*Verbena officinalis* L.). Indeed the idea of convales-cence is also an important idea within Western herbal medicine, but is increasingly difficult to achieve in our modern Western lifestyles.

Tilia presents us with many possibilities to support the process of convalescence by suggesting a sweating (diaphoresis) cure for our infec-tions (not easy if you are still on the go), and by suggesting convalescent and therefore immune system 'tonic' effects by relaxation of our digestive and nervous systems. By relaxing the peripheral circulation

Note: The concept of tonic

Tonics have the ability to provide 'the pan-optimisation of functionality of biological systems'. They may support discrete or individual systems, or provide overall support for the totality of the living being.

—Mary Tassell

From a traditional Western herbal medicine viewpoint, and in particular from the physio-medical approach, a tonic was able to trophically restore nutrition and therefore the function of an organ, a tissue, or an area of the body by optimising both circulatory and vasomotor function to that area. Improving the elimination of waste products of normal metabolism was also a key method of providing a 'tonic' effect. The concept of vitality was also fundamental in the assessment of a person's wellbeing and capacity to manage and eliminate disease processes, and herbal therapy was also aimed at enhancing innate vitality.[9]

Tilia takes pressure off the heart and so acts as a 'tonic' to the heart and circulation. No wonder lime blossom was Maurice Messegue's first and favourite bathing herb to use for aiding deep recovery!

Insomnia

This is another potential use for Tilia tea or tincture. Due to its safety, long-term use of Tilia—perhaps combined with chamomile (*Matricaria chamomilla* L.) or lavender (*Lavandula angustifolia* Mill.) for example could prove beneficial to those with a tendency to insomnia. In fact we find that Tilia can be a useful ingredient in sleep mixtures for women experiencing sleep disturbance and night sweats.

Headaches

Headaches are one of those key symptoms that it is difficult to offer good advice about before more is known about the case. Headaches can be related to just about any other part of the body and occasionally are a sign of more serious disease. Tilia can be very helpful in reducing the frequency of headaches caused by nervous tension or by insomnia for instance. But headaches that do not respond to treatment, herbal or otherwise, should be investigated thoroughly for their origin.

Methods of preparation and use

The flower and bract are usually made into an infusion and taken as a drink either hot or cold.

It is also traditionally used as a bathing herb and can be used for young children or in pregnancy with complete safety. A foot bath is a fabulous way to experience Tilia as an external preparation, and a foot-bath is a common and significant ritual across the world. Tilia flowers can be made into a tincture, which should be left to macerate for long enough to produce a reddish, syrupy consistency. The bark is anti-inflammatory, astringent and demulcent, and has been used to make anti-inflammatory poultices.

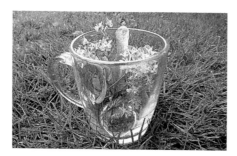 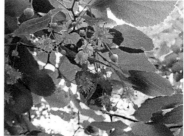

Cautions and care

Tilia is extremely well tolerated and not associated with any particular side effects or concerns.

Summary

Tilia is an under-investigated but extremely commonly used herb of great service to the lay-person and practitioner alike. It is well-tolerated, moistening, softening, generally soothing and is complementary to many other nervous system herbs such as *Melissa officinalis* L., *Valeriana officinalis* L. or *Passiflora incarnata* L. It also combines well with other herbs (for example elderflower) for common colds especially with fever. It is complementary to and commonly used to improve poor peripheral circulation (with for example hawthorn *Crataegus spp*). It is slow acting and can be taken in large doses over long periods of time.

Lavender (Lavandula angustifolia L.)

Lavender is mainly familiar to us for aiding relaxation and sleep. Time spent in contemplation with this familiar garden friend, might remind us of its semi-evergreen upright habit. This inner strength can help melt away our own resistance to change, clear melancholy and restore clarity. The joyful aroma seductively banishes any liverishness and reduces inflammation and spasm, even in acute situations.

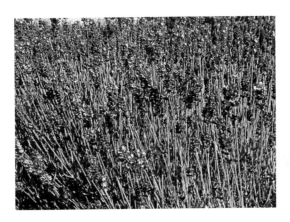

Classification

Lavender is a member of the touchy-feely Lamiaceae family. Who cannot resist brushing their fingers through lavender, rosemary, mint, thyme and many other Lamiaceae plants? This family are largely aromatic plants whose volatile oils contribute enormously to their antspasmodic effects. These volatile oils act as sedatives and relaxants, anti-catarrhals and febrifuges, stomachics and expectorants and their constituents have been greatly studied. Research has confirmed traditional use for many of these aromatic plants as endocrine (hormonal) regulators, and as powerful antimicrobials.

Basic botany

Barker[1] states that seven lavenders are detailed in the Flora Europaea and three of these are regarded as significant to human needs for medicine and perfumery. These are the 'true' lavenders (often derived from *Lavandula angustifolia* Mill.), 'spike' lavender (*Lavandula latifolia* Medic.)

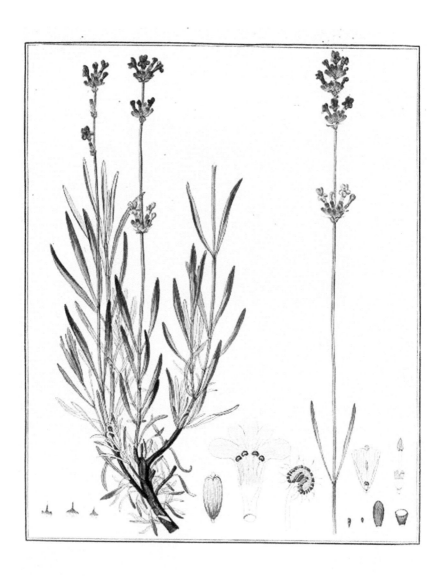

and 'French' lavender (*Lavandula stoechas* L.). There are many cultivars and dwarf forms that are popular horticulturally. Lavender has been one of the most popular herbs of ancient medicinal usage. Both herbs have antiseptic and spasmolytic capacity, although lavender should be regarded as having a more sedative and less stimulating edge than rosemary.

Lavandula angustifolia Mill., (also known as *Lavandula officinalis* Chaix and *Lavandula vera* DC) is very commonly used in Western herbal medicine and will be described here.

- **Leaves** small, simple, opposite and entire. Foliage is grey/green.
- **Stems** erect, square cross-section, hairy.
- **Flowers** Blue/purple in colour. The petals/sepals are fused into a cup or tube, which is bilaterally symmetrical The flowers are arranged on loose spikes.
- **Habitat** dry, stony places in the Mediterranean. Prefers sunny, well-drained open position on chalky soil.[21] Similar to rosemary (*Rosmarinus officinalis* L.) it is also capable of growing in arid limestone outcrops in Europe, as well as the northern wetter climates.
- **Parts used** flowers, flowering spikes and upper leaves.
- **Harvesting** collect on a hot sunny day, earlier rather than later.

Main constituents

Much (but not all) of the research on lavender involves specifically the investigation of the essential oil, and its use in aromatherapy, internally or externally. It is important to not reduce lavender to only its essential oil, which although valuable and reliably medicinally active, is only part of the story.

Essential oils are made by most members of this family, in the epidermal glands of the leaves. Accumulation of monoterpene glycosides (iridoids) including linalool, caffeic acids and other acids are known to have pharmacological importance as antivirals and anti-inflammatory agents. Mild bitters and therapeutic tannins are found in the whole plant. Miscellaneous triterpenes such as ursolic acid, and flavonoids such as luteolin are also found.

Main therapeutic actions confirmed by research

Antispasmodic

Like other members of this family, lavender is thought to affect GABA receptors as well as calcium channels and thus exhibits sedative, antispasmodic and anxiolytic effects.[22,23]

Antidepressant

Studies have shown antidepressant activity and a decrease in autonomic nervous system arousal, and patients have responded well to lavender essential oil when monitored for wellbeing whilst undergoing difficult medical procedures. Lavender tea has also been used to good effect alongside orthodox drugs in the treatment of depression.[24,25]

Cholagogue and choleretic

Bitters within the whole lavender leaf and flower act as antispasmodics to the gall bladder and exert an anti-inflammatory effect within the gall bladder itself, within the duodenum where bile acids are secreted, and also in the liver which may serve to counter possible 'backflow'—or hepatobiliary damage.

Although stimulating bile flow has been one of the traditional strategies of Western herbal medicine in aiding adequate elimination, modern research on plants such as lavender and to a greater extent, turmeric (*Curcuma longa* L.), artichoke (*Cynara scolymus* L.) and other traditional choleretics and cholagogues such as the *Berberis* species, has shown that actually there may be many other effects taking place.[2] Lavender in particular may have a relaxing and anti-inflammatory effect in the 'enterohepatic' cycle, thus correcting this flow from the liver into bile duct into gall bladder into the gut, it is possible to influence not just the local area, but also chronic constipation, migraine, acne rosacea, inflammatory bowel disease, dysbiosis, chronic skin diseases, and autoimmune diseases.[2]

You may remember in Chapter 5 we explored the idea of ideal digestion from an ancient humoural perspective. This suggested that over-activity of digestive fire (choler) as well as under-activity (leading to phlegm or melancholy) can be influenced by food and by herbs. *Lavandula officinalis* L. could be seen as correcting digestive fire and therefore resulting in a carminative effect, reducing spasm, but aiding the function of the gut, its nervous system and its microbiome.

As also explored in Chapter 5, much of what we call allergy today is strongly linked to a disordered microbiome. Once again, lavender can play a valuable role here both in controlling overreactions of the skin (topically), and by correcting dysbiosis internally.

Anxiolytic and antispasmodic via the nervous system

Lavandula sp is often used for anxiety, headaches, migraine, nausea, vertigo, flatulent dyspepsia, colic and insomnia.[24,26,27] The linalool content of the essential oil has been identified as having specific action here on the central nervous system, via inhalation.[28] It should be remembered though that this is only part of the picture in terms of lavenders overall mechanisms of action. Headaches and migraine of a 'liver' origin (a Western herbal medicine concept), will respond well to lavender, or to other relaxing herbs with a liver/gall bladder/digestive effect.

Lavender also exhibits diuretic and diaphoretic potential suggesting a peripheral circulatory relaxation effect. Therefore it may be included in treatments for hypertension in agitated individuals, coughing fits, asthma, and following trauma.

This relaxing circulatory effect can result in longer-term regeneration and therefore lavender can be considered as a 'tonic' for the nervous system.[29]

Anti-inflammatory, vulnerary, rubefacient

Externally lavender can be used as a rubefacient in a similar way to rosemary (*Rosmarinus officinalis* L.). This technique involves application of the herb to the skin either with massage, or by heat and is ideal for rheumatic pain, or joint pain as it brings circulation to the area. Wonderfully, and seemingly paradoxically, lavender can cool inflammation and irritation such as swollen insect bites. It may also be applied to infected wounds and bruises, and Barker notes that he has even:

> *Used the essential oil successfully for infections of bone which have become resistant to massive doses of anti-biotics.*
>
> —Julian Barker[21]

One study showed improved healing of episiotomy scars with applications of lavender.[30]

Methods of preparation and use

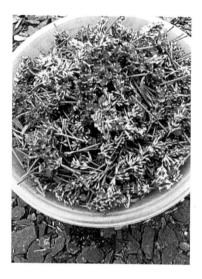

Lavender harvesting.

Lavender may be taken as a tisane, and is surprisingly pleasant to drink even when feeling nauseous or 'headachy'. The infusion can be applied to the skin hot or cold as a compress, to calm inflammation. It works wonders on insect bites, and is ideal for those who do not react in expected ways, for example, in the overreactions of allergy often seen in the case of diabetics. Lavender may be administered as an inhalation, avoiding oral administration. This can be extremely useful in certain circumstances.

Lavender is often distilled into an essential oil where there will be a removal of some of its constituents, and a concentration of others. Lavender essential oil (organic and high quality) can be applied undiluted to the skin, avoiding the eye area. Lavender can be made into a tincture, and used in herbal mixtures. Many possibilities of external application are possible including baths, ointments, plaisters, creams, oils and so on. You might want to try this simple recipe and treat your skin to a soothing and healing lavender and oatmeal wash.

Lavender and oatmeal bath sachet

Ingredients:

- A small glass jar or a muslin square or bag (see notes below)
- Five parts oatmeal (organic oats or oat flakes will do)
- One part dried organic lavender flowers

If you do not have oatmeal to hand, grind your oat-flakes or oats in a clean, dry food processor. Stir in the lavender flowers and mix gently. Place into a clean dry glass jar for use later and label.

Place a handful of the lavender oat mixture into a muslin bag or make your own muslin pouch. Muslin can be purchased from a haberdasher and sometimes from kitchen shops. Maybe you have some old cotton sheets that can be re-purposed into squares of approximately 20 centimetres squared. You will need some cotton string to tie the square. Simply place the oatmeal and lavender onto the centre of the square, gather the four corners and tie securely.

To use: Place your muslin bag into bath water whilst it is running. Allow the oatmeal and lavender to soften and squeeze gently from time to time to release the milky lavender—oat juice. Apply the pouch directly as a poultice if necessary.

Cautions and care

Lavender is extremely well tolerated and, despite extensive research (particularly of the essential oil), is not associated with any particular side effects or concerns.

Summary

One of our best-loved aromatic plants, lavender possesses hugely beneficial medicinal properties and can be used both internally and externally. Its key actions involve antispasmodic, anti-inflammatory and anxiolytic activity, making it of huge benefit for chronic conditions where pain, stiffness and inflammation are at play. Its relaxing and calming actions also mean that it can be employed where restlessness, headaches and insomnia are an issue. Backed up by plenty of research, safe and effective, lavender often forms an indispensable part of the herbal dispensary.

Nettle (Urtica dioica L.)

The presence of nettles almost everywhere, even in the most industrial of locations, reminds us of nettle's long association with humankind and its willingness to stay with us. It weaves its way into the fabric of the Earth, and also within us, getting right down to cellular level and helping the flow of nutrients in, waste products out. A tonic for every fibre of our being. Thank you nettle for your smarting reminder of our nature!

Classification

Nettles are members of the Urticaceae family, a tropical and temperate family of herbs and shrubs that includes the Stinging Trees of Australia, as well as the humble but very useful pellitory of the wall (*Parietaria diffusa* Mert & Koch) found on city walls and cliffs alike, throughout Europe.

Basic botany

Dull green, unbranched perennial 30–150 centimetres herb covered in stinging hairs. Spreads vigorously by tough yellowish rooting shoots forming patches of either male or female plants.

- **Leaves** opposite, saw-toothed, cordate; stipules—four. Covered with stinging hairs.
- **Flowers** nettles have male and female flowers on separate plants. The male flowers grow in small loose clusters near the top of the plants. The female flowers grow in long catkin-like clusters.
- **Habitat** a ubiquitous plant often found at boundaries, near buildings and walls, ditches, riverbanks and stream sides. Areas associated with habitation. Found everywhere.
- **Parts used** leaves and stems, roots (specific for benign prostatic hyperplasia), seeds and fibres.
- **Harvesting** harvest leaves in early spring before flowering. If nettle tops are repeatedly cut they will produce new shoots which you can harvest throughout the summer months. Use scissors to cut and lift into harvesting bag. Wear gloves if you are concerned about being stung. Harvest roots primarily in autumn, although they may be harvested any time.

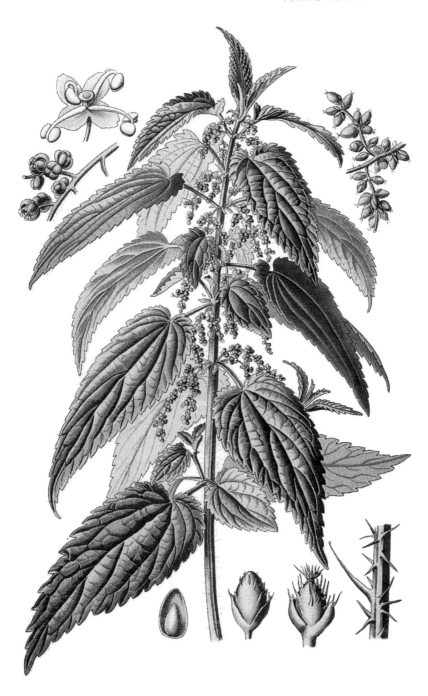

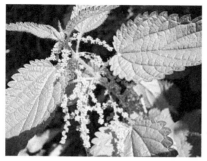
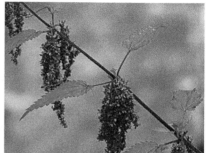

Male nettle flowers.   Female nettle flowers.

Main constituents

In the leaves and stinging hairs:

- Flavonol glycosides, especially rutin.[31]
- Sterols, scopoletin, chlorophyll in high yields, carotenoids.
- Vitamins including C, B group, and K. Protein.
- Various minerals, and a rich source of silicon.
- Plant phenolic acids.
- Amines are found within the stinging hairs (including histamine, serotonin, and acetylcholine). Amines are a common compound found in the structure of hormones. Hormones are made from three key compounds—either: amines, peptides or steroids.

NB: The hairs are effectively fine silicon glass needles. You can see very clearly the stinging needles in this picture below of nettle in frost.

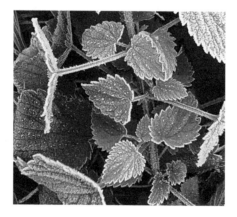

Nettle's stinging hairs dissolve in tinctures and with heat, during the preparation of an infusion or a soup, for example.

In the roots:

- Sterols and steryl glycosides including sitosterol, and lignans—all now thought to act as selective oestrogen receptor modulators.
- Lectin (agglutinin).
- Phenylpropanes, polyphenols and polysaccharides.
- The coumarin scopoletin.

Main therapeutic actions confirmed by research

Astringent and haemostatic

Rutin, a flavanol glycoside, is a well-known blood vessel integrity enhancer, and Vitamin K is thought to be responsible for the styptic action of nettle leaf.

Nettle is a traditional remedy for nose bleeds, and also as part of a strategy for excessive uterine bleeding. We have found that it can result in reduced menstrual bleeding in cases where it was excessive. Also anecdotally, it been identified as the ingredient in a herbal prescription that stopped mild but persistent haematuria (blood in the urine). This is interesting because pellitory of the wall (*Parietaria diffusa* Mert & Koch) is a close relative of nettle and is used traditionally across Europe to arrest kidney stone formation and also treat the results of kidney stone problems; bleeding, inflammation and reduced kidney function.

As we can see nettle is used in traditional phytotherapy to stop bleeding, but it also has a traditional use for 'building blood' or increasing the vigour of the blood via not just iron, and nutrients, but in a more dynamic and vitalistic sense. With such an abundance of nutrients including chlorophyll that can be transformed into blood products, there is a strong theoretical mechanism behind that concept—and it has been suggested that nettle may be haemopoietic—aiding the growth of new healthy red blood cells (erythrocytes).[32]

Many modern phytotherapists would agree that nettle is a gentle and subtle adaptogenic agent. It allows improved elimination yet also acts as a nutrient and supportive agent. Adaptogens improve our capacity to adapt and to cope with changes. Those changes may be internal or external, but at all stages of life we are called upon to adapt to change. Wellbeing can increase our likelihood of adapting successfully.

Essentially, adaptogens help us to live with greater mental and physical endurance and vitality, while mitigating the cost of stressors and building our reserves through enhancing our regenerative (anabolic) capacities.
—Donald Yance[33]

Diuretic

Nettle is a traditional herb included in treatments for gout, and so the diuretic action has the addition of a tendency to eliminate uric acid.

In addition nettle is often considered to be a 'tonic' for the eliminative organs of the kidney and liver. Antioxidant activity and improved liver function have also been demonstrated (under laboratory conditions). Thus it was considered a prime ingredient in herbal mixtures regarded as 'blood purifiers' (older words that describe this would be aperient or depurative). Nettle is used worldwide as an effective skin 'tonic' and is often a base ingredient of prescriptions aimed at easing burns, skin rashes, urticaria, eczema, acne and other skin conditions. One preliminary study showed antibacterial and anti-inflammatory effects from a herbal preparation for acne, that included nettle.[34]

Increasing activity of the kidney is a key concept of Western herbal medicine in the treatment of arthritis and rheumatism. Nettle has a long history of use as an anti-arthritic and this could suggest one mechanism of action.

Anti-allergic and anti-inflammatory

Nettle leaf is supported by clinical trial data as being useful in treating allergic rhinitis.[35-37] These studies demonstrate that nettle leaf acts as an anti-inflammatory with a broad activity, including the inhibition of pro-inflammatory prostaglandins. Much of the data on the capacity of nettle to act as a general anti-inflammatory comes from an array of research papers looking at specific compounds found in abundance in nettle such as the phenolic and caffeic acids, and flavonoids.

It has been demonstrated that other mechanisms have further anti-inflammatory effects and can reduce symptoms of colitis. As a vulnerary to digestive membranes, there is an increased likelihood that the microbiome will be better established. This in turn is likely to reduce allergic conditions, and improve immunity generally.

Numerous positive studies have been conducted on nettle with regard to reducing painful arthritis symptoms. Some have focussed on the counter-irritation effects of the application of the stinging plant over the joints affected (ouch!), whilst other studies have involved the more commonly used approach of taking nettle extract internally.

Antiscorbutic

Due to high levels of vitamin and amine derivatives, it is likely that nettle acts to increase vitamin C levels. Its anti-inflammatory effect on the digestive mucosa and enhancement of liver and kidney function may also increase the capacity to absorb minerals. In Chapter 2 we considered the effect of tannins and how excessive tea drinking could potentially inhibit the absorption of iron. Drinking nettle tea may help reduce the consumption of regular tea and also provide a rich source of vitamin C and iron at the same time. As you may remember, vitamin C enhances the absorption of iron across the wall of the gut. Thus fabulous nettle provides us with an excellent example of pharmacokinetic synergy, where one substance acts on another to alter its movements, and influences its final concentration in our systems.

Nettle is safe and ideal for consumption as a food or as a medicine in pregnancy. Nettle is also considered to be a mild galactagogue meaning it has the capacity to improve breast milk production and quality.

Antioxidant and apoptotic effects

Recent research investigating nettle extract and its effect on breast cancer cell lines, found in vitro anti-proliferative effects, indicating a potentially valuable role for nettle in the treatment of breast cancer.[38] Antioxidant effects supported by increased catalase production have also been proven by research.[39]

Mildly hypoglycaemic

Data on nettle and its capacity to reduce blood glucose levels and act as an antidiabetic agent are contradictory, but may have more to do with design problems of the research itself. Recent research however, appears to be underpinning the concept of a potentially important role for nettle in the management of type two diabetes.[40,41]

Nettle has shown antifungal activity—useful in cases where patients are diabetic or exhibiting glucose intolerance and thus prone to fungal infections.[42]

Benign prostatic hyperplasia (BPH)

BPH involves the benign enlargement of the prostate gland in men. There have been some positive studies showing that nettle root can have good effects in men with BPH.[43,44]

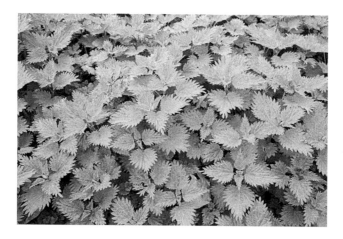

Methods of preparation and use

Nettles can be prepared as a delicious and fortifying food. Nettles are best gathered before flowering and in the early spring. Collection of the upper leaves and soft stems is ideal. Nettle seed can be collected later in the year and incorporated as a high protein food. Nettle roots should be harvested in the very early spring before the plants have grown more than a few centimetres in height. Nettles can be made into an infusion from the fresh nettle tops or by drying them and storing them for later use.

Nettle tincture can be prepared or, using a juice extractor, a nettle juice can be made in the spring. Some companies sell a bottled nettle juice for medicinal use (e.g., Salus UK, Phytoproducts UK). Now you have been amazed by the sheer versatility and healing powers of humble nettle, you may wish to self-medicate at some point using the simple recipe below.

Mixed wild leaves pesto

Ingredients:

- Fresh wild nettles 1 cup
- parmesan cheese (grated) 1 cup
- walnuts 1/3 cup
- wild garlic leaves 1 cup
- parsley/coriander 1 cup
- extra virgin olive oil 1/2 cup
- lemon juice (optional)
- sea salt and pepper

Blend all the ingredients in a food processor and keep in a sealed jar in the fridge. Use on pasta, as a salad dressing, on roasted vegetables or fish. Keeps well for 48 hours. In the winter months, swap the green leaves for soft kale leaves or watercress—it's lovely!

Cautions and care

Nettles are extremely well-tolerated and are not associated with any particular side effects or concerns. Nettle stings are of course another story!

Summary

The central role of this food-like herb in herbal medicine shows itself at all stages of life.

It is of great value as a re-mineraliser. But also has a quality recognised in traditional herbal medicine as being a 'blood builder'— meaning more than just nutrition, but also the formation of blood and its capacity to nourish cells and ultimately the tissues bathed in the products of blood, such as joints and skin.

> *This is a plant whose therapeutic use is difficult to convey by its physiological actions alone.*
>
> —Julian Barker[1]

Nettle can be added as an adjunct to prescriptions due to its capacity to be both nutrient and cleansing at the same time. Like chamomile, it can be used in combination with almost any herb and can be taken throughout pregnancy, or in more complex and serious medical scenarios. Possible exceptions are where a person is balanced on a cliff edge with say—liver or kidney failure, or (as ever) when taking anticoagulants like warfarin or a modern version thereof.

We have used nettle however as a stabilising influence in weaning people off multiple conventional medications (within a professional, therapeutic, mutually agreed on setting). Nettle can stabilise and improve allergic and atopic conditions such as eczema, asthma and hayfever.

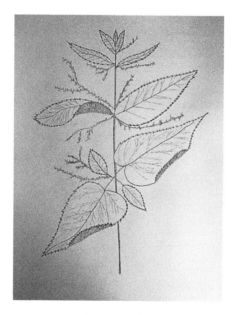

Line drawing of Nettle.

Bibliography

Please find listed below some resources which you may find useful if you wish to compare folklore and traditional uses with the modern-day uses listed above.

Allen, D. and Hatfield G., *Medicinal Plants in Folk Tradition: An Ethnobotany of Britain and Ireland*. 2004: Timber Press.
Baker, Margaret, *Discovering the Folklore of Plants*. 1996: Shire Publications Ltd.
Cheij, R. *The MacDonald Encyclopedia of Medicinal Plants*. 1984: MacDonald.
Grigson, Geoffrey, *The Englishman's Flora*. 1974: Paladin Books.

MacCoitir, Niall, *Irish Wild Plants. Myths, Legends and Folklore*. 2008: Collins Press.

Millican, W. and Bridgewater, S., *Flora Celtica: Plants and People in Scotland*. 2006: Birlinn Ltd.

Vickery, Roy, *A Dictionary of Plant Lore*. 1995: Oxford University Press.

Wood, Matthew. *Herbalism: Basic Doctrine, Energetics and Classification*. 2004: North Atlantic Books.

References

1. Barker, J., *Notes toward a therapeutic model of phytotherapy in Britain*. British Journal of Phytotherapy, 1991. 2(Spring): pp. 38–46.

2. Mills, S., *The Principles and Practice of Modern Phytotherapy*, K. Bone, Editor., Churchill Livingstone.

3. Heinrich, M. et al., *Fundamentals of Pharmacognosy and Phytotherapy*. 2012: Churchill Livingstone.

4. Walker, A. et al., *Promising hypotensive effect of hawthorn extract: A randomized double-blind pilot study of mild, essential hypertension*. Phytotherapy Res. 16: pp. 48–54.

5. Walker, A. F. et al., *Hypotensive effects of hawthorn for patients with diabetes taking prescription drugs: a randomised controlled trial*. Br J Gen Pract, 2006. 56(527): pp. 437–443.

6. Zorniak, M., B. Szydlo and T. F. Krzeminski, *Crataegus special extract WS 1442: up-to-date review of experimental and clinical experiences*. J Physiol Pharmacol, 2017. 68(4): pp. 521–526.

7. Orhan, I. E., *Phytochemical and pharmacological activity profile of Crataegus oxyacantha L. (hawthorn)—A cardiotonic herb*. 2016: Curr Med Chem.

8. Wang, J., X. Xiong and B. Feng, *Effect of crataegus usage in cardiovascular disease prevention: an evidence-based approach*. Evid Based Complement Alternat Med, 2013. 2013: p. 149363.

9. Priest, A. and P. LR., *Herbal Medication: A Clinical and Dispensary Handbook*. 1982: C. W. Daniel.

10. Jayachandran, K. E. A., *Crataegus oxycantha extract attenuates apoptotic influence in myocardial-ischaemic-reperfusion injury by regulating Akt and HIF-1 signaling pathways*. Journal of Cardiovascular Pharmacology, 2010. 56: pp. 526–531.

11. Quettier-Deleu, C. et al., *Hawthorn extracts inhibit LDL oxidation*. Pharmazie, 2003. 58(8): pp. 577–581.

12. Dalli, E. et al., *Crataegus laevigata decreases neutrophil elastase and has a hypolipidemic effect: a randomized, double-blind, placebo-controlled trial*. Phytomedicine, 2011. 18(8–9): pp. 769–775.

13. Bernatoniene, J. et al., *The effect of crataegus fruit extract and some of its flavonoids on mitochondrial oxidative phosphorylation in the heart.* Phytother Res, 2009. 23(12): pp. 1701–1707.

14. Swaminathan, J. K. et al., *Cardioprotective properties of Crataegus oxycantha extract against ischemia-reperfusion injury.* Phytomedicine, 2010. 17(10): pp. 744–752.

15. Holubarsch, C. J. et al., *The efficacy and safety of Crataegus extract WS 1442 in patients with heart failure: the SPICE trial.* Eur J Heart Fail, 2008. 10(12): pp. 1255–1263.

16. Fuchs, S. et al., *The Dual Edema-Preventing Molecular Mechanism of the Crataegus Extract WS 1442 Can Be Assigned to Distinct Phytochemical Fractions.* Planta Med, 2017. 83(8): pp. 701–709.

17. Holubarsch, C. J. F., W. S. Colucci and J. Eha, *Benefit-Risk Assessment of Crataegus Extract WS 1442: An Evidence-Based Review.* Am J Cardiovasc Drugs, 2018. 18(1): pp. 25–36.

18. Pittler, M. H., R. Guo and E. Ernst, *Hawthorn extract for treating chronic heart failure.* Cochrane Database Syst Rev, 2008(1): p. CD005312.

19. Tassell, M. C. et al., *Hawthorn (Crataegus spp.) in the treatment of cardiovascular disease.* Pharmacogn Rev, 2010. 4(7): pp. 32–41.

20. Lavagna, S. M. et al., *Efficacy of Hypericum and Calendula oils in the epithelial reconstruction of surgical wounds in childbirth with caesarean section.* Farmaco, 2001. 56(5–7): pp. 451–453.

21. Barker, J., *The Medicinal Flora of Britain and Northwestern Europe.* 2001: Winter Press.

22. Yeung, K. S. et al., *Herbal medicine for depression and anxiety: A systematic review with assessment of potential psycho-oncologic relevance.* Phytother Res, 2018. 32(5): pp. 865–891.

23. El Alaoui, C. et al., *Modulation of T-type Ca2+ channels by Lavender and Rosemary extracts.* PLoS One, 2017. 12(10): p. e0186864.

24. Schuwald, A. M. et al., *Lavender oil-potent anxiolytic properties via modulating voltage dependent calcium channels.* PLoS One, 2013. 8(4): p. e59998.

25. Nikfarjam, M. et al., *The effects of lavandula angustifolia mill infusion on depression in patients using citalopram: a comparison study.* Iran Red Crescent Med J, 2013. 15(8): pp. 734–739.

26. López, V. et al., *Exploring pharmacological mechanisms of lavender.* Front Pharmacol, 2017. 8: p. 280.

27. Sayorwan, W. et al., *The effects of lavender oil inhalation on emotional states, autonomic nervous system, and brain electrical activity.* J Med Assoc Thai, 2012. 95(4): pp. 598–606.

28. Ota, M. et al., *(-)-Linalool influence on the cerebral blood flow in healthy male volunteers revealed by three-dimensional pseudo-continuous arterial spin labeling.* Indian J Psychiatry, 2017. 59(2): pp. 225–227.

29. Hoffman, D., *Medical Herbalism: The Science and Practice of Herbal Medicine*. 2003: Healing Arts Press.
30. Vakilian, K. et al., *Healing advantages of lavender essential oil during episiotomy recovery: a clinical trial*. Complement Ther Clin Pract, 2011. 17(1): pp. 50–53.
31. Francišković, M. et al., *Chemical composition and immuno-modulatory effects of Urtica dioica L. (Stinging Nettle) Extracts*. Phytother Res, 2017. 31(8): pp. 1183–1191.
32. Bone, K. and S. Mills, *Principles and Practice of Phytotherapy: Modern Herbal Medicine*. 2nd ed. 2013: Churchill Livingstone.
33. Yance, D., *Adaptogens in Medical Herbalism*. 2013.
34. Kılıç, S. et al., *Efficacy of Two Plant Extracts Against Acne Vulgaris: Initial Results of Microbiological Tests and Cell Culture Studies*. 2018: J Cosmet Dermatol.
35. Bakhshaee, M. et al., *Efficacy of supportive therapy of allergic rhinitis by stinging nettle*. Iran J Pharm Res, 2017. 16(Suppl): pp. 112–118.
36. Roschek, B. et al., *Nettle extract (Urtica dioica) affects key receptors and enzymes associated with allergic rhinitis*. Phytother Res, 2009. 23(7): pp. 920–926.
37. Mittman, P., *Randomized, double-blind study of freeze-dried Urtica dioica in the treatment of allergic rhinitis*. Planta Med, 1990. 56(1): pp. 44–47.
38. Fattahi, S. et al., *Antioxidant and apoptotic effects of an aqueous extract of Urtica dioica on the MCF-7 human breast cancer cell line*. Asian Pac J Cancer Prev, 2013. 14(9): pp. 5317–5323.
39. Wolska, J. et al., *[The influence of stinging nettle (Urtica dioica L.) extracts on the activity of catalase in THP1 monocytes/macrophages]*. Pomeranian J Life Sci, 2015. 61(3): pp. 315–318.
40. El Haouari, M. and J. A. Rosado, *Phytochemical, Anti-Diabetic And Cardiovascular Properties Of Urtica Dioica L. (Urticaceae): A Review*. 2018: Mini Rev Med Chem.
41. Bouchentouf, S. et al., *Identification of phenolic compounds from nettle as new candidate inhibitors of main enzymes responsible on type-II diabetes*. 2018: Curr Drug Discov Technol.
42. Broekaert, W. F. et al., *A chitin-binding lectin from stinging nettle rhizomes with antifungal properties*. Science, 1989. 245(4922): pp. 1100–1102.
43. Safarinejad, M. R., *Urtica dioica for treatment of benign prostatic hyperplasia: a prospective, randomized, double-blind, placebo-controlled, crossover study*. J Herb Pharmacother, 2005. 5(4): pp. 1–11.
44. Ghorbanibirgani, A., A. Khalili and L. Zamani, *The efficacy of stinging nettle (Urtica dioica) in patients with benign prostatic hyperplasia: a randomized double-blind study in 100 patients*. Iran Red Cres Med J, 2013: pp. 9–10.

CHAPTER SEVEN

Swimming upstream: common conditions and therapeutic considerations

Introduction

This chapter is the first of four chapters demonstrating the herbal approach to the treatment of specific commonly seen conditions. When writing these chapters one of the questions we wished to address was: 'What is the evidence for the herbal approach?'

This is not as straightforward to answer as it may seem for a number of reasons.

We hope that it is becoming more obvious to you that there exists a substantial body of research now underpinning the use of whole plants and how they work on a pharmacological level. The weight of evidence for the effectiveness of herbs was one of the reasons that Western herbal medicine was identified as a complementary therapy suitable for Statutory Self Regulation in the 1990s. We have used a small amount of this research where appropriate throughout the text of this book.

What is less obvious is the effectiveness of the Western herbal philosophy of practice, specifically the person-centred approach to treatment. This is generally not something that research has focussed on for too many reasons to discuss here.

Over the following chapters exploring pathophysiology and therapeutics, we consider key conditions that people most commonly present with when visiting their medical herbalist or their doctor.

We begin by outlining the current conventional understanding of each of these conditions from a pathophysiological view, and then describe what conventional treatments are recommended and used for these conditions. Using case studies to illustrate the phytotherapist's approach, we then dive into the therapeutic rationale and regimens of Western herbal medicine. This encompasses some of the key standpoints of Western herbal medicine protocol, the macro-physiological view, and an assessment of vitality and constitution.

We wish to draw attention to the differences between a conventional medical approach and that of the Western medical herbalist. Some similarities are inevitable; modern physiological advances to our understanding are also shaping the herbalists' practice. But due to the nature of plant medicines, their complexity, and their capacity for tonification, tissue integrity enhancement and resilience-building it is not possible for the herbalist to be working with plants as if they were 'drugs' alone. Also, fundamentally the herbalist's standpoint on health, vitality and dynamism within the human body leads to unique differences in the understanding and interpretation of pathophysiology, and also to therapeutics; the application of plants as medicines.

This can, and has, made it difficult to convey to the public how herbalists practice, and explains why it is difficult to talk about what herb may be good for a particular condition. It explains the success of retail outlets selling herbs, vitamins, minerals and other non-herbal supplements; they are operating from a conventional standpoint of health, disease and the application of medicine to disease. The strength of phytotherapy lies in its truly person-centred not disease-centred approach.

Understanding the physiological processes in detail and from a broader viewpoint (macrophysiology), gives a whole and complex approach to observing functions that are taking place (or not!) and is a key feature of phytotherapy. This is because treatment is aimed at restoring these functional processes, which can sometimes be best achieved by taking a step back and looking at a person's case from a distance. To do this requires taking a detailed case history.

Whole Body Listening

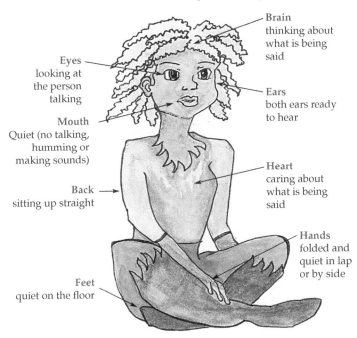

Brain
thinking about
what is being
said

Eyes
looking at
the person
talking

Ears
both ears ready
to hear

Mouth
Quiet (no talking,
humming or
making sounds)

Heart
caring about
what is being
said

Back →
sitting up straight

Hands
folded and
quiet in lap
or by side

Feet
quiet on the floor

Identifying what is happening that is 'out of synch' and then using herbs to try and 'nudge' these diverse processes back into a normal function is a key strategy of the medical herbalist. Choosing herbs that will affect and improve function is sometimes done physiologically but sometimes energetically (and often both!). For example, stimulation of circulation, relaxing and tonifying the nervous system, could all be seen as being functional corrections, but the herbalist might also observe energetically that this specific person is too 'dry' and therefore might also benefit from herbs that are circulatory, tonic to the nervous system—*but also moistening*.

The evidence for the herbal approach? As practitioners we see the evidence regularly. The inclusion of the case studies detailed in Chapters 7, 9, 10 and 11 will, we hope, give you some idea of what is achievable when patient, practitioner and plant work together. We will now look at how the medical herbalist looks at the process of menopause, and provides help for women experiencing troublesome symptoms at this time. In Part 2, we look at how a medical herbalist approaches the diagnosis of migraine in an individualised way.

Part 1. Menopause and peri-menopause

Definition—What is the menopause?

Menopause is defined as the cessation of menstruation for at least 12 months at the end of the reproductive phase of life due to ovarian failure (no bleeding should occur after 2 years). This conventional definition of ovarian failure is meant to be factual and un-emotive, but it is interesting to reflect how such language has fed into our conventional beliefs about menopause and the sole focus of treatment—hormone *replacement*. The word failure in itself immediately brings negative connotations to a totally natural process.

There is no reliable hormone marker to conclusively prove menopause, although lowered oestrogen and raised follicle-stimulating hormone (FSH) levels are often seen, but we will describe some of the hormonal changes in more detail later on. The average age for menopause is 51.8 years (but 47–56 is common).

The peri-menopause (also known as the climacteric) is the phase of progressive 'ovarian failure' that commences up to 5 years before. Ovarian function can be erratic and intermittent, even post-menopausally.

Post-menopause is the remaining phase of life following menopause.

This could be looked at as being unburdened from monthly hormonal upheaval and can also be seen as an opportunity to experience a time of good health.

Premature menopause is defined as women whose menopause occurs before the age of 40. This is thought to be approximately 1%, and for 1 in 1000 women this will be before the age of 20. Ovarian failure tends to be earlier in women who smoke, who have had a hysterectomy (ovaries preserved), or ovarian tissue surgery, and occurs surgically for women who have had an oophorectomy (ovaries removed).

The menopause is a natural physiological event, and like menarche, it is a transition from one stage of life to another. Although this time of life is a cessation of fertility, a healthy balanced climacteric should not be dominated with negative symptoms. Studies show that up to 25% of women do not experience troublesome symptoms at menopause, however the majority of Western women do,[1] and when these symptoms become severe or prolonged the term menopausal syndrome has been suggested.

For most women experiencing mild to moderate menopausal symptoms, there will be no pathological process found. This puts menopausal symptoms in the category of 'functional conditions'. Other examples of functional disorders include irritable bowel syndrome (IBS). So a functional disorder is a medical condition that impairs the normal function of a bodily process, but where every part of the body looks completely normal under examination, dissection or even under a microscope. This can present very real problems for conventional medicine in terms of identifying treatment strategies that do not have an identified 'pathology'. Herbal medicine is ideally suited to helping people with functional conditions because dealing with the optimisation of function is where plant medicines excel.

Menopausal syndrome

Menopausal syndrome is the term applied to women experiencing serious and life-altering symptoms at menopause, often with complicating factors. This may include hot flushes and night sweats, mood swings, global anxiety and palpitations, but to a level that is intolerable and may also involve pathological changes such as hypertension, thyroid dysfunction and severe depression. This scenario requires robust herbal medicine interventions in partnership with an experienced practitioner and may require conventional treatment options too.

Causes and symptoms: pathophysiology of menopause and menopausal syndrome

We need to start right at the beginning to clearly understand what happens and why symptoms may occur in the way that they do. We looked at the female reproductive system in chapter three, but now we will revisit it in more detail here. Women are born with a finite number (approx 1 million) of primordial follicles in their ovaries. Each primordial follicle has the potential to mature during the monthly cycle. Maturation of primordial follicles each month releases oestrogen, and follicles either become the ovulated 'egg' or provide background hormones to support ovulation. They have usually depleted to a critical number (about 1000) by age 50, which means that ovarian hormone levels change dramatically from the mid-40s into the mid-50s in a woman's life.

Following menarche (the onset of monthly menstrual periods), the ovary matures up to 20 follicles per month, one of which will move to the 'antral stage' and become the 'egg' or ovum that is ovulated. The follicles collectively provide a background 'chorus' of hormones (oestrogen and progesterone), that causes thickening of the endometrium (lining of the womb).

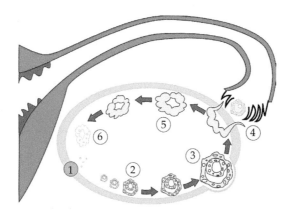

Diagram of follicle maturation in the ovary.

This all occurs in the first half of the cycle as a result of hormones secreted by the pituitary gland (which you may recall is in the sensory/emotional centre of the brain). The pituitary gland produces follicle-stimulating hormone (FSH), stimulating the maturation of the hormone-producing follicles, and then, to encourage ovulation, it secretes luteinizing hormone (LH).

It is also important to know that ovulation leaves behind a small area of tissue in the ovary known as a yellow body (corpus luteum). This produces progesterone for about 2 weeks, putting a brake on the endometrial breakdown and therefore menstrual bleeding (and allowing a window for fertilisation of the newly ovulated ovum (egg)). The corpus luteum also acts as an inhibitor to the pituitary gonadotropins FSH and LH. As the corpus luteum runs out of progesterone, bleeding will start if fertilisation has not occurred, or if the corpus luteum is insufficient.

There are many other processes involved in this deceptively simple cycle, involving lots of biofeedback mechanisms. As a result, explaining the menstrual cycle and what may be happening during natural life changes (menarche and menopause) or during imbalances (such as pre-menstrual syndrome (PMS), ovarian cysts, irregular bleeding) can be very difficult and there can be a tendency to try and over-simplify things into 'too much' or 'too little' oestrogen or progesterone.

For our purposes it is worth noting the following biofeedback loops due to their potential to wreak havoc at peri-menopause.

During the last 2–5 years before menopause the number of follicles available and therefore proceeding to the antral stage falls, and so there are fewer and fewer available for final maturation. This process, influenced by so many other wellbeing factors, can be erratic and so symptoms can occur in episodes and then seemingly disappear, only to return later. Sometimes one ovary is more dominant or functional than the other, and symptoms can appear to alternate monthly.

> **Note:** This means there is less oestrogen and progesterone at peri-menopause. However these two hormones are dancing partners, and work best when balanced with each other. Sometimes, they are out of balance with each other during the peri-menopause, and this can lead to symptoms such as lighter or heavier menstrual bleeds.

The functionality of ovulation can be affected, and as a result circulating levels of inhibin (from the corpus luteum) decrease, leading to elevated levels of pituitary gonadotrophins and therefore FSH. FSH can be measured by blood test to suggest if symptoms may be due to climacteric change.

> **Note:** Elevated gonadotrophins may be one cause of many of the emotional symptoms experienced by some women at peri-menopause. These are often referred to as being like PMS, and women often comment they felt similarly at menarche (when their periods first started).

Gonadotrophin Releasing Hormone also known as GnRH is released by the hypothalamic region of the brain and travels via the blood vessels to the pituitary gland where it can stimulate the release of the anterior pituitary hormones (also known as gonadotrophins) FSH and luteinizing hormone (LH). It is interesting to consider here for a moment the other hormones produced by the pituitary also known as the 'master-gland', or as the 'conductor of the hormonal orchestra'.

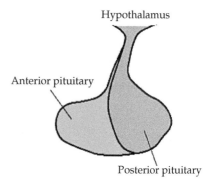

- Prolactin, which acts on the breasts to induce milk production.
- Adrenocorticotropic hormone, which stimulates the adrenal glands to secrete steroid hormones, principally cortisol.
- Growth hormone (GH), which regulates growth, metabolism and body composition.
- Thyroid stimulating hormone (TSH), which stimulates the thyroid gland.
- Gonadotrophins (LH and FSH) that stimulate the ovaries and testes.
- Oxytocin a hormone secreted during labour but also known as the 'love' hormone for its role in our emotional feelings of connection and attachment to others.
- Antidiuretic hormone (ADH) affecting kidney excretion of urine and thirst.

Note: Changes to any of these hormones can result in symptoms familiar to women with menopausal syndrome.

Also worth a mention!

Although not fully understood, melatonin (secreted by the pineal gland) is also secreted in significant quantities by the gut. In fact our large intestine secretes more than 400 times more melatonin in our gut than in our bloodstream. In relation to gut function, melatonin is not subject to diurnal variations, but has a role to play in gastro-intestinal motility, inflammation and pain.[2] In a recent research paper by Tordjman et al., melatonin has been described as an endogenous synchroniser and a chronobiotic molecule, acting via the hypothalamus to stabilise body rhythms. This powerful molecule is a down-regulator of the GnRH gene and has specific actions on LH pulsatile secretions. On top of all this, it influences neuroendocrine rhythms such as body temperature cycles.[3]

It is not hard to see how dysregulation of melatonin secretion can play into many of the symptoms experienced by women at the menopause. There have also been links made between the functioning of the melatonin cycle with inhibition of breast cancer via oestrogen receptor sites (ER-alpha cancers in particular).[4] Dysregulation of melatonin production in the gastrointestinal tract may lead to disrupted motility, compromised bowel function and subsequent poor metabolism of hormones, which will impact on reproductive health.

> **Note:** Thus we can link the gut, sleep and oestrogen receptors all in one go! Many women experience sleep problems at menopause and digestive imbalance is extremely common too.

Getting back to our description of what happens leading up to menopause …

As antral follicle numbers fall critically for recruitment, ovulation occurs unpredictably so that oestrogen production and menstrual cycles become erratic. This transitional phase of progressive ovarian shutdown (failure) is a major part of peri-menopause. This can lead to erratic bleeding patterns, and seemingly paradoxically this can mean menstruation can get less frequent and less heavy (less follicular maturation) or more heavy and frequent (corpus luteum failure).

> **Note:** Fluctuations in hormone homeostasis can lead to compensation by the body, and one response may be an increase in corticosteroid hormones from the adrenal glands. This can be one factor in the increase of fat deposition around the abdomen, but may also feed into feelings of anxiety and palpitations. It can also lead to interference of thyroid hormone transport mechanisms, potentially leading to eventual exhaustion of the thyroid gland. Hypothyroidism is one potential complication of menopause.

As cyclic ovarian activity slows and then ceases, so does menstruation, and the endometrium itself atrophies, but the basement membrane of the endometrium remains and is capable of regeneration in the presence of administered oestrogens (HRT). Conventionally, hormone replacement therapy seeks to negate the effects of lowered oestrogen (oestradiol).

Lowered oestrodiol can lead to

- Atrophy of the lower genital tract and urinary tract (common embryological origin). This sometimes causes recurrent urinary tract infections.
- Lactobacilli, supported by oestrogen levels, use their glycogen stores to produce lactic acid, thus keeping the pH suitably low, and preventing urinary tract infections (UTI's). Drops in oestrogen at menopause affect this process, reducing native populations of lactobacilli and leading to a more alkaline environment, which can also cause recurrent UTI's.
- Vulva and vagina lose collagen and tone, and have reduced blood flow, possibly affecting orgasm.
- Vaginal shortening, loss of normal rugae, thinning of the stratified epithelium.
- Vaginal dryness as a result of reduced secretions can lead to superficial dyspareunia (painful sexual intercourse).
- Uterus and cervix atrophy and shrink in size.
- Supporting pelvic ligaments weaken can, potentially leading to uterovaginal prolapse.
- Atrophic changes to urethra and muscles of the bladder may lead to urgency and frequency; loss of tone in the bladder, and structures supporting the bladder neck may result in stress incontinence.

Presented in this way, menopause sounds like a disaster and serves to exaggerate the need for supplementation with oestrogens once produced by the ovary.

Acute menopausal syndrome

Acute menopausal symptoms can be brought on by surgical removal of the ovaries, and are thought to be neuroendocrine in origin—unsurprisingly there is an element of 'shock' involved. Severe symptoms for some women or for women who are not yet at the average menopausal age, should be considered for conventional hormone replacement to prevent extreme symptoms and outcomes (such as bone loss) that exceed normal menopausal change.

Hot flushes and sweats (known as vasomotor symptoms) disturb normal sleep patterns, disrupt REM sleep, (a kind of sleep that is characterised by rapid eye movements) and produce psychological symptoms similar to sleep deprivation syndrome. (e.g., difficulty in making decisions, poor short-term memory, anxiety, loss of confidence, mood changes, esp. irritability).

The cause is thought to be in part due to the changes in hormone homeostasis affecting thermo-receptors (temperature regulators), giving different temperature readings for core body temperature and peripheral body temperature. Our core body temperature (Tc) is defined by an upper temperature, above which sweating may be induced to cool us, and a lower temperature, below which shivering may be induced to warm us up. Between these upper and lower temperatures is the thermo-neutral zone, a range of temperatures wherein our internal environment is comfortable and sweating or shivering do not occur.

Hormonal imbalances (remember GnRH and Melatonin are involved here) may disrupt this situation. As you may expect, the hormonal dynamics of this are quite complex at menopause, but a simplistic summary would read something like this:

- Noradrenaline (a sympathetic nervous system neurotransmitter) acts to narrow the width of our thermo-neutral zone.
- Serotonin opposes the action of noradrenaline.
- Oestrogen helps keep serotonin levels raised.
- When oestrogen levels fall, the serotonin in our bodies also falls.
- This results in a rise in noradrenaline levels, which results in a narrowing of our internal thermo-neutral zone and consequently flushes and/or sweating are triggered.[5]

Joint aches and pains (arthralgia) especially of the balls of the feet, but potentially anywhere may occur. Also pins and needles, and increase in reports of carpal tunnel syndrome. Vaginal dryness and atrophy can lead to urinary tract infections and/or genital discomfort. Loss of sexual desire is reported. The brain has E2 (oestrogen) receptors, which may account in some part for the often-experienced emotional symptoms and brain fog, and also loss of sexual desire. Mood changes and tearfulness, or a feeling of increased PMS, is common at peri-menopause.

It is important to address other midlife concerns and causes of symptoms such as the loss of fertility, unwarranted anxiety about the loss of femininity and ageing. Children may be leaving home, parents may be ageing or dying. Depression and suicide are increased in this phase of life.[6]

Conventional approaches to treatment

In the UK, the current guidelines of practice for doctors for treating women at menopause are to be found at the National Institute of Health and Care Excellence (NICE) website. The guidelines recommend HRT and also some herbal medicines as being effective in relieving symptoms for women. HRT can be offered as a risk/benefit ratio. After the 'Million Women Study' in 2000 when the trial was halted due to unprecedented levels of breast cancer directly linked to HRT use, further trials have focussed on whether certain types of HRT carry less risk.

Transdermal applications (patches and creams) have been found to carry less risk of breast and endometrial carcinoma. So-called bio-identical oestrogen and progesterone combined are recommended for women who have not had a hysterectomy, and un-opposed transdermal oestrogen is recommended for those who have no uterus or ovaries. This is because all these versions of oestrogen supplementation are proliferative (to the endometrium and breast tissue) in effect.

Other treatments that may be offered include antidepressants and clonidine (an adrenergic agonist drug that reduces vasospasm). Clonidine acts to reduce noradrenaline levels, which may also impact hot flush rates. Testosterone therapy and cognitive behavioural therapy (CBT) are also 'allowed' (despite a lack of evidence for the benefits of testosterone).

Isoflavones, black cohosh (*Actaea racemosa* L. synonym *Cimicifuga racemosa*) Sage, (*Salvia officinalis* L.) and St John's wort (*Hypericum perforatum* L.) are all recommended by NICE, although with the caveat that there is no knowledge of safety and efficacy (a rather excessively dismissive and erroneous comment, since they are non-proliferative).

Problems surrounding the conventional treatment of the menopause include the massive concerns still surrounding the use of HRT and breast cancer. HRT is contraindicated for women who have a family history of breast cancer. HRT tablets have been linked to increased risk of developing a blood clot. Some women experience side effects such as nausea, bloating, breast tenderness and headache as a result of taking HRT. For some women the side effects are so pronounced that they cease to take HRT. The numbers for which this is the case are not recorded. Menopausal symptoms are a common reason for women to consult a medical herbalist.[7]

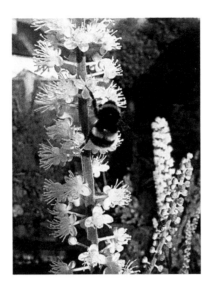

Black cohosh flowers.

Western herbal medicine's approach to treatment

It is worth repeating here that menopause is a natural physiological event, and like menarche, it is a transition from one stage of life to another. Western herbal medicine differs in its approach to conventional medicine in that it seeks not only to replace what is missing via artificial means, but to help support many different body systems to rebalance and adjust to the new status quo, thus optimising good health generally.[8] The whole approach of the medical herbalist was demonstrated to relieve perceived symptoms in one patient-centred study.[9]

This transition may be supported by a good diet to help optimise gut function and support the hormonal shifts that are occurring at this time. A good diet can serve a dual purpose here: it can supply the body with plant-based compounds that can interact with different cell receptors and provide relief from menopausal symptoms. Also, a good diet will help support gut function, so crucial to hormone conjugation in the gut and of course, long term health more

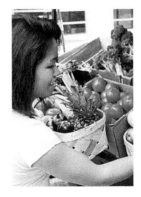

generally. This whole approach epitomises the grey area between food and medicine, as medicinally active phytochemical compounds in common plant-based foods take centre stage. It also highlights the fact that medical herbalists can use plants for women transitioning through menopause, whilst not necessarily using plants that interact with oestrogen receptors at all.

As a direct result of research into soy isoflavones and the reputation of soya in reducing the incidence of breast cancer and menopausal symptoms in women from countries with a very high soy-based diet (such as Japan), a new oestrogen receptor site (ER2 or ERβ) was discovered and this has transformed our understanding of menopause. ERβ is expressed preferentially in normal breast and ovarian tissue and most strongly expressed in the ovary and prostate. It protects against 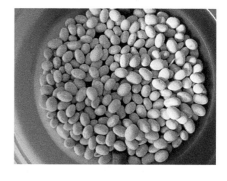 breast cancer development, promotes greater bone density, gives cardiovascular protection, and helps reduce menopausal symptoms.

Compounds found in many plant foods, not just soya, but all beans, (including lentils and linseeds) can be used by our body in all sorts of beneficial ways for women and men, and medicinal plants traditionally used for women's health can have a positive impact on women at menopause.

Significantly for the herbalist who is focussed on the health and ecosystem of the body as a whole—all post-menopausal hormones may go through a conversion in the gut by microbiota, in the peripheral fatty tissues of the body, and also in the liver cell. The health of these diverse tissues therefore may be significant in the experience for all women at menopause transition and beyond.

Oestrogen receptors (ERs)

There are two main types of oestrogen receptor: ERα alpha ('classical'), and ERβ beta (only discovered in 1996 by Kuiper et al.). Originally it was thought that soy and other herbal medicines used successfully at menopause must contain replacement oestrogen, which would explain their efficacy. Thus they were called phyto-oestrogens. The truth is more complex (of course!).

Most phyto-oestrogens, especially isoflavones, have higher binding affinity to ERβ rather than ERα. This significantly pro-

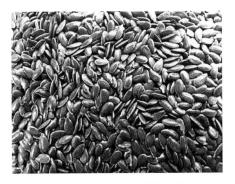

tects breast tissue from excessive oestrogen effects caused by the more powerful ERα. This explains population studies showing considerably lower rates of breast and prostate cancers in people with high isoflavone diets. The two receptors are opposite and complementary, like Yin and Yang. *So, oestrogens can stimulate in one tissue, and be depressant (or antagonist) in another.* Phyto-oestrogens from traditionally used medicinal plants are now therefore called Phyto-SERMs (selective oestrogen receptor modulators).

Compared with oestradiol (the most potent oestrogen), Phyto-SERMs have a limited biological role and are capable of achieving only some of the consequences associated with endogenous oestrogens, such as symptom reduction e.g., hot flushes, (a typical effect mediated by ERβ). Unlike oestradiol none of the Phyto-SERMs trigger the full range of oestrogen-like actions because of their preferential activation of ERβ. For example, they do not stimulate ovulation, endometrial (womb lining) proliferation, and therefore do not re-start menstruation after menopause, which are more typical ERα related effects.

So, are plant oestrogens safer? Potential negative effects of Phyto-SERMs have been studied, and ruled out. Soy formula fed to infants for example, showed no significant developmental or reproductive differences between these infants and those fed cows formula.[10] Phyto-SERMs may have pro- or anti-oestrogenic effects (agonist or antagonist) depending on the physiological environment.

In other words—when post-menopausal women (who are relatively oestrogen-deprived) consume isoflavones, an oestrogen-like, and symptom reducing effect is observed by activation of ERβ receptors. However women of childbearing age may gain helpful anti-oestrogenic effects again by activation of ERβ and thus countering ERα mediated effects of oestrogen.

So basically, plants containing what were once called phyto-oestrogens have been shown to act selectively in different circumstances, providing extra oestrogenic effects in those who are deprived, and a dampening of oestrogenic effects in those who have too much. In herbal medicine terms this is a classic example of an **amphoteric** *action.*

Four main types of plant-derived selective oestrogen receptor modulators (SERMs) have been identified

- Isoflavones, coumestans and lignans collectively known as phenolic phyto-oestrogens; found in many commonly eaten foods especially beans and pulses, but also many medicinal plants.
- Triterpenoid and steroidal saponins found largely in medicinal herbs.
- Phytosterols including beta-sitosterol. Beta-sitosterol is found in nut oils and avocado oil and is being investigated for its potential to reduce benign prostatic hyperplasia.
- Resorcyclic acid lactones are rare contaminants of plant material stored in damp conditions.
- An exception to this would be the phytoestrogen 8-prenylnarengenin (8-PN), a prenylated flavonoid found primarily in hops, and considered to be one of the most potent phyto-oestrogens ever discovered. Historically women working in hop fields reported menstrual cycle disturbances during hop harvesting, and hop baths have traditionally been utilised as a treatment for some gynaecological conditions. Research in 2018 revealed that 8-PN, unlike most Phyto-SERMs binds preferentially to ERα. Nevertheless, hop has not been demonstrated to cause proliferation of breast or endometrial tissue. ERα is predominant in bone tissue leading to speculation that some benefits may be derived in cases of menopause-derived osteoporosis.[24] This piece of research, whilst interesting of itself, is another example of one specific active constituent being focussed on as opposed to the whole plant, and therefore does not give us a complete picture of the overall benefits of hops.

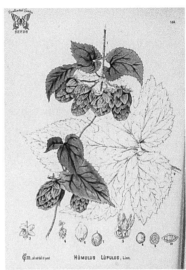

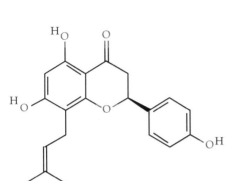

Structure of 8-prenyl-naringenin.   Hop (*Humulus lupulus* L.)

Lots of Phyto-SERMs are still being identified and studied—it is a dynamic area of research. So far points to consider include:

- Most appear to require conversion by gut bacteria in at least two stages and this has been found to be highly variable—person to person.
- Antibiotics significantly reduce plasma levels of isoflavones. (They are also responsible for interfering with melatonin production in the gut).
- Successful binding of oestrogen at the receptor site is another important variability factor. Oestrogen receptor sites are found in a wide variety of body tissues including the prostate, the brain, bone, intestine and the heart.

Oestrone—a weak oestrogen synthesized from cholesterol.

Summary

Focussing solely on *replacement* of hormones once present during the fertile/menstrual stage of a woman's life, distracts from the crucial role played by other parts of our body in hormone homeostasis. The herbal approach may involve an array of herbal medicines that positively impact the immune system, digestive system, nervous system and so on, and reduction of infection, inflammation, and other 'stressors' will improve many women's experience of the transition of menopause.

Conventional research has focussed largely only on the Phyto-SERMs and their isolated use in large trials (see NICE guidelines). So, whilst the medical herbalist may include a variety of Phyto-SERM containing foods and herbs for a woman experiencing menopausal symptoms, this will be nowhere near the complete picture.[25]

Also worth noting is that after menopause, weaker oestrogen made in our body is produced by conversion (in the liver) of androstenedione, secreted by the adrenal cortex, to oestrone by peripheral tissues (such as fat tissue). Thus liver support, adrenal support, and healthy fat intake are all aspects of a woman's health to be considered by a herbal approach.

Successful management of the climacteric will involve some key features in herbal medicine, such as

- Restoration of quality sleep.
- Reduction of stressors such as chronic pain or recurrent infection.
- Improvement of gut function and therefore the microbiome, enhancing the conversion of Phyto-SERMs in the gut, and also supporting serotonin and melatonin levels.
- Support of liver function and therefore hormone conjugation and excretion.
- Thyroid support.
- Blood sugar metabolism support.
- Nervous system support.
- Antispasmodics for the vascular system.
- Use of a personalised approach and of complex mixtures, which allows great flexibility within a single prescription for an individual.

Menopausal symptoms—two comparative case studies

Case 1

A 54-year-old woman, whose menstruation had stopped 18 months ago, and who had been experiencing poor sleep and hot flushes with mood swings. She was busy running the family home, and helping with her husband's business, but she was becoming increasingly irritable, and occasionally angry and argumentative, which she disliked intensely.

This lady was of normal weight for her height. She exercised regularly (at the gym), but had hypertension for about 2 years, treated with nifedipine (a calcium-channel blocker drug). She was quite red in the face, and almost 'raced through' her consultation, fidgeting her legs throughout. Her blood pressure at the first consultation was 160/98 mmHg. Her husband worked long hours and she managed the home and household entirely.

> **Definition—*Nifedipine*:** Nifedipine is a calcium-channel blocker drug that alters the inward displacement of calcium ions through the slow channels of active cell membranes. This influences the myocardial cells (the cells within the specialised conducting system of the heart) and the cells of vascular smooth muscle. Thus, myocardial contractility may be reduced, the formation and propagation of electrical impulses within the heart may be depressed, and coronary or systemic vascular tone may be diminished.

Her menses through her life had been regular and unproblematic. She had used HRT initially when her periods stopped, but she experienced a number of unpleasant effects (spotty skin, more moodiness, breast tenderness), so she decided to stop and had not used it now for 11 months.

Primary symptoms included

- Falling asleep easily, but waking around 4am in the morning, difficult/impossible to get back to sleep.
- Moody, irritable and even angry at times.
- Hot flushes in the early hours of the morning and through the day.
- Hypertension, despite medication.

Significant background factors

- Mild constipation—incomplete daily bowel movement, some abdominal bloating and occasional indigestion. This was despite a diet with a daily variety of vegetables, whole grains and legumes, nuts and seeds.
- Occasional headaches—relieved by drinking more water.
- Worried about son, who was just going off to university.

Treatment plan

The herbal medicine prescription, aimed at soothing and calming nervous system and circulatory stress, contained yarrow (*Achillea millefolium* L.), motherwort (*Leonurus cardiaca* L.), cramp bark (*Viburnum opulus* L.), and lime flower (*Tilia cordata* Mill.). Also aimed at reducing vasospasm it was intended to reduce the heat and flushes, and also, hopefully, the blood pressure. Valerian (*Valeriana officinalis* L.) and hops (*Hummulus lupulus* L.) taken just before bedtime were calming and relaxing herbal medicines that could help support hormone balance ultimately. The key factor here was also to please drink more water. Stop, pause and drink, slow down, and breathe.

Rationale

Although mood swings and hot flushes are common symptoms for women to experience at menopause, there is something distinctly 'Hot' about this patient. From a Western herbal perspective, this 'heat' is coming from the liver, and so herbs that reduce heat in the liver (such as bitters), and soothe and moisten the nervous system (heat is eventually drying), would be ideal.

- Lime flower and valerian could be seen as moistening, whilst yarrow and hops both contain therapeutic bitters.
- Yarrow and valerian can have gentle corrective actions on the digestive system, particularly where heat and tension exist.
- Cramp bark and motherwort, both muscle relaxants, should help reduce flushes, irritability and blood pressure.
- This persistent theme of addressing liver function in traditional herbal medicine, is interesting, now we understand the crucial role of the liver in conjugating and metabolising hormones especially post-menopausal. Water is a necessary part of liver metabolism, and dehydration will exacerbate feelings of 'stress'.

At the first follow-up consultation, 6 weeks later

This lady had noticed her sleep had been subtly better, she still often woke around 4am had a mild flush of heat, then seemed most often to fall back to sleep again with ease. She felt a little better during the day as a result, and had taken more care to drink more water as advised. The daytime hot flushes had disappeared altogether, and she was often less irritable. Her blood pressure this time was 150/94 mmHg, and she was still taking nifedipine.

At the second follow-up, 6 weeks later

Now free of hot flushes and sleeping well almost every night. Her mood was more even and 'more like my old self', she also noticed her digestive system was working really well, and was less sluggish. She had run out of night-time herbal medicine, but had continued with the daytime one. Her blood pressure was 140/88 mmHg. She was still taking nifedipine. We agreed we would review her blood pressure in a further 6 weeks to see if there had been any further improvement.

Case 2

A 53-year-old woman presented with menopausal symptoms and erratic menstruation that had been building up over the last 2 years or so. Menses were much lighter but the cycle had shortened from 28–30 days to 20–21 days, and the pre-menstrual symptoms seemed to fill all the space in between. She felt tired and heavy, lacking in mental clarity and cognition. She had dull headaches frequently through the week, and found it difficult to fall asleep. As soon as she lay down in bed she would get several hot flushes with palpitations. She also experienced numerous hot flushes throughout the day, but felt cold in between. Her blood pressure was 120/70 mmHg. She was not taking conventional medicines and was fearful of taking HRT as there was a family history of breast cancer.

Primary symptoms

- Shortened menstrual cycle (20–21 days).
- Pre-menstrual tension for most of the time.
- Foggy-headed, lack of concentration and clarity of mind.

- Dull regular headaches.
- Difficult to get off to sleep.
- Hot flushes, palpitations.

Significant background factors

- A long history of irritable bowel syndrome. Often with loose urgent bowel movements with bloating and abdominal discomfort.
- She had some stress in her life, mainly to do with work, and feeling foggy-headed was adding to her work-related fears.
- She had a happy home life but felt too tired to exercise.
- Her diet was increasingly based on sweet treats to give her a boost, but she used to eat very well, and had in the past liked to cook.

Treatment plan and rationale

This lady is showing signs of depletion, and lack of energy, possibly also depleted in terms of vitamins and minerals (such as iron). Energetically, this depletion is related to the adrenal glands and adaptogenic herbs are used to tonify and rejuvenate. Depletion of this type can exacerbate anxiety and fear, and cause difficulty getting off to sleep (and thus interferes with one major restorative mechanism). If we become tired and depleted we are more likely to crave sweet things, putting further stress on the hormonal orchestra, and we might feel less like exercising which might otherwise help reduce anxiety.

The herbs

A tonic restorative prescription was devised for use during the day: Oats (*Avena sativa* L.), chamomile, (*Matricaria chamomilla* L.), motherwort (*Leonurus cardiaca* L.), chaste berry (*Vitex agnus-castus* L.), wild yam (*Dioscorea villosa* L.) and fennel (*Foeniculum vulgare* Mill.). At night, a tea of passion flower (*Passiflora incarnata* L.), oats (*Avena sativa* L.), lemon balm (*Melissa officinalis* L.) and chamomile (*Matricaria chamomilla* L.) was given.

Herbal medicines such as lemon balm, motherwort and chamomile, can have a soothing and repairing (nervine) effect on the nervous system, whilst also acting as anti-inflammatory, antispasmodic and carminatives to the digestive system. Lamiaceae family herbs are often described as warming, but are *as warm as normal health should be*, so if

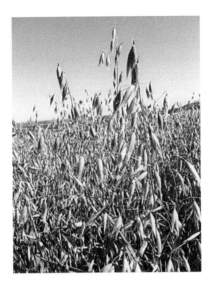

Oat flowers (*Avena sativa* L.)

they are effective at reducing inflammation they could result in a cool-ing to normal effect.

Tonic adaptogens such as oats can be used both in the day and at night as they are not over-stimulating, and wild yam can be seen as a tonic adaptogen, antispasmodic to the digestive system and as hormone support at peri-menopause and menopause. Tension can reduce nourishment of tissues and organ systems, and so nourishment can be required even where there can be 'excess'—such as in this case.

Chaste berry was used here to try to lengthen and regulate the men-strual cycle, and relieve pre-menstrual symptoms, and in combination with

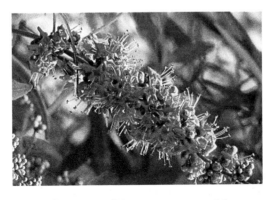

Chaste Tree (*Vitex agnus-castus* L.)

a tonic like wild yam, may additionally help improve ovarian function until there are no more follicles to mature. Modern research has confirmed many of the traditional uses for chaste berry, and also the selective oestrogen modulating effects of herbs such as wild yam. Aromatics like fennel give ease from wind and bloating, but also aid the microbiome, and in the case of fennel itself have a supportive hormonal balancing role too.

Diet and lifestyle

Suggestions were to eat more cooked root vegetables with green parsley and watercress chopped on top. Also to use aromatic herbs such as mint, basil, coriander leaf and dill in salads and as fresh chutneys (see note below). If craving sweet, try a teaspoon of molasses in hot water, or oat milk with some cinnamon or nutmeg mixed in, which may be drunk as a nourishing pick-me-up. Although these suggestions contain foods with high vitamin and mineral content (e.g., iron, calcium), they are also energetically and constitutionally suited to this lady. The gentle aromatic sourness from the chutney and fresh aromatic/green herbs helps restore vitality, and capacity for assimilation. The sweet nourishing drink supports the emotional heart, and is tonic to the nervous system.

Raw chutney

Stimulate all of your taste receptors with this magnificent raw chutney inspired by the fabulous Madhur Jaffrey and her book *World Vegetarian* 1998. Ebury Press.

100 g fresh grated coconut (or 75 g dried desiccated coconut soaked in 150 ml hot water for 30 minutes).

1 teaspoon quality sea or rock salt

1 teaspoon honey or dark cane sugar

1 teaspoon tamarind paste

2 tablespoons lemon juice plus the finely grated zest

1–2 fresh hot green chillis chopped finely

2 medium shallots (finely sliced and soaked in the lemon juice)

100 g fresh coriander leaves, chopped

2.5 centimetres peeled fresh root ginger finely chopped

Half a teaspoon of cumin seeds toasted in a dry frying pan

Put all of the ingredients into a blender and grind to a fine paste. add water to help the process if needed. Scrape into a serving dish and drizzle over some raw hemp seed oil (or similar). Serve with vegetable rice or any dish to enliven all of your taste receptors!

First 6-week review appointment

Feeling much better in her digestive system—it had been 'like a miracle'.

She was also experiencing normal healthy daily bowel motions for the first time she could remember.

- Having less pre-menstrual symptoms, and almost no headaches.
- Still feeling tired, although sleeping a little better, but was hopeful this would improve further.
- Loving the oat milk with cinnamon, and was preparing a vibrant meal most days now.

A further 8 weeks on

Last two menstrual cycles were 26–27 days long, a big improvement, and she was still feeling much better in herself in between. Her digestion was still great, and she was now sleeping a little better. She still felt tired, but was wondering about starting some yoga or pilates classes, and was aware she was not doing any exercise at all. She was eating much better however, and she felt very motivated to continue to do so.

Third follow-up 8 weeks later

Last two menstrual cycles were 26 or 27 days, and the bleed itself was getting lighter and fewer days. No pre-menstrual symptoms, no headaches, good digestion and energy-returning. Sleep mostly good and now enjoying 2–3 yoga classes per week.

What evidence is there for the herbal approach?

It is not difficult to find research underpinning the use of specific herbs to treat specific symptoms experienced by women during the menopause.

Examples of this include the use of liquorice root to lessen hot flushes,[11] the use of black cohosh to lessen the effects of hot flushes,[12] the use of fennel to alleviate menopausal symptoms,[13] etc. As we all know by now, this is only half of the story and is not a true reflection of how herbalists work.[9] More human studies in real-life situations are much needed.

Combining conventional and herbal treatments

Many of the dietary and self-help recommendations we present below would be appropriate even alongside a conventional hormone replacement approach. However it is true to say that in this particular case women tend to choose either one mode of treatment or the other and are less inclined to combine the two. Indeed, when a patient is taking HRT, the implications of this for their system are so powerful that often the subtler, more tonic and supportive effects of herbs can be 'drowned out' by large doses of synthesised hormones. In this event, if a patient is also desirous of herbal support, the focus of the treatment would change to helping the system deal with the significant drug load without it impacting detrimentally on their health in the long term.

Self-help: the kitchen pharmacy

An important aspect of herbal medicine lies in its ability to allow people to help themselves. Here are a few hints and tips that can be done by anyone, and which may help alleviate things.

At this time possibly more than ever it is important to go back to basics and think about making sure that your diet is healthy, you are getting sufficient rest, regular exercise and enough time for relaxation and enjoyment.

- Do what you can to minimise stress in your life, and allow yourself time to relax. Avoid stimulants such as caffeine and refined sugar.
- If you are a smoker, do your best to quit. The body uses precious vitamins and minerals in its efforts to detoxify the products of smoking, thus depleting the system.
- Specifically use whole soy products rather than supplements or extracts.
- Exercise regularly (but not excessively). Regular exercise has been associated with a reduction in symptom severity.[14]
- Maintain positive friendships.

Menopause and diet

- Include dietary phyto-oestrogens in your diet as far as possible, i.e., tofu, tempeh and ground linseeds. Eat a wide range of grains, seeds and pulses.
- Eat plenty of fresh fruit and vegetables.
- Make sure you are well hydrated.
- Avoid too much coffee and other stimulants (stimulants include caffeine, refined sugar and alcohol).
- Include fermented foods where possible (ie kimchi, sauerkraut) to support a healthy gut microbiome.
- Fresh watercress, parsley, and sprouted seeds are both full of important vitamins and minerals, and they are living foods—full of vitality; eat lots.

You can help support a tired nervous system with gentle nervous system tonic herbs such as passion flower, oats, St John's wort and rosemary. A medical herbalist will not only have access to a large selection of beneficial medicinal plants, but may also make useful suggestions as to what ones may be most appropriate for that specific individual.

You can lend a helping hand to your liver and adrenal glands with dandelion root and liquorice root respectively—although many other possibilities are available. The liver and digestive system are involved in key processes of post-menopausal hormone production; this is why liver support in the form of herbal medicines is such a fundamental part of the herbalists' approach. Nettle (a gentle liver tonic) will also be a great herb to take as a tea at this time, as its vitamin and mineral content will provide valuable support for those depleted at peri-menopause.

We spoke of SERMs earlier. Perhaps a herbal tea of red clover, Calendula and motherwort will provide welcome and delicious backup here. Finally, you might wish to try this lovely recipe for a 'Menopause Cake'. Who says medicine can't taste good *and* be effective!

Recipe for menopause cake

4 ozs/100 g soya flour
4 ozs/100 g wholemeal flour (replace with more oats for a wheat-free loaf)
4 ozs/100 g rolled oats
4 ozs/100 g linseeds (flaxseed)

2 ozs/50 g pumpkin seeds
2 ozs/50 g flaked almonds or walnuts or any other nuts
2 ozs/50 g sesame seeds
2 ozs/50 g sunflower seeds
two pieces of finely chopped stemmed ginger (optional)
8 ozs/225 g raisins or dates or cranberries
½ teaspoon nutmeg
½ teaspoon cinnamon
½ teaspoon ground ginger
15 fl oz/425 ml soya milk
1 tablespoon malt extract

Method

Put all the dry ingredients into a large bowl. Add the soya milk and malt extract, mix well and leave to soak for about 30 minutes to 1 hour. Heat the oven to 190°C/375°F/gas 5. Line a small loaf tin with baking parchment. If the mixture ends up too stiff (it should have a soft dropping consistency), stir in some more soya milk. Spoon the mixture into the prepared tin and bake for about 1 to 1 and a half hours. Test with a skewer to check its cooked properly. Turn out and cool. Eat one thick slice of menopause cake a day.

Red flags

Night sweats

Relatively common in menopause but may also be caused by infections such as Lyme disease or tuberculosis. Lymphadenopathy may also cause night sweats. Ask about recent travel abroad, persistent cough or possibility of tic bites. Also ask about any unusual swellings that may involve lymph glands (in the neck for example)

Menorrhagia (heavy periods)

Also fairly commonly experienced during menopause as a result of hormone imbalance. Any menorrhagia which is unresponsive to treatment should be referred for further investigation, to eliminate pathological causes. Also any bleeding occurring after menstruation has stopped for 1 year.

Low mood

Mood related symptoms are again not uncommon. Be aware of the possibility of underlying clinical depression.

Conclusion

Patients seeking help in dealing with symptoms surrounding the menopause represent a fairly significant proportion of our work as consulting medical herbalists. The health scares which continue to surround HRT, and the paucity of other available options in terms of orthodox medicine results in many women washing up at our doorsteps 'when all else has failed'.

Over-the-counter remedies will only ever be helpful to a relatively small percentage of women due to the complex nature of menopause, and its susceptibility to being impacted by the stresses and strains that many women experience in this changing stage of life. It is supremely amenable to help and support however when that help and support is tailored to the needs of the individual. Tonic herbs are of particular use here, as the need to support the system as a whole is often the key to success.

There really is no substitute for a full herbal medicine consultation, the opportunity to be heard, and to reflect on our health and wellbeing as a complete whole. This may be the first time a woman has had the opportunity to properly consider and address her broader health concerns so thoroughly.

Part 2. Migraine

What is a migraine?

> **Definition—Migraine:** Ancient Greek of *hemi* meaning half and ancient Greek of *kranion* meaning skull = *hemikranion*. Late Latin users used the word hemicranias to describe a headache or pain in the head involving half of the head only. The common pronunciation of this word in old French was *migraigne*. 14th-century Middle English used the word megrim. In 1777 this was then re-spelt in English to give us migraine.

The modern-day definition of migraine

Migraine = a severe, recurring, throbbing headache, often (but not always) unilateral, and worsened by movement. Headache can last between 4–72 hours. Visual disturbances may precede a migraine (approx. 1/3 of cases) and nausea and vomiting may accompany it.

Other symptoms may include:

- Visual disturbances—flashing lights, zig-zag patterns or blind spots
- Numbness or a tingling sensation/pins and needles, often starting in one hand and moving up the arm to the face, lips and tongue
- Dizziness
- Transient aphasia (difficulty speaking)
- Photophobia, phonophobia
- Mood changes (depression or elation)
- Skin hypersensitivity
- Food cravings
- Repetitive yawning
- Loss of consciousness (rare)

It is not uncommon for migraine and sinusitis to be confused, and a misdiagnosis made. Both conditions can present with nasal and sinus congestion, nausea, facial pain and pressure, moderate to severe headache, pulsing/throbbing pain and headache made worse by physical activity. Establishing the presence or absence of an underlying sinus infection or predisposition towards 'sinusy' conditions can be helpful. Of course the two conditions may co-exist.

The phenomenon of migraine is something that the herbalist encounters on a regular basis, either as the primary reason for the consultation, or as a symptom uncovered during the consultation process. In terms of prevalence, the Migraine Trust (founded in 1965) have published the following figures:

- Migraine is the third most common disease in the world (behind dental caries and tension-type headache) with an estimated global prevalence of 14.7% (that's around one in seven people).
- Migraine is more prevalent than diabetes, epilepsy and asthma combined.
- Migraine affects three times as many women as men, with this higher rate being most likely hormonally-driven.

- Research suggests that 3000 migraine attacks occur every day for each million of the general population. This equates to over 190,000 migraine attacks every day in the UK.
- More than three-quarters of migraine sufferers (migraineurs) experience at least one attack each month, and more than half experience severe impairment during attacks.

There are currently seven main types of migraine, as classified by the International Headache Society. Very simply they are:

- Migraine without aura—*common migraine* the most frequent
- Migraine with aura—*classic* or *complicated migraine*
- Migraine *without headache*
- Migraine with brainstem aura—*basilar type migraine*
- *Hemiplegic migraine* (can cause temporary paralysis)
- *Retinal migraine* (very rare, may cause loss of vision in one eye)
- *Chronic migraine*

Migraine sufferers themselves will tend to describe their migraine more in terms of circumstances linked to or associated with how they experience them, therefore common terminology also includes menstrual migraine, weather-related migraine, morning migraine, abdominal migraine etc.

> *I got a bad migraine*
> *That lasted three long years*
> *And the pills that I took*
> *Made my fingers disappear.*
> —David Bowie, Time Will Crawl, Glass Spider Album

Causes and symptoms: pathophysiology of migraine

Although a specific classification system has been developed the actual cause of migraine is unknown. Extensive research has uncovered a number of mechanisms involved in the aetiology of migraine including the following:

Blood vessels, the trigeminal nerve and neuropeptides

Disorders of nervous tissue function can be initiated by a number of metabolic mechanisms, including hypoxia (low oxygen) and blood glucose balance. The brain consumes energy at ten times the rate of tissues in the rest of the body. Its only source of fuel is glucose. Nervous system tissue can be vulnerable to disordered function as a result of hypoglycaemia.

Disordered function results in self-propagating waves of cellular depolarisation spreading across the brain at a rate of 3–5 millimetres/minute, a phenomenon called cortical spreading depression (CSD). CSD is thought to be responsible for the migraine aura itself. Cerebral blood flow (CBF) is reduced as a result of this. Transient vasoconstriction of blood vessels in the brain then results in rebound vasodilation leading to pain.[15]

Blood vessels of the meninges are more receptive to pain that those in other areas of the body due to rich nerve supply via the trigeminal nerve. The trigeminal nerve may also release vasoactive neuropeptides, which enhance the pain further. Nitrous oxide (NO) and bradykinin are involved in this, and they produce an inflammatory response around the innervated blood vessels.

It has been noted that serotonin (5HT) levels fluctuate during a migraine. Serotonin is involved in many processes in the body, including sleep, mood, memory and hormone regulation. Bradykinin and other prostaglandins are produced from serotonin. Some effective drugs in the treatment of migraine work via interaction with serotonin receptors.

The experience of hypersensitivity of the skin reported by some sufferers is thought to result from trigeminal nerve involvement. It is widely accepted that there is a genetic predisposition to migraines but the triggers can vary from person to person. Stress is often cited as a leading trigger for migraines. One hypothesis for this is that prolonged or excessive sympathetic nervous system stimulation results in overload, which alters the balance of the relative concentrations of neurotransmitters in synaptic clefts, resulting in excessive vasodilation.

Excessive sympathetic nervous system stimulation in the digestive tract will then lead to nausea and sickness, as well as a slowing of the digestive processes, resulting in pain relief medications not being properly absorbed. Remember serotonin, the neurotransmitter that fluctuates during migraines? It should be noted here that approximately 90% of the body's serotonin is located in the gut! Finally, there is a very definite relationship between migraines and hormonal fluctuations, however direct mechanisms of action remain unclear as experiences vary enormously.

There is no specific diagnostic test for migraine. Diagnosis is dependent upon the taking of a full case history and identifying an underlying pattern of symptoms. The International Classification of Headache Disorders (produced by the Headache Society and recognised as an official classification by the World Health Organization) recommends that diagnosis of a headache as migraine is dependent upon the following criteria:

- The presence of any two of the following headache symptoms: unilateral, throbbing, worsened by movement, severe or moderate.
- And the presence of one of: nausea/vomiting, photophobia and phonophobia.

Interesting Fact: Crocodile medicine

Dating back to at least 1200 BC, the Ebers papyrus is a compilation of ancient Egyptian prescriptions and medical treatments. One treatment for shooting pains in the head is consistent with what we now call migraine.

A strip of linen was used to tie a clay crocodile holding grain in its mouth to the head of the patient.

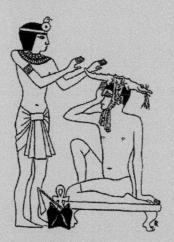

The names of the gods that were believed to be able to cure illness were written on the linen strip. Interestingly it is now thought that this technique could have worked, as compressing the scalp may have helped constrict dilated blood vessels that were contributing to the pain.

Artwork produced by migraine sufferers gives us a very real and unique insight into some of the neurological symptoms that people experience. There is a very specific type of zig-zag pattern called a scintillating scotoma, which has been reproduced in artworks.

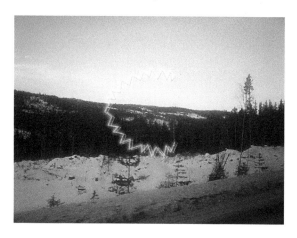

These jaggy, zig zaggy lines have also led them to be called fortification spectrum, after the battlements of a castle. Scintillating scotomas (which we think sounds like a type of nocturnal mongoose) are thought to be caused by the aforementioned CSD, and can constitute an aura which may or may not result in a migraine.

Interesting Fact: Lewis Carroll

Lewis Carroll was a migraine sufferer (migraineur) and it is thought that his invention of the disappearing Cheshire cat may have originated in the visual auras he suffered, which gradually disappeared.

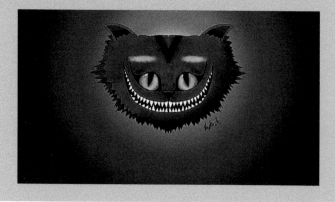

Conventional approaches to treatment

The National Institute for Health and Care Excellence (NICE) clearly state on their website that there is no cure for migraine. They currently recommend the following treatment strategy:

- Identify and minimise/avoid triggers. (This may include the patient keeping a migraine diary for at least 8 weeks.)
- Pain relief medicines.

Common conventionally accepted triggers for migraine include amine-containing foods such as chocolate, alcohol and cheese. Stress is recognised as another trigger, and research shows that most migraines are experienced at the weekend.[16] Stress management techniques may therefore be recommended by a GP within an orthodox framework for the treatment of migraine.

Pain relief medications include a class of drugs called triptans, which work via serotonin receptors on blood vessel walls and nerve endings to block the release of inflammatory neuropeptides. They can be highly effective at aborting a migraine, but are contra-indicated in cardiovascular disease and many conditions involving the circulatory system, due to their interactions with blood vessel walls. Paracetamol or Aspirin may be offered with or instead of a triptan.

Dealing with nausea and vomiting

Medications such as triptans can be administered as a nasal spray or via subcutaneous injection, which can be helpful if nausea or sickness prevents oral administration. Anti-emetics such as metoclopramide, domperidone, or prochlorperazine are also recommended (even in the absence of nausea and vomiting).

NB: Gabapentin and pregabalin (both triptans) are two examples of medications that list aphasia (impairment of language and speech) as a potential side effect.

Prophylaxis (longer-term prevention)

Drugs for long-term prophylaxis may also be offered, and include:

Topiramate   An antiepileptic drug with a complex mechanism of action, involving blockage of voltage-dependent

	sodium and calcium channels. The relevant mechanisms of action responsible for efficient migraine prophylaxis remain unclear.
Propanolol	A beta blocker commonly used for a number of disorders. (Works at the level of beta receptors to block the actions of adrenaline.)
Amitriptyline	A tricyclic antidepressant, with a number of pathways including blocking serotonin reuptake inhibition.
Tolfenamic acid	A cyclooxygenase (COX) inhibitor, preventing the formation of certain prostaglandins.
Naproxen	A COX inhibitor
Diclofenac.	A COX inhibitor

Painkiller habituation

Currently the NHS Choices website advise patients against taking pain killers for more than 10 days in a month in the long term. Regular pain killer use can engender something called an analgesic overuse headache, meaning that when you stop taking the painkiller you get a headache. This can make migraines difficult to treat. NICE guidelines do not recommend prophylactic treatment in younger adults (age 12–17) unless supervised by a specialist.

NICE guidelines for the treatment of migraine also include the option of ten acupuncture sessions. It may often be the case that individual doctors develop their own particular strategies working inside this framework, and some may also consider a more broad-based approach, involving more focus on dietary and lifestyle changes and possibly even the use of some more 'complementary' strategies (ie the inclusion of feverfew in the treatment strategy).

Currently, due to the perspective that this is not a 'curable' condition in terms of orthodox management, treatment is largely symptomatic and is aimed at minimising the impact of migraine on daily life. Thus complete resolution is rarely achieved. The potential for painkiller habituation and rebound headaches to occur is also a factor.

Western herbal medicine's approach to treatment

Ancient Greek doctors who followed the humoural approach to medicine, saw migraines as an excess of yellow or black bile: choler or melancholia. Thus a rebalancing of the internal environment was central to treatment.

Michael McIntyre, former president of the National Institute of Medical Herbalists sees migraine as:

> *a restorative attempt by the body, mind and spirit (vis medatrix naturae)*
> *to achieve reparation of a substantially disordered internal economy.*
>
> —Michael McIntyre

This can be seen as a form of internal 'early warning system' by which the body protects itself from further damage by shutting the system down. He goes on to say that migraines can be seen to have a logic of their own, and describes them as,

> *A prayer for nutrition, rest and restoration.*

Masking of pain with painkillers may therefore be counterproductive in the long term, as it prevents the body from addressing an underlying threat to health, and does not allow the body to be heard. As always the treatment of migraines should centre upon the individual. The multifactorial nature of both the physiological pathogenesis of migraine and of the factors surrounding individual cases makes it very amenable to the flexible nature of herbal treatment. A few of the more common scenarios underlying migraine presentation will now be described:

It is often (but not always) the case that migraine sufferers are driven people. They can be over-achievers who demand much of themselves and have a high work ethic. In these cases, people tend to judge themselves on what they have not achieved rather than what they have achieved. Thus their cup will never 'runneth' over.

There may often be an element of 'running on empty': where constantly pushing their systems (and their adrenal glands in particular) can lead to long-term depletion of resources. Over-achievers can often end up promoted to a level where they are struggling to keep up. They often neglect themselves by missing meals, by minimising leisure time, taking work home etc. When people who fall into this category do relax (at the weekend for example) the system can crash in terms of internal reserves. They are in deficit; demand exceeds supply.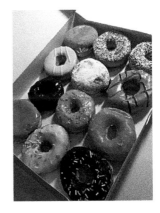

Possibly one of the key issues here is diet. Migraines may be triggered by either missing meals or by eating foods with high sugar content.

Remember in the anatomy and physiology section we talked about nervous tissue and red blood cells as specifically needing glucose as their main energy source. Drops in blood sugar level in a stressed person who has either missed a meal or has eaten a refined sugar snack, and thus induced an insulin spike in the system, can present as a migraine trigger. The other word in that sentence is stress of course.

The chronic stress that many people are under can result in high levels of fight-or-flight substances coursing through our bodies with no way for us to burn them off. This can also present as a trigger, and, of course, many of these chemical mediators will act to raise the blood sugar levels, so that we have the energy to either fight or run.

Adrenaline stimulates glucose release from the liver; simultaneously, growth hormone and cortisol levels rise, causing body tissues (muscle and fat) to be less sensitive to insulin. More glucose is available in the bloodstream. In the case of the sugary snack eater, an input of refined sugar plus a metabolic rise in blood sugar due to chronic levels of adrenaline is going to result in a massive insulin spike, and subsequent glucose crash. In the case of the 'meal misser' low glucose will reap its own effects.

The bottom line is maintenance of stable blood sugar will pay dividends for many migraine sufferers. This means taking the time to relax and eat good quality food, and not to skip meals. Eliminating refined sugar from the diet of migraine sufferers can result in significant improvements. The role of hormones as migraine triggers is also a key factor to treatment. Recording exactly where in the menstrual cycle migraines occurs will dictate what is needed to resolve them.

For example, during the luteal phase of the menstrual cycle, a woman's basal body temperature rises. This represents an extra drain on resources as energy has to be supplied to both brain and uterus. Cravings for chocolate etc. can thus be explained. Migraines occurring pre-menstrually usually require hormonal balancing.

Some general strategies—fitting the treatment to the patient

- Assess stress levels.
- Assess diet and nutritional status.
- Determine when/how/if your patient is able to relax.

Herbs with useful mechanisms of action pertaining to the pathophysiology of migraine generally would include:

Ginkgo biloba L. (maidenhair tree)—improves restricted cerebral blood flow, thus optimising the availability of oxygen and glucose to nervous system tissue.

Bitters are really useful when a patients' migraines show a definite link with poor digestion. Happily bitters will also help address blood sugar imbalances. Directly linked to this of course, is the tendency to constipation. Constipation can significantly impact on conditions such as migraine, as the system becomes sluggish and some patients report a sense of feeling 'toxic'. Improving bowel function can sometimes be all that is needed to ameliorate a tendency towards migraines in some people. Lovely bitters can help with this, and dandelion root *Taraxacum officinalis* radix L. is a great example of a herb which works on this level to improve bile flow, keep gut peristalsis healthy and support the gut microbiome.

But of course we do not want to fall into the trap of simply prescribing according to identified pathophysiological actions. We need to dig deeper for optimal success. For example nervines and tonic herbs can be crucial to treatment and need to be selected according to the individual case history of the patient.

Speaking of the patient, let's look a little more closely at patient constitutions, and how they impact our treatment plans.

- Red-faced, loud, irritable people (choleric presentation).
  Overuse of stimulants may be part of the picture—caffeine, alcohol etc.
  Use cooling, bitter, relaxing herbs. The herb feverfew (*Tanacetum parthenium* (L.) Sch.Bip.) has a history of use as a warm infusion for purging choler. It is a bitter herb, and is probably the best-known herb today in use for the treatment of migraines. Those red-faced, irritable choleric types may well benefit from this.
- Fatigued, pale people with low blood pressure. Depleted people. Circulatory stimulants, warming tonic herbs, digestive tonics.
- Tense, uptight people. May complain of a headache, which feels like a tight band around the head. This may involve chronic underlying stress and present with anxiety. Relaxing nervines, circulatory support.

- Menstrual migraines. Establish where in the cycle they are occurring. Treat accordingly. Follicular phase: nourish ovaries and vital reserves. Luteal phase: stimulate luteal phase, nourish the uterus. Pre-menstrual phase: regulate menstruation. Post menstruation: building and blood nourishing herbs. Address depletion. Rebalance circulation.

So we can see now why the question 'what can I take for my migraine??' does not have a straightforward answer!

Pain relief

It is a general belief that orthodox medicine has 'superior firepower' when it comes to pain relief. This has come about, at least in part, by the exclusive use of the mono-chemical approach that uses 'high strength' and 'targeted' phrases which engender faith in their efficacy. Whilst there is no doubt that orthodox medications can be highly effective in terms of pain relief, the herbal medicine arsenal is deceptively gentle but at the same time can significantly alleviate discomfort as well as tackling pain directly.

Useful herbs for this purpose would include:

Pulsatilla vulgaris Mill.	*Matricaria chamomilla* L.
Filipendula ulmaria (L.) Maxim.	*Lavandula officinalis* L.
Piscidia erythrina (L.) Sarg.	*Viburnum opulus* L.
Salix alba L.	

Gelsemium sempervirens (L.) J.St.-Hil. (Practitioner use only. Schedule 20)

Probably the best-known herb in terms of migraine relief is *Tanacetum parthenium* L.

Mrs Grieves Modern Herbal (first published 1931) does not mention feverfew for the treatment of migraine at all, rather describing it as an aperient, carminative bitter and a general tonic.

Bone and Mills explained this oversight when they wrote:

> In 1973, at the suggestion of a friend, Mrs Anne Jenkins of Wales started taking three fresh leaves of feverfew each day in an attempt to rid herself of severe and recurrent migraines. After 10 months, Mrs Jenkins headaches had vanished and did not return so long as she kept taking feverfew. Her enthusiasm rapidly led to an epidemic of feverfew users.
>
> —S. Mills and K. Bone[17]

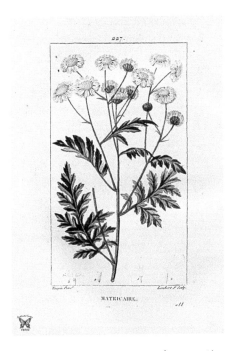

Feverfew (*Tanacetum parthenium* L)

It is certainly true to say that its reputation for migraine relief has totally overshadowed its longer history as a gentle, cleansing nervine. As with so many medicinally active plants the mechanisms of action of feverfew seem to involve multiple pathways. They have been shown to include:

- Decrease in vascular smooth muscle spasm
- Inhibition of prostaglandin synthesis/anti-inflammatory actions
- Blockage of platelet granule secretion (blood thinning properties)

The sesquiterpene lactone content (specifically parthenolide) has been cited as an important active constituent in many of these actions. Flavonoids and volatile oils are also present, as are coumarins.[18] Interestingly feverfew has also been found to contain melatonin, a hormone which we discussed in the first half of this chapter. Chronic migraine headaches have been associated with low circulating levels of melatonin.[19]

Okay, so we have a few more things to think about. Let's take a look at a case history to see how some of these concepts can be put into practice:

Migraine case study

A 57-year-old gentleman presented with a combination of chronic mouth ulcers and long-term skin problems which had worsened in recent times. The skin presented as a number of raised, red lumps, primarily on his torso, which he had been experiencing for years. The mouth ulcers tended to move around in his mouth but were often located on the tip of his tongue and around his lips. He did not wear dentures. Mouth and skin problems often happened at the same time.

He was a long-term sufferer of migraines, which he had noticed could be triggered by missing a meal. Alcohol was also a trigger and he felt he had a low tolerance for alcohol. He first experienced migraines in his mid-30s at a stressful time in his life concerning his marriage.

Primary symptoms included:

- Visual aura. Flashing lights
- Temperature changes. Could be rapid
- Severe headache. Intense pain
- Vomiting

He noticed that mouth ulcers sometimes accompanied the migraines. A bad migraine would occur approximately once every 2 months and he needed 2 days to recover from them. He also experienced what he called headaches around once every 10 days, which he described as a dull throb. He had tried taking feverfew (*Tanacetum parthenium* (L.) Sch. Bip.) in the past, which he believed helped at the time.

Significant background factors:

This gentleman suffered a sports injury to his lower back, resulting in occasional bouts of serious pain, which were almost always associated with low mood. His back had not been a problem in recent years, but he still experienced anxiety or depression from time to time. He felt that this was related to his eyes—possibly eye strain. He was getting his eyes checked regularly and wore reading glasses. He described himself as a warm person in terms of circulation etc. He described both his sleep and appetite as reasonable, and he did get hungry before meals. His diet was good, and he had recently reduced his coffee intake to 2 cups a day.

Treatment plan and rationale:

1) **Calming nervines**
   Stress certainly played into the initial onset of migraine and, in the longer term, anxiety appeared to underpin many of the problems presented. Allowing the sympathetic nervous system to relax can take the strain off the adrenal glands and lessen the impact of fight or flight chemical mediators.
2) **Improving gut function and integrity of mucous membranes**
   Although diet and appetite were both good mouth ulcers were an indication of potential inflammatory processes occurring further down the GI tract. Mouth ulcers were causing the patient significant distress, and therefore attention to mucous membrane integrity was one of the focuses of treatment. Skin health generally usually has close links to digestive function also. Headaches and migraines often respond well to liver support.
3) **Cleansing and cooling**
   Mouth ulcers, red raised lumps on skin and migraines all have the common feature of inflammation underlying them. Gently encouraging system detoxification and using anti-inflammatory herbs will allow the body to start to address these issues.

This gentleman came across as a mix of choleric and melancholic temperaments. Herbs were chosen for their cooling and relaxing properties.

The herbs

The first prescription included the deceivingly gentle but extraordinarily healing herb chamomile (*Matricaria chamomilla* L.). This was chosen for its gentle bitter actions, its calming and soothing properties and its anti-inflammatory effects, all of which would be of benefit to this patient. The herb wood betony (*Stachys betonica* L. syn. *Betonica officinalis* L.) was also used. Herbalist and author Christopher Menzies-Trull describes this herb as useful for 'neuralgic and ischaemic conditions affecting the head'. It is also a supportive liver herb and has gentle nervine properties.[20] Culpepper, in The English Physician, describes it as being for 'those that have continual pains in their heads, although it turn to phrensy'. It is bitter and cooling.[21] A third herb included in the first prescription was holy thistle (*Carbenia benedicta* L.). Another bitter and excellent liver herb, it has a reputation for 'pushing out eruptions' and as a depurative (blood cleanser). A mouthwash was also prescribed using sage (*Salvia officinalis* L.), marigold (*Calendula officinalis* L.), marshmallow (*Althaea officinalis* (radix) L.) and comfrey (*Symphytum officinale* (fol) L.) tinctures.

First follow-up 3 weeks later:

Compliance: No problems taking the medicine

Headaches/migraines: Headaches are possibly starting to be less frequent. A bit early to say regarding the migraines.

Mouth ulcers: Still getting mouth ulcers, but they are healing much more quickly. Also some do not actually develop fully.

Skin: A few less raised red lumps. No big ones have developed in the last 10 days. They are not as painful. Some are starting to develop on his legs (new).

Anxiety: Has been 'through the roof' in the morning. Has woken feeling really anxious in last few weeks, and feeling listless. These both improve as the day goes on. (**NB**: This gentleman was getting married within the next month and was anxious about the whole build-up to the event).

Miscellaneous: He had started taking a prebiotic supplement to help support gut flora.

Treatment plan:

Due to increasing levels of underlying anxiety, the calming adaptogenic herb ashwaganda (*Withania somnifera* (L.) Dunal.) was added to the prescription, as was the cooling adrenal tonic herb borage (*Borago officinalis* L.), wood betony, chamomile and holy thistle remained in the mix.

Second follow-up, 4 weeks later:

Mouth ulcers: None for the last 10 days. Not unusual to experience a good patch, but it was unusual to not have one when he has been so stressed. Has been keeping up with mouthwash.

Migraines: The odd headache, no longer every 10 days. No bad migraines since the first visit.

Anxiety: Still experiencing some in the morning but receded somewhat.

Skin: Not as bad as was on the first visit. Still not very good though.

Treatment plan: Slight change to main mix = addition of figwort (*Scrophularia nodosa* L.) a cooling and anti-inflammatory lymphatic, skin herb.

Third follow-up 7 weeks later:

Recent healthcare concerns. This gentleman had suffered a number of tick bites in recent months, and had been experiencing night sweats and pustules on the arms and legs. He was prescribed a 10-day course of doxycycline, a tetracycline antibiotic, and felt that he was now around 75% recovered from what was diagnosed as probable Lyme disease.

Mouth ulcers: Much better. Can sometimes feel one starting to form, but it doesn't come to anything.

Migraines: Had almost forgotten about them!

Generally feeling very well in himself.

Treatment plan

Given the most recent healthcare challenge, this patient was now prescribed 2 weeks worth of a strong anti-infective mix, and then the main mix was modified to include longer-term support for the immune system. The initial anti-infective mix included purple coneflower root (*Echinacea purpurea* (L.) Moench., and wild indigo (*Baptisia tinctoria* (L.) R.Br.).

Fourth follow-up 8 weeks later:

This gentleman was happy to report he felt very well.

Mouth ulcers: None. Occasionally feels one starting to form but they don't come to anything.

Migraines: Experienced a few instances of 'was that a migraine or not?' where he had a shift in perception of colour changes and some temperature shifts, but nothing more.

Skin: Not bad at all. A few pimply spots but nothing alarming or distressing.

Current Situation:

This gentleman has now been consulting his herbalist (with one 5-month break) for nearly 2 years.

In his own words:

'In that time I can only remember one "full-blown" migraine … with all the symptoms (terrible headache, nausea, vomiting, temperature fluctuations, lights and other things!) and about 3 or 4 minor ones (lights and sometimes hot flushes). Prior to that I was getting one migraine every 5 or 6 weeks, been this way for years. At the moment none at all, and not had one since the spring (mid-May) and that was a minor one'.

He is currently still taking herbal medicine with regard to another healthcare issue, which is on-going.

Summary

It is often the case that patients come for a consultation about a situation other than migraines, although they are a sufferer of them. It can then come as quite a surprise to people to learn that in fact significant improvements, if not complete resolution, can be achieved in the case of migraines by looking at the individual picture. They may have lived with sporadic migraine for some time, under the impression that 'nothing can be done' and it is only when they request help for something else that it becomes apparent that the migraines can be improved upon. It is possible therefore to view migraines as a kind of red flag, thrown up by the body that imbalances in the system are leading to neurological disruption. Those imbalances or perturbations can vary enormously.

In this gentleman's case, stress and anxiety undoubtedly played a considerable role in the aetiology of the migraines. It is our view that the mouth ulcers and skin complaint that he also presented with were different aspects of that same underlying disruption. Words like eruptive, volcanic, hot can be applied to all of these symptoms, emphasising the need for cooling and soothing herbs in terms of the energetics involved.

Again this case demonstrates the medium-term length of treatment required for herbs to have a beneficial effect. The correction of broad-based, chronic imbalances is rarely something that can be achieved quickly. Patience and faith are required.

> **Note:** Traditionally, heat in the 'blood' from excess activity in the liver was seen as the aggravating factor in any 'inflammatory' complaint presenting with heat and redness. Using herbs with an affinity for 'liver cooling' in such instances is an example of the energetic use of herbs in Western herbal practice. Aphthous ulcers, for example, are considered by medical herbalists to often be of 'liver origin'. Metabolically, the liver is of course the source of most of our body heat, and it is central to many inflammatory responses. Nevertheless, abnormal liver function tests may not be forthcoming, as these are often only found where acute liver cell death is occurring, and so, we are using the term 'liver' here but as an energetic red flag, not necessarily a currently 'measurable' pathological red flag.

What evidence is there for the herbal approach?

Research into the use of herbs in the treatment of migraines has shown variable results overall, which it may be said is unsurprising when the interventions are not targeted to specific underlying imbalances. One randomised, double-blinded, placebo-controlled trial by Kamali et al.[22] looking at a combination of three herbs (*Viola odorata* flos L.—sweet violet, *Rosa damascina* flos L.—damask rose, and *Coriandrum sativum* semen L.—coriander seeds) combined with propranolol (a beta blocker), reported significant improvements in the test group, compared to the control group (who also received the propranolol). It is interesting to note that all three herbs used here are aromatic plants with digestive and antispasmodic actions. The potential benefits of coriander seeds *Coriandrum sativum* semen L., were also investigated by Delavar et al., who concluded that syrup of coriander seeds was effective at reducing duration and frequency of migraine attacks, and also at decreasing pain severity experienced by the migraineur].[23] Traditionally coriander seed is constitutionally cooling to the liver.

Combining conventional and herbal treatments

Many migraine sufferers are taking regular pain killers for their migraines when they first consult a herbalist. This does not pose a significant problem for the herbalist, who can work around these drugs, and put supportive herbs in place to correct underlying imbalances. Ultimately it usually becomes possible to reduce the dependence upon pain killers, as duration, frequency and severity of symptoms all recede.

Self-help: the kitchen pharmacy

It is tempting to state that migraines are such a complex scenario, and their origins are so variable in people, that self-help is limited in its scope. However there is nothing that cannot be helped. The basic tenets of self-care can often significantly reduce the intensity and duration of a migraine. Some of these we have already touched on in terms of self-help at menopause.

Reduction in stress levels is a really key one here, and most of us know where the stress comes from in our lives, and to what extent it is possible to minimise it. For stressful situations in life that are not easily resolved, make sure you are getting all the support available to you. Allowing time out for ourselves for a walk in the country, a read of a book or magazine, or even a doze on the sofa can seem selfish, and we often choose to give these things a low priority in favour of 'other commitments', but we do this at our peril. If we do not recognise the intrinsic value of self-care, we can often ultimately pay the price.

Remember Michael McIntyre's concept of what a migraine really is? Let's remind ourselves, because it's worth repeating:

> A prayer for nutrition, rest and restoration.

Keep well hydrated—often the body's cries for water go unheard and unrequited, leading to system overload. Keeping hydrated can help keep the dreaded constipation at bay also. Eat well. Don't skip meals. Don't eat junk food, processed food etc. (you know the drill). Bitter foods (such as dandelion and sorrel leaves, radishes, cresses, and rocket), which cleanse and support digestive and liver function, would be really helpful.

Taking bitters before a meal would also be a good strategy—ask your herbalist for these, or try some Angostura bitters in sparkling water.

Nettle tea can be of real value, as it is cleansing (remember the old concept of a depurative), nutritious and balances out blood sugars. For migraines with nausea, chamomile tea works well for some, ginger tea for others. You can always chop fresh ginger into a cup of chamomile tea.

Feverfew has been used, with varying degrees of success as a prophylactic in the treatment of migraine. The most common strategy is to eat three fresh leaves every day (be prepared for the bitterness). For those of us with sensitive systems it would be advisable to wrap the leaves in bread before eating. This minimises the possibility of developing a mouth ulcer from the contact of these strong bitter leaves with sensitive mucous membranes lining the mouth. You will note from the story concerning Mrs Jenkins that she took the feverfew for 10 months. Sticking with something and having faith is often really necessary!

NB: Make sure that you are really comfortable identifying this easily grown and common plant. Do not use the leaves of variegated feverfew as the variegations are caused by a viral infection of the plant.

Treat the underlying cause wherever possible. If you do not have a fairly good idea what this is, a consultation with a herbalist may be a jolly fine idea.

Red flags

When treating patients with migraines and/or recurring headaches, they are often long-standing and pre-diagnosed. Signs to watch out for that, require further investigation include:

- A first-time headache, occurring after the age of 50 (possible stroke/bleed/tumour)
- A first headache soon after pregnancy (vulnerability to thrombosis)
- Headache with fever and or photophobia and a stiff neck (check for meningitis)
- Any states of altered consciousness or focal neurological signs (such as weakness in one arm/leg, muscle spasm or altered gait). (Rule out a space-occupying lesion)
- Headache with red-eye, dilated, non-reactive pupil (possibly acute angle-closure glaucoma)
- Any headache that is not improving with treatment or is getting worse despite it

- Unusual headache in a patient on anticoagulants (rule out a bleed due to over anti-coagulation)
- Constant headache, always in the same location—never goes away

If you have any doubts about what you are dealing with, always refer.

Conclusion

Looking at the case studies presented in this chapter, a number of points become apparent.

- Herbal medicine can help in cases where people do not respond well to conventional drugs.
- Herbal medicine can help in cases where a clear diagnosis has not been obtained.
- Herbal medicine can work effectively alongside orthodox drugs. It may act to enhance the actions of orthodox drugs or it may result in a reduction in dosage of orthodox drugs needed to achieve the desired effect. Herbal medicine may also act to help the body effectively deal with orthodox drugs, thus minimising the potential for side effects to be experienced.
- Herbal medicine can act to normalise physiological function generally, thus achieving unexpected benefits for the patient.
- Herbal medicines can act as prebiotics and probiotics, normalising gut flora and optimising health.
- Symptoms may fluctuate during treatment, but people do tend to respond well to herbs, particularly if they are prepared to take them over the medium term/long term.
- Herbal medicine does not tend to fall under the category of the 'quick fix'. To really address underlying imbalances time may be needed. Improvement is usually steady, however.

Benefits can be achieved by the application of some basic principles, such as:

- A good understanding of current knowledge regarding the underlying physiological processes underpinning illness is crucial to treatment.

- This knowledge is then coupled with an ability to 'stand back' from the patient and regard them as a unique individual. Observation of the 'macrophysiology' of the patient, their symptoms, their constitution, the energetics underlying the dynamic of their wellbeing can provide vital information regarding the tailoring of treatment to suit that patient and that patient alone. Redressing the balance, and nudging diverse physiological processes back to normal function is a key strategy to treatment.
- Herbs are chosen with regard to both their mechanisms of action on a pharmacological level, and on their suitability for the individual patient, based on the constitution, (the need for warming, cooling, moistening or drying).

Ultimately patient-centred treatment requires a rational and intelligent approach combined with intuition and a genuine feel for both people and plants. This is where the potential for resolution rather than management lies.

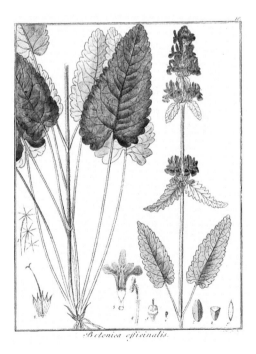

Wood betony (*Stachys betonica* L.)

Bibliography

McIntyre, Michael, *Mastering Migraine—Making Meaning of the Message.* Notes From a 1-day Seminar. November 2008: Regents College London.

Romm, Aviva, *Botanical Medicine for Women's Health.* 2010: Churchill Livingstone Elsevier.

Stevenson, Clare, *The Complementary Therapists Guide to Conventional Medicine.* 2011: Churchill Livingstone Elsevier.

Trickey, Ruth, *Women, Hormones and the Menstrual Cycle.* 3rd ed. 2011: Melbourne Holistic Health Group.

References

1. Sassarini, Jennifer, and M. A. Lumsden, *oestrogen replacement in menopausal women. Age and Ageing,* 1st July 2015. 44(4): pp. 551–558.
2. Chen, C. Q. et al., *Distribution, function and physiological role of melatonin in the lower gut.* World J Gastroenterol, 2011. 17(34): pp. 3888–3898.
3. Tordjman, S. et al., *Melatonin: Pharmacology, functions and therapeutic benefits.* Curr Neuropharmacol, 2017. 15(3): pp. 434–443.
4. Hill, S. M. et al., *Melatonin: an inhibitor of breast cancer.* Endocr Relat Cancer, 2015. 22(3): pp. R183–204.
5. Freedman, R. R., *Menopausal hot flashes: mechanisms, endocrinology, treatment.* J Steroid Biochem Mol Biol, 2014. 142: pp. 115–120.
6. Blumel, J. E. et al., *Quality of life after the menopause: a population study.* Maturitas, 2000. 34(1): pp. 17–23.
7. Barnes, J., *Traditional herbalists' prescriptions for common clinical conditions: A survey of members of the UK National Institute of Medical Herbalists.* Phytotherapy Research, 1998. 12: pp. 1099–1573.
8. Denham et al., *What's in the bottle? Prescriptions formulated by medical herbalists in a clinical trial of treatment during the menopause.* Journal of Herbal Medicine, 2011. 1: pp. 95–101.
9. Green et al., *Treatment of menopausal symptoms by qualified herbal practitioners: a prospective, randomized controlled trial.* Family Practitioner, 2007. 24: pp. 468–474.
10. *Concerns for the use of soy-based formulas in infant nutrition.* Paediatr Child Health, 2009. 14(2): pp. 109–118.
11. Nahidi, F. et al., *Effects of licorice on relief and recurrence of menopausal hot flashes.* Iran J Pharm Res, 2012. 11(2): pp. 541–548.
12. Mehrpooya, M. et al., *A comparative study on the effect of 'black cohosh' and 'evening primrose oil' on menopausal hot flashes.* J Educ Health Promot, 2018. 7: p. 36.

13. Rahimikian, F. et al., *Effect of Foeniculum vulgare Mill. (fennel) on meno-pausal symptoms in postmenopausal women: a randomized, triple-blind, placebo-controlled trial.* Menopause, 2017. 24(9): pp. 1017–1021.

14. Trickey, R., *Women, Hormones and the Menstrual Cycle* 2011: A&U.

15. Vinogradova, L. V., *Initiation of spreading depression by synaptic and network hyperactivity: Insights into trigger mechanisms of migraine aura.* Cephalalgia, 2018. 38(6): pp. 1177–1187.

16. Guidotti, M. et al., *Symptomatic or prophylactic treatment of weekend migraine: an open-label, nonrandomized, comparison study of frovatriptan versus naproxen sodium versus no therapy.* Neuropsychiatr Dis Treat, 2013. 9: pp. 81–85.

17. Bone, K. and S. Mills, *Principles and Practice of Phytotherapy: Modern Herbal Medicine.* 2nd ed. 2013: Churchill Livingstone.

18. Pareek, A. et al., *Feverfew (Tanacetum parthenium L.): A systematic review.* Pharmacogn Rev, 2011. 5(9): pp. 103–310.

19. Murch, S. J., C. B. Simmons and P. K. Saxena *Melatonin in feverfew and other medicinal plants.* The Lancet, 1997. 350: pp. 1598–1599, doi: http://www.esalq.usp.br/lepse/imgs/conteudo_thumb/Melatonin-in-feverfew-and-othe-medicinal-plants.pdf.

20. Menzies-Trull, C., *Herbal Medicine: Keys to Physiomedicalism Including Pharmacopoeia.* 2003: The Faculty of Physiomedical Herbal Medicine (FPHM).

21. Culpeper, N., *Culpeper's Complete Herbal.* 1995: Wordsworth Press.

22. Kamali, M. et al., *Efficacy of combination of Viola odorata, Rosa damascena and Coriandrum sativum in prevention of migraine attacks: a randomized, double blind, placebo-controlled clinical trial.* Electron Physician, 2018. 10(3): pp. 6430–6438.

23. Delavar Kasmaei, H. et al., *Effects of Coriandrum sativum syrup on migraine: a randomized, triple-blind, placebo-controlled trial.* Iran Red Crescent Med J, 2016. 18(1): p. e20759.

24. Štulíková, K., *Therapeutic Perspectives of 8-prenylnaringenin, a potent phytoestrogen from hops.* Molecules. 2018 Mar; 23(3): pp. 660. Published online 2018 Mar 15. doi: 10.3390/molecules23030660.

25. Ralph, A. and G. Webley, *A Prospective audit of Pragmatic herbal treatment of women experiencing menopausal symptoms using Measure Yourself Medical Outcome Profile (MYMOP2) questionnaires.* Journal of herbal Medicine, May 2019.

CHAPTER EIGHT

Native healers: five more key plants from the Western herbal tradition

Y*ou may wish to read this chapter in conjunction with the section on the lymphatic system, which we covered in Chapter 3.*

Introduction

In this third *materia medica* chapter taking an in-depth look at five magnificent plant protectors, we will cover plants used for the lymphatic and respiratory systems, as well as herbs with wide-ranging, general applications. During our journey we will cover all the main topics surrounding these plants that were considered in Chapters 4 and 6, and we will also explore concepts such as emmenagogues and the use and value of mucilaginous herbs. We will pause to take a moment to consider the concept of the energetic properties of herbs in a bit more detail, and we will look at the preparation of oxymels, medicinal preparations made from honey and vinegar, which have been in use for thousands of years. (Sekanjabin is an Iranian version of this ancient form of medicine, and is a syrupy, minty drink, still used today). Let us make a start with the magnificent herb thyme.

Five magnificent plant protectors

Thyme (Thymus vulgaris L.)

It is as though the full force and energy of a whole tree has been packed into the tiny leaves and stems of this incredibly reliable plant protector. Thyme has the capacity to restore order, and even stays on to mop up the aftermath.

Classification

Thyme belongs to the mint family, also known as the Lamiaceae. Mostly found in the Mediterranean, they are usually small shrubs or herbs. The mint family includes such familiar plants as motherwort (*Leonurus cardiaca* L.), wood betony (*Stachys officinalis* L.) and marjoram (*Origanum vulgare* L.).

The thymes themselves are very variable and prone to hybridisation, making classification a difficult task.[1] Wild thymes found in the UK include *Thymus praecox* Opiz, *Thymus praecox* subspecies brittanicus, and Breckland or creeping thyme (*Thymus serpyllum* L.). These latter species are often found on grazed pasture and cropped grassland areas, and are variable in their aromatic scent. Barker notes that a species of thyme (*Thymus capitatus* L. Hoffman & Link in all likelihood), may have been brought north by the Romans due to its use in religious observance.[1]

Basic botany

An erect grey-ish green aromatic sub-shrub (often woody below) 10–30 centimetres in height. Semi-evergreen, and widely cultivated, it is familiar as a culinary and garden plant, and is loved by bees.

- **Flowers** flowers are whitish-to pale purple and are female or hermaphrodite. The flower calyx is bell-shaped, usually two-lipped, hairy in the throat. Corolla has a straight tube and protruding stamens. Some of the flowers form a distinct whorl, and there is a tendency for the flowers to crowd the top of the stems, and become interrupted below.
- **Leaves** neat linear elliptical evergreen leaves, only a trifle longer than the flowers, sit directly on the stem.

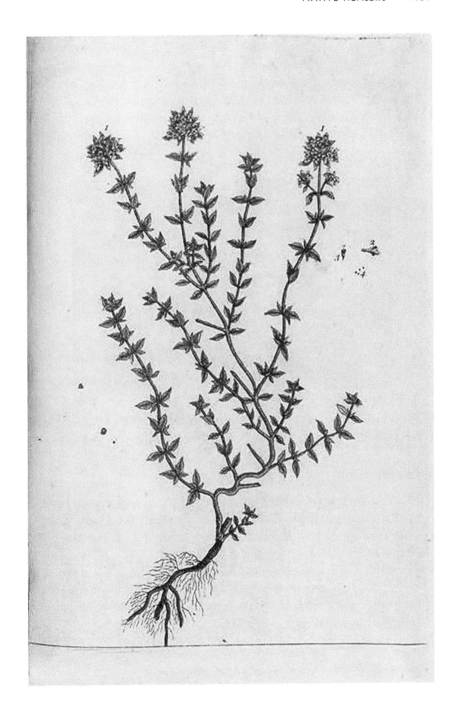

- **Habitat** native to the Western Mediterranean from Spain to the heel of Italy. There are some 70 species of thyme in Europe, mostly from the Mediterranean, and very few native to northern Europe.[1,2] Thymus species prefer dry slopes and rocks but will adapt to cooler climates (*Thymus vulgaris* L. is also known as winter thyme).
- The word thyme is derived from the ancient Greek word 'thuein', meaning to offer incense/burn or sacrifice (to burn for the sake of the Gods).

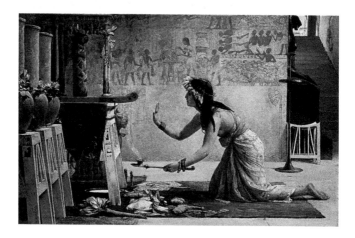

- **Parts used** flowering herb and the uppermost leaves with their small flexible stems (not woody). Harvested just before or during flowering.

Main constituents

- *Volatile oils*: The volatile oil of thyme has been investigated as the main therapeutic agent of which the major component is thymol.[3]
- *Other compounds*: Carvacrol (see below), 1,8-cineole, borneol, thymol methyl ether and alpha-pinene.
- *Carvacrol*: A phenolic monoterpene with intrinsic antimicrobial and antifungal activity, possibly produced by the plant to protect itself from pathogenic microbes. It is found in thyme and oregano species and also black walnut leaves and hulls.

Note: Remember—extrapolation of the properties of single constituents may not represent the true nature biologically when used as the whole plant.

It is recognised that plants containing such compounds are used extensively in many societies on the globe, and research about such practices can be found in journals that specialise in primary research in ethnomedicine (such as the *Journal of Ethnopharmacology*).

The chemicals produced by plants are exceptionally diverse and complex in structure, and are likely to have been developed over millennia to have the capacity to bind to their protein and DNA targets. Thus plant antibacterials are very different in shape and chemistry to existing conventional antibacterial chemotypes (often derived from other microbes) such as the antibiotics erythromycin and tetracycline.

Tetracycline structure

Erythromycin Structure

Carvecrol Structure

This makes herbs like thyme a valuable resource, especially since there may be other mechanisms of action beyond what is currently understood about them.[3] This is an interesting thought in an age of increasing bacterial resistance, and one that has exercised researchers.[4] Performance as an antimicrobial and for antioxidant activity has been demonstrated for thyme.[5,6]

Other interesting constituents within thyme include:

Flavonoids (apigenin, luteolin, thymosin and others) and polyphenolic acids (labiatic acids, rosmarinic and caffeic acids). All the above constituents are considered to contribute to anti-inflammatory and antimicrobial effects.

Main therapeutic actions confirmed by research

Anti-infective agent

Thyme has marked antimicrobial activity (see above) especially with the tissues of the respiratory system such as the sinuses, and the lungs and associated structures.[7] In recent research Sakkas and Papadopoulou state that:

> The thyme oil antimicrobial effect is also attributed to carvacrol and thymol, and its antimicrobial spectrum is wide, including bacteria (Aeromonas spp., B. cereus, B. subtilis, E. faecalis, L. monocytogenes, methicillin-resistant S. aureus, S. epidermidis, S. enteritidis, S. Typhimurium, Helicobacter pylori, E. coli, E. coli O157:H7, Y. enterocolitica, K. pneumoniae, Shigella spp., Campylobacter jejuni, and P. aeruginosa) and fungi (C. albicans, C. tropicalis, C. glabrata, C. krusei, C. parapsilosis, S. cerevisiae, dermatophytes, Fusarium spp., and Aspergillus spp.).

They go on to explain the mechanism of action of essential oils as anti-microbials by saying:

> The essential oils, particularly those rich in phenolics, have the potential to alter both the permeability and the function of the cell membrane proteins by penetrating into the phospholipids layer of the bacterial cell wall, binding to proteins and blocking their normal functions.
>
> Because of their lipophilic nature, essential oils and their compounds can influence the percentage of unsaturated fatty acids and their structure.

Ultimately they conclude:

> However, because of the variety of molecules present in plant extracts, their antimicrobial activity cannot be accredited to a single mechanism but to a number of diverse mechanisms at various sites of the bacterial cell outer and inner components, affecting the functions of cell membrane, cytoplasm, enzymes, proteins, fatty acids, ions, and metabolites.
>
> —P. C. Sakkas and C. Papadopoulou[6]

This last comment cuts through to one of the central recurring themes of whole plant medicines, that plants operate at a multiplicity of levels to exert their effects, and that studying compounds in isolation will not tell you about the whole plant.

Thyme also has some activity on the urinary and digestive tissues.

Expectorant

The capacity to expel and propel mucous up and out of the alveoli into the bronchioles and the bronchi and out of the body via the throat or stomach is a vital and *vitalistic* (having sufficient vitality) function. The mucous itself is produced by goblet cells within the mucous membranes of the lungs, and the mucous should be just the right consistency to entrap pathogens and cellular debris and yet also to be able to flow up and out of the body, expelling the results of inflammation and infection along the way.

True expectorants achieve this through mechanisms as yet unclear, but which involve the adequate and effective but not excessive muscular spasm of the lung tissues and also via the mucociliary escalator; some herbs being quite specific in this regard (*Pimpinella anisum* L.). Indeed, some old-fashioned 'sweets' trace their origins to the pharmacists' herbal store-cupboard for this reason—such as aniseed twists, cough candy and so on.

Western herbal medicine recognises that herbal medicines can:

a) thin excessively thick mucous. (*Sambucus nigra* L. (flowers), *Plantago lanceolata* L.)
b) can thicken excessively watery mucous (*Hyssopus officinalis* L., *Plantago lanceolata* L.)
c) can dry up excessively copious mucous (*Euphrasia officinalis* L.)
d) can soothe a deficient and dry mucous membrane (*Althaea officinalis* L. (leaf)).

This allows the medical herbalist to respond to a patient's acute or chronic infection with incredible diversity and with a uniquely individualised approach.

You will note that *Plantago lanceolata* L. has been cited here both to thicken watery mucous and to thin excessively thick mucous. This is another excellent example of an amphoteric action—the moving of the body back into balance in whatever direction is needed. Ribwort plantain, and greater plantain (*Plantago major* L.) are great lung tonics, restoring and stabilising normal function.

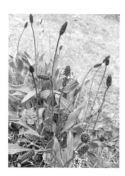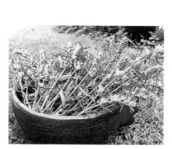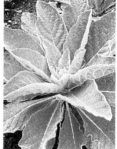

Classic pulmonary herbs, ribwort plantain, hyssop, and mullein.

Western herbal medicine recognises a number of pulmonary expectorants some more stimulating or sedating in their temperament (*Thymus vulgaris* L., *Hyssopus officinalis* L., *Prunus serotina* Ehrh., *Verbascum thapsus* L.,

Glycyrrhiza glabra L. and so on). Once again this allows the herbal prescription to be adapted to the person, or even to the phase of the infection process.

The above actions, confirmed by research, underpin the words written of Thyme in Culpeper's Complete Herbal (1653):

> *It is a noble strengthener of the lungs, as notable a one as grows.*

Antioxidant

Thyme is not simply an anti-infective expectorant, but a powerful antioxidant reducing oxidative stress on vulnerable cells. As such it makes for a superior medicine for use with infection and inflammation whether acute or chronic, and in preventing the acute becoming chronic! There is a huge array of scientific papers on the antioxidant effects of *Thymus vulgaris* L.[8–10] Some indicate that the antioxidant effects accelerate wound healing, others demonstrate that there is less DNA damage as a result of infection, where thyme is used.

Anti-inflammatory

The polyphenol content of *Thymus sp.* has been cited as central to providing valuable anti-inflammatory actions. This anti-inflammatory action is demonstrable for amounts commonly used in cooking (food as medicine!).[11]

Note: Energetic qualities. We have been looking at 15 different medicinal plants in detail. Each one has a long history of traditional use and most of them have modern research available for either their constituent parts or the whole herb used as a medicinal agent.

Another way of assessing whether a herb might be appropriate for a specific person uses a system of 'energetics'. Most traditional systems of medicine have a system of energetics. Traditional Chinese medicine places herbs within a framework of Yin and Yang, and of Organs and Elements. Ayurveda similarly has a dynamic energetic system of Doshas, and Elements. Humoural traditions also incorporate Elements and Organ systems.

Each of these systems also considers the vitality as animating the cells, tissues, organs and the whole body. We would like to introduce two key energetic concepts for your consideration. These come from the Western herbal tradition and have their roots in the eclectic and Physio-medical traditions, but are also echoes of the ancient Greek and Unani traditions and also must owe some thanks to the First Nations and Native traditions of the Americas where European settlers picked up and developed these themes, before returning them back to Europe.

The first concept is whether a herb can be considered as stimulating or relaxing.

The second concept is whether a herb can be considered to be moistening or drying.

Thymus vulgaris L. can be seen as Stimulating and Drying. Why? Firstly, We are using the terms Stimulating or Relaxing rather than the more ancient terms Hot and Cold. This is because Hot and Cold can be confusing when thinking about the human body and the processes of disease. For example—when you consider that coldness and subsequent stagnation can lead to inflammation—which by definition is Hot!

Let's look at the terms in a bit more detail ...

The stimulating (Hot)/sedating (Cold) polarity is active and drives all change, action and manifestation. Hot denotes a high level of energy or activity. Hot activates, excites, expands, disperses, moves and circulates. Cold is more sedative and demonstrates a low level of energy or activity. Cold slows down, sedates, contracts, congeals and obstructs.

One of the key herbs in physio-medicalism was cayenne pepper (*Capsicum minimum* Robux). Adding this spicy plant was seen to add vitality by stimulating circulation and therefore increasing flow, reducing stagnation, improving elimination and clearing the way for the body to send in its own healing mechanisms to the affected area.

The Dry, astringent (constricting)/Moist (relaxing) polarity is often referred to as passive because it is usually secondary to the active, primary stimulating/sedating qualities. In other words, heating things eventually drives away moisture. These Dry/Moist qualities refer to the relative level of moisture present in a system. You may also recall the way that tannins (drying) cause puckering of the membranes of the mouth and the constriction and congealing of proteins when tannins are added to milk for example.

Thymus vulgaris L., is an expectorant, the essential oils are highly phenolic and powerfully antiseptic. It is an upright, evergreen herb, capable of withstanding wide temperature variation. The capacity to be an expectorant is quite stimulating. There is stimulation to the nervous innervation of the bronchial tubes that encourages a more productive cough. Thymus also dries up excessive mucous secretions, and helps expel them via expectoration. This drying quality can also be seen as making the mucous membranes more resilient. Members of the Lamiaceae family share the quality of astringency. Astringents are drying and have the effect of increasing resilience by closing any 'gaps' that are allowing 'leakage' or not maintaining an effective boundary for a body tissue: in this case, the boundary between the lung and the outside world. The lungs in Chinese medicine are called the Precious Organs for this reason.

Ultimately this astringency and stimulation increases vigour, vitality and resistance. But since mucous membranes must be kept moist, this also suggests that overuse of *Thymus vulgaris* L. alone could eventually result in *excessive* dryness. The addition of a moistening herb may be required alongside thyme, especially if the person is already 'very dry' or if they will need to use thyme over a longer period of time.

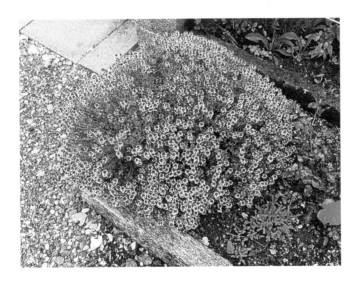

The application of this well-known culinary herb as a heroic medicine

Some people feel a natural inclination to steer clear of seeing the doctor and avoid taking conventional medicine under any circumstances. This strategy can result in doing nothing at all, however. It is disappointing to hear that a person has suffered unnecessarily with a nasty chest infection, or sinusitis, for example, and finally been so ill that they just 'had to take antibiotics', when they could have used herbal medicine instead.

We have found that certain plants, like *Thymus vulgaris* L., particularly in combination with other soft and gentle herbs, can perform fantastically well for even quite serious infections. They really are the heroes of herbal medicine. We do advise you work alongside a medical herbalist if you can; but it is also possible to monitor symptoms and signs (such as fever, and malaise) and persist with sufficient dose and frequency of dose, to treat infections successfully at home.

In Chapter 9 we will identify some key 'red flag symptoms', or things to be watchful for when treating respiratory tract infections, that may require conventional medical intervention. But with plenty of common sense, and judicious use of 'heroic' doses of herbs, much can be achieved.

We often come across cases where a person has had three courses of antibiotics to clear a chest infection, and still feels unwell. It may be that a person will need to take herbs like *Thymus vulgaris* L. for 3–6 weeks, rather than antibiotics for 3–4 weeks; but with careful monitoring, and realistic observation of improvements, it will be possible to avoid antibiotics in most cases.

Peter Holmes describes thyme as warming and drying, pungent, bitter and astringent. He ascribes benefits of it for melancholic and phlegmatic temperaments.[12] One of the most recent pieces of research regarding the antimicrobial actions of *Thymus sp.*, was conducted by de Oliviera et al.[13] and tested its effectiveness against *Candida albicans*, *Staphylococcus aureus*, *Enterococcus faecalis*, *Streptococcus mutans* and *Pseudomonas aeruginosa*. This piece of research also tested the potential for *Thymus* to damage healthy cells from a cross-section of tissue types. The research concluded that:

> *T. vulgaris* L. *extract was effective against all biofilms, promoted high cell viability, anti-inflammatory effect and presented no genotoxicity.*

The effectiveness of *Thymus vulgaris* L. in reducing lung inflammation and in acting as a cytotoxic agent in pulmonary cancer cell lines was also demonstrated in research by Oliviero et al. in 2016.[7]

Finally a spot of housekeeping.

Because of its great antiseptic properties, thyme oil can be used to make a simple and effective disinfectant spray for work surfaces, which is also kind to the environment.

Methods of preparation and use

Oxymels

Oxymels are a traditional preparation comprising of vinegar (acetic acid) mixed with honey. Often the oxymel was used for its expectorant properties. Both vinegar and honey have preservative properties, so this is a useful way of keeping herbs for use at a later date.

Vinegar itself can be seen to have healthful properties especially if it is made by a natural fermentation process such as apple cider vinegar (you can buy this 'with the mother'), or perhaps a wine vinegar made from a 'mother' but not pasteurised. As we saw in Chapter 4, it is possible to preserve dried herbs in a vinegar solution. These can be used internally or externally.

It is also possible to use honey as a preservative for herbs. Dried lavender flowers, sage leaves, bitter orange peel, and, of course, thyme, can be pressed into a jar of honey and used at a later date. Good quality raw honey also has health benefits and can improve the taste of any other medicine—including a vinegar! Herbal honeys can also be used internally or externally.

Thyme oxymel preparation

Cover 1 tablespoon of dried thyme with 5 tablespoons of organic cider vinegar. Leave to soak, in a closed jar for up to 1 year, but at least 2 weeks—keep in a cool or cold place whilst this is happening.

Strain off the dried herb by using a tea strainer or similar and collect the now 'infused' vinegar. Now add 4–5 tablespoons of good quality honey (ideally one that states the flowers the bees have fed on, and has not been heat extracted). Stir well, and keep in a labelled jar.

Either take small doses 'off the spoon', to ease a sore throat or cough, or add to hot water and sip through the day. You can add powdered cinnamon, ginger, nutmeg or lemon zest to your honey and leave it in, so that when you mix the honey with the vinegar you have two herbs not one!

Cautions and care

There have been no reports of any harmful effects to the baby with the use of the herb thyme in pregnancy. There is one reference from 1913 that reports an irritant paste used by doctors to procure an abortion, that included soap, potassium iodide and among other things, thymol (remember thymol is an extract of *one* compound found in the essential oil of thyme). This could account for the caution often cited for *Thymus vulgaris* L. and other herbs with a relatively high phenolic essential oil component, to not use in pregnancy.[14]

In the laboratory, some phyto-oestrogenic activity was demonstrated.

> *It is always worthwhile seeking the advice and on-going professional support of a qualified medical herbalist if pursuing treatment whilst pregnant.*

We have found it is possible to safely use many antimicrobial herbs, such as thyme during pregnancy, however, unfamiliarity of plant medicines can lead to anxiety for users, and there is unlikely to be professional support from conventional practitioners at this time.

Summary

This familiar culinary Mediterranean plant can pack a powerful punch when it comes to anti-infective properties. Its warming and drying energies, combined with its anti-inflammatory, expectorant and anti-infective qualities, make it a go-to herb for cold, damp conditions such as chest infections, especially where mucous needs shifting from the chest. Traditionally it is often used alongside moistening herbs such as liquorice to offset the possibility of inducing an over dry state due to high (heroic) doses or longer-term use. Its aromatic properties are great also for enhancing digestion.

Yarrow (Achillea millefolium *L.*)

The diffusive structure of yarrow leaves and flowers signifies how it can diffuse out from our centre to affect our circulation, its output and return. Yarrow really does remind us of the interconnectedness of our whole physiology.

Classification

Yarrow is a member of the Asteraceae family and grouped into the 'sneezeworts'. Sneezewort itself (*Achillea ptarmica* L.) hints at possible uses of these plants to help you if you have a cold and are sneezing, and perhaps also as a curiosity—that some herbs cause sneezing, a property seen as beneficial and known as a sternutatory. Another yarrow, *Achillea ligustica*, is recorded as being employed by wild birds in greening their nests to protect against pathogens.[15]

The name *Achillea* comes from the ancient story of how Achilles staunched the wounds of his soldiers with this plant—as taught by Chiron, the Centaur.

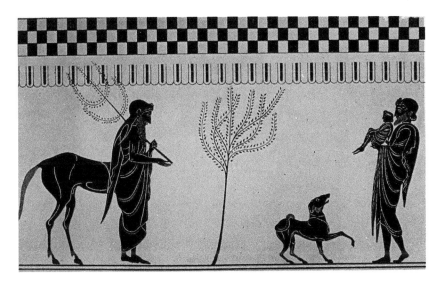

Chiron the centaur and his pupil of medicine Achilles.

Basic botany

An erect perennial herb (8–60 centimetres in height).

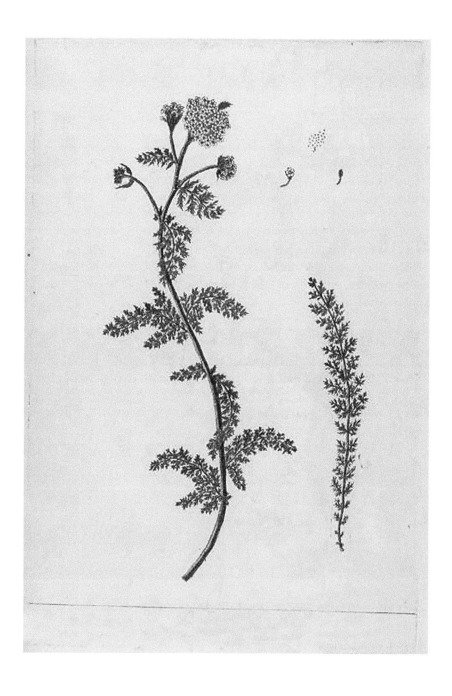

- **Leaves** dark green feathery leaves, pinnately divided.
- **Stem** a somewhat woolly unbranched stem.
- **Flowers** the flower heads sit close in a flat-topped cluster, neat as a white brooch.[1] Often creamy or even pink. Flowers are approximately 4–6 millimetres in diameter with a yellowish centre and whiteish rays. Yarrow flowers later in the year July–October, although may persist into November and beyond if the weather is mild.
- **Habitat** a common and persistent wild plant of grassy banks and roadsides, hedgerows, grassland and coastal areas.

The plant releases a warm aroma when rubbed. It is a stoloniferous plant—meaning it forms underground stolons that allow it to spread and form patches. We have observed it can form a neat ring when allowed to do this unimpeded.[2]

Parts used

Uppermost leaves and flowering tops are harvested when the plant is in full flower. This plant is almost always used after drying due to the potential for photosensitivity, and dermo-sensitivity (although this is rare). Used by every herbalist, possibly more than any other herb, this herb is often called 'the herbalists herb'. Its value as a medicinal plant is also reflected in the fact that it is repeatedly cited as a key herbal medicine in surveys done on medicinal plants across the globe.[16-19]

> If you consult old herbals you would get the impression that it can be used for almost anything and, as a result, wonder how it can be used for specific ills in a reliable way. The 'cure-all' reputation of yarrow owes in great part to a very complex set of ingredients that give it strength but also safety. This is because of the inter-relationships between them and the buffering effect, as in all plants, of the so-called 'inert' matrix of cellular material.
>
> —Julian Barker[1]

Main constituents

- Resins and volatile oils including cineole, pinene (as does thyme), limonene, thujone, caryophyllene
- Yarrow, like chamomile yields chamazulene, and also achilleine (a glycol-alkaloid), balchanolide

- Flavonoids and flavoneols including luteolin, quercetin, apigenin and kampherol
- Triterpenes
- Sterols
- Organic acids (achilleic acid, phenolic acids, ascorbic acid)
- Polyacetylenes
- Cyanogenic glycoside (very small amounts)
- Sesquiterpene lactones have been investigated and are thought to be a key active ingredient.

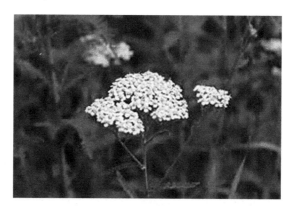

Yarrow (*Achillea millefolium* L.)

Main therapeutic actions confirmed by research

Anti-pyretic and diaphoretic

The use of herbs with a profound diaphoretic action is globally considered by herbalists to aid elimination of viral infections, and improve the febrile response. Yarrow is a classic example, but also boneset (*Eupatorium perfoliatum* L.), and cinnamon (*Cinnamonum verum* J. Presyl), ginger (*Zingiber officinale* Roscoe) and linden blossoms (*Tilia species*) are all well known. Use of fever suppressants such as sedative anti-inflammatories are considered to prolong the cold/flu process.

Anti-inflammatory

Yarrow is used worldwide for a number of inflammatory complaints, and seems to have what appear to be contradictory actions. The mechanisms of action of its anti-inflammatory effects continue to be investigated.[20] One theme we have explored in this course already, is that by improving 'flow' and the natural function of things, inflammation can be reduced or prevented, and the natural healing processes of the body can begin to exert their effects.

The flavonoids apigenin, kaempferol and luteolin have been identified as having anti-inflammatory properties which may benefit chronic neurodegenerative disorders such as multiple sclerosis, Alzheimer's disease and Parkinson's disease.[21]

Spasmolytic

Like other herbs with volatile oils that are antispasmodic (*Matricaria chamomilla* L., *Nepeta cataria* L. and *Thymus vulgaris* L.), yarrow has a great antispasmodic capacity within the digestive and circulatory systems. Thus as an antispasmodic to the peripheral circulation (and enabler of diaphoresis), yarrow can reduce vasospasm (such as with hot flushes), and is useful in fever management. It can be useful in anxiety syndromes where flushing is apparent, or where nosebleeds occur.

It is also spasmolytic to the digestive system and acts as a carminative, and so has a role in reducing nervous dyspepsia, colic, flatulence, IBS and even gastritis. Herbs with these significant digestive properties are usually taken before meals to enhance the digestive cascade. Sometimes, if a person has become too unwell, it is worth taking after meals, until sufficient vigour has been achieved, and a before-meal dose can be tolerated.

Haemostatic

Yarrow has a reputation for stopping internal and external bleeding, and many herbalists have anecdotal examples of how the use of yarrow in an emergency situation has proved effective. The astringency aspect is well documented in traditional literature, for use with nosebleeds, but also bleeding wounds (internal and external).

With its capacity to improve the portal circulation and act as a venous tonic, *Achillea millefolium* L. can be helpful to painful, itchy or bleeding haemorrhoids. It has also proved useful for excessively heavy menstrual bleeding, and yet paradoxically can also be used in scanty blood flow at menses.[22] Some authors suggest this is due to the levels of azulene in the plant, but also it is a possibility that ensuring venous tone to the pelvic basin may improve the function of the uterus and associated tissues. Although Achillea does contain a small amount of therapeutic tannin, the haemostatic action is thought to be due to other constituents such as the flavonoids and the alkaloid achilleine.[22]

Hypotensive

Yarrow has a gentle amphoteric action on the whole circulatory system and can therefore prove useful in many cases of high blood pressure, or reduced circulation. It is usually used as an adjunct to other herbs more directly associated with the circulatory system (such as *Crataegus sp.* and *Tilia sp.*) and herbs of the nervous system for this purpose.

Aromatic bitters

As an aromatic bitter, yarrow performs a multitude of digestive functions and stimulates the digestive cascade, but also provides gentle relief at the same time. Bone and Mills, even suggest its usefulness in dealing with acute viral hepatitis, and value its role as a supporter of liver function.[23] It has performed well as a hepatoprotective in laboratory studies.[22]

Emmenagogue

The use of yarrow as a menstrual regulator and corrector herb may stem from a variety of possible effects, including its capacity to tone the veins. It is not seen as an abortifacient—which is another possible use of the term emmenagogue—literally—to stimulate menses. However, caution should be exercised if used in pregnancy, and other less stimulating herbs can be used. It is considered amphoteric as a gynaecological herb.[22]

Note: **Emmenagogues.** Emmenagogues should be seen as herbs that not only stimulate menstrual flow but, as renowned herbalist David Hoffman puts it:

> *In a wider sense they indicate a remedy that normalizes and tones the reproductive system.*[24]

Vapour baths and hot fomentations of herbs were used and promoted by many herbals for easing distressing symptoms of dysmenorrhoea (period pain). This condition was seen to arise from a deficiency of circulation and warmth, and herbs considered as emmenagogues would have been included in the hot compresses and baths. Commonly used would have been mugwort (*Artemisia vulgaris* L.), tansy (*Tanacetum vulgare* L.) and hops (*Humulus lupulus* L.), but also yarrow (*Achillea millefolium* L.) and thyme (*Thymus vulgaris* L.), as both of these herbs were considered to be warming and increasing of the circulation.

Yarrow in particular was considered by the eclectic physicians and in the physiomedicalist tradition, as repairing the venous tone and as a strengthener of the portal circulatory system. Lack of venous tone was cited as one common cause of dysmenorrhoea because the pelvis has a whole network of veins crowding the gynaecological organs.

The consultant gynaecologist and obstetrician who works collaboratively with Anita (The Integrated Gynaecology Clinic), was taught by her professor to observe the apparent dilation of such veins and how patients complaining of chronic pelvic pain, or regular dysmenorrhoea had venous congestion that was observable at laparoscopy.

John Stevens, an associate of Coffin in 19th-century England, used 'injections' into the vagina of warm mugwort and yarrow to ease pelvic pain, and this approach echoes the methods of Dioscorides, Trotula and Parkinson.[25]

The term emmenagogue was originally used to describe the effect of bringing on menstruation. This ties in with ideas across medical practice, that any form of provoked elimination was good. Throughout history there have been populist movements for elimination by any means—vomitoriums (a practice of vomiting to purge from ancient Rome), blood-letting (popular in Europe), and others. Although we have frequently discussed using herbs to gently encourage and improve elimination of normal waste products of metabolism, we do not wish to advocate any of these more radical elimination therapies.

In modern herbalism you may find the term emmenagogue is also confusingly applied to herbs that are much less cathartic in their action and instead are more supportive, allowing a return to normal menstruation. Such herbs are positively fertility-enhancing. Misunderstanding about the meaning of the word emmenagogue has therefore led to inaccuracy about whether a herb is broadly supportive of uterine function, and safe to use in pregnancy, or is likely to induce abortion.

In this way raspberry leaf (*Rubus ideaus* L.) was, and still is, incorrectly seen to be a profound stimulator of labour, rather than the gentle uterine tonic it really is. We have found it to be hugely supportive in pregnancy where there is uterine weakness, and also for mild to moderate prolapses of the vaginal walls or to ease heavy or painful menstruation. You may like to follow our plant tasting method for raspberry leaf, and use your own senses to observe how this plant may have efficacy in this regard.

Always ask a herbalist before using herbs in pregnancy.

Methods of preparation and use

Yarrow is such a flexible and useful herb. It is virtually indispensable in the modern-day herbalists' dispensary. It also makes a fine medicinal dancing partner, combining well with other herbs. Using yarrow as part of a tea blend is a particularly good way to utilise this plant. Add other herbs according to the outcome you are trying to achieve. This will also help to offset its slightly bitter taste, which may be off-putting if drank without other accompanying herbs. Aerial parts of the herb are used, and it is an easy herb to dry and keep for use all year round. Please see below for notes on drying herbs.

Suggested tea blends incorporating yarrow could include:

Cold and flu tea: One part yarrow to two parts elderflower, peppermint, limeflower and eyebright.

Circulatory tonic tea: Equal quantities of yarrow, hawthorn, lime flower.

Note: Drying herbs for later use. Pick your leaves, flowers or flowering herb after the dew has dried if possible. Hang in small bunches in a well-ventilated place, out of direct sunlight if possible and transfer to an airing cupboard or similar to fully dry. This may take several days. Herbs can also be laid flat on trays or shelves with a mesh to allow air circulation. Commercially, herbs can also be freeze-dried. A dehydrator can help dry herbs that may not dry quickly enough without aid.

Dehydrators can also be used to dry fruit and foods. You will note that a dehydrator will dry something to a moisture level of your choosing. In other words, you can remove 60 or 90% of the moisture. When drying herbs, the moisture not adequately removed will potentially cause spoiling and moulds can form. This is almost always extremely undesirable and not only will make your medicinal herb ineffective and possibly harmful—it is very sad to watch all your hard work go off!

Once you have successfully dried your herb, store in a cool dry place in a sealed container that will not condensate or get damp. Store in the dark or in a dark coloured container to protect from light. Don't forget to label the jar!

Interesting Fact: I Ching

In the market place of every Chinese town there were a few I Ching priests who would throw coins for you, or take the yarrow stalks, and get answers to your questions, but then it was forbidden.

—M.-L. Von Franz[26]

Traditionally in China yarrow stalks were (and still are) used in the divinatory process called the *I Ching* (*Book of Changes*). Ordinary people were banned from using the *I Ching* in Communist China. In 1960 however, Mao considered reducing some of the socialist political pressures exerted on the people of the country. He considered two options; increase the rice ration (they were constantly hungry) or allow the *I Ching* to

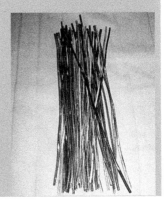

be used again. All sources he consulted told him that the people would choose the *I Ching* over more food. The *I Ching* was allowed for a year or two before being subsequently banned again.

Cautions and care

The Asteraceae family is known for its potential for causing sensitivity reactions (although this is rare in practice). It is advisable not to use this herb during pregnancy or lactation without professional advice. No negative effects in human pregnancy have been reported or found for this herb. There are animal studies that have demonstrated some negative effects during rat gestation. These studies, using very high doses (and rats!), may be extremely limited in their relevance and it may not be possible to extrapolate any clinically useful data.

Summary

Yarrow—the herbalists' herb, ancient cure-all—is a modern aid to many maladies, appropriate to acute and chronic medicine. Warming, bitter yarrow, corrects the circulation, and supports liver function, digestion and the pelvic organs. Due to its complex constituents, complex actions and overall amphoteric effects it can be applied to almost any situation and demonstrates the complexity found in plant medicines.

Dandelion (Taraxacum officinale *aggr. F. H. Wigg)*

The worldwide herb with consistent international use as a dermatological agent. Dandelion, restoring order to disorder, we explore the triple aspects of this lionine medicinal plant. It reaches into multiple processes and has protective and tonic effects that are impossible to trace in a linear way.

Classification

Dandelion belongs to the Asteraceae family, also known as the Compositae. We have met this family before, in Chapter 6, when we looked at the fantastic healing properties of marigold (*Calendula officinalis* L.). For historical reasons you will find that some families have two accepted names. In this case, Compositae is derived from the Latin and refers to the composite nature of the flower itself (or inflorescence), which is composed of many tiny flowers usually in a disc-like arrangement. Asteraceae is derived from the word Aster in Latin, meaning star, and comparing the flowers to a star, whose rays are represented by the tiny flowers that comprise the capitulum. You will remember that the capitulum is a flower head, which is masquerading as a single flower.[1]

You may also notice that after the usual Latin binomial *Taraxacum officinale* there are the letters 'aggr'. This is the shorthand version of the word aggregate and refers to the fact that dandelions are in fact a number of very closely related species of plants that are treated as one species.

Basic botany

A well-known 'weed' across the world, and yet due to the capacity to produce viable seed without necessarily going through a sexual process, the biology of dandelion is very complex and best left to the experts, and dandelions themselves.

- **Leaves** long (5–40 centimetres), narrow, lobed and green (never spotted). The lobes point back towards the base of the plant, which forms a basal rosette. The leaves are known as *'dent-de-lion'* (lion's tooth) in France, from where our English word 'dandelion' comes. *Taraxacum* may possibly refer to eyesight (from the Arabic), or (from the Greek)

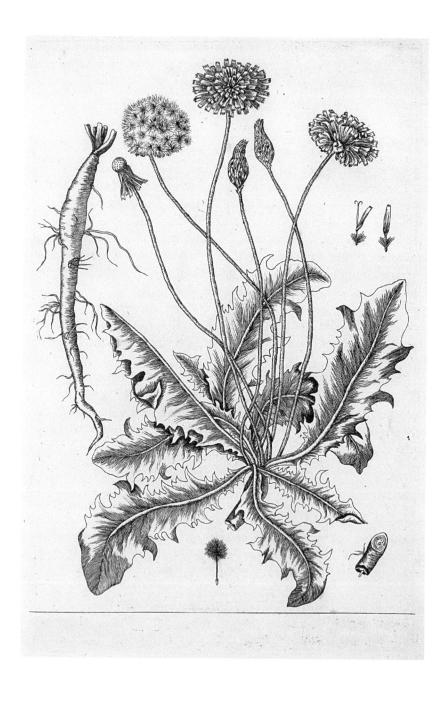

medicinal cure. Barker[27] attributes all of these names to a possible esoteric meaning of 'teeth' and 'sight', of heraldic or Cabbalistic origin.

- **Flower heads** a mid-yellow, and flat-topped or slightly convex when open. All the florets are rayed, the inner ones being shorter than the outer ones. Flower bracts are dark green—even bluish in colour, and the outer bracts are recurved but not horned.
- **Flower stems** succulent and hollow, (containing a useful, but poisonous milky latex). Similar in length to the leaves, never branched, and bear a solitary terminal capitulum (2.5–7.5 centiemetres diameter).
- **Root** an orange-brown tap-root, under the basal rosette of leaves.
- **Habitat** ubiquitous plant of waysides, paths, fields and gardens.

The large and conspicuous 'clock' (called a pappus) is formed of many straight, feathery hairs, joined to the fruit by a thin stalk. These individual hairs are called pappi. This is familiar to children all over the world who have invented games associated with the time and how many puffs it takes to blow away all of the seeds.

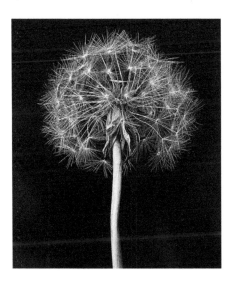

Once all the pappi have been dispersed a pale green-whitish capitulum is left, bare and dimpled. This earned the plant the name of 'priests crown' during the Middle Ages (Elliot, 1995).

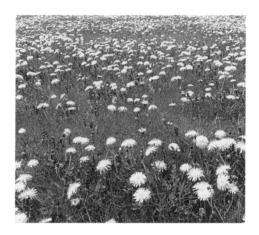

Dandelion (*Taraxacum officinale* aggr. F.H. Wigg)

Parts used

The leaves are gathered fresh as a nutritious food and bitter salad leaf. According to Doug Elliot[28] this plant is rivalled only by *Chenopodium* species in its nutritional content. The leaves are also gathered separately from the roots (and flower stems) for medicinal use—ideally they are gathered in spring before flowering. In the Northern Hemisphere, this is often before 21st April when flowering begins.

The flowers are used to make wine, and syrups. The flower stems produce a milky latex that can be applied externally to warts. The root, once an official medicine (*officinale*), is still used by medical herbalists

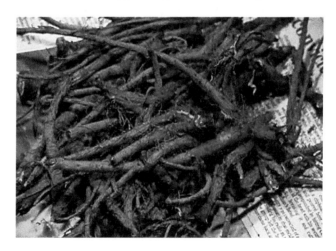

and may be combined with the leaf, or used independently. The long orangey coloured tap roots are carefully dug from the ground in early spring as the leaves are starting to sprout, alternatively they can be found in the autumn if they can be correctly identified from their leaves. Ideally the root has time to build up its stores between flowering.

The root was an official medicine in the United States Pharmacopeia from 1831–1926, and remained in the National Formulary until 1965.[28]

Main constituents

- *Bitters*: A bitterness value is determined for drugs according to their degree of bitterness compared to quinine as the standard. Thus plants with extremely bitter tastes (assessed organoleptically-by tasting), such as gentian (*Gentiana lutea* L.), and centaury (*Centaurium erythraea* Rafn.—another herb named after Chiron!), are more bitter than dandelion. Terpenoids and bitter sterols such as taraxacin and taraxacerin are responsible for the bitter taste as some of the sesquiterpene lactone compounds listed below.

- *Flavonoids*: The ubiquitous flavonoids luteolin, apigenin and quercetin,[29] which all have antioxidant properties.

- *Mydriatic alkaloids and Triterpenes*: Taraxasterol is a pentacyclic triterpene, which has demonstrated anti-inflammatory and anti-microbial properties.

- *Sesquiterpene lactones*: Including eudesmanolides, tetrahydoridentin, taraxacolide-0-β-glucopyranoside, 13-dihydrolactucin, ixerin D, germacranolide acid, taraxinic acid, β-glucopyranoside, ainslioside, 13-dihydro-taraxinic-acid β-glucopyranoside.[30]

- *Phenylpropanoid*: The phenylpropanoid caffeic acid is present in leaf, roots and flowers, as is its ester, chlorogenic acid.[29] Chlorogenic acid is found in coffee, and dandelion roots continue to be used as a coffee substitute.

- *Guaianolides*: Lactucin and lactupicrin which are structurally similar to matricin—a guanolide found in *Matricaria chamomilla* L.—another Asteraceae family member.

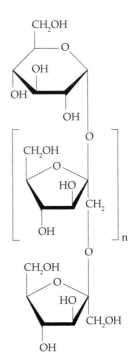

The structure of inulin.

- *Inulin*: a polysaccharide (polyfructane) with antidiabetic properties which helps to sensitise the body to its own insulin. Inulin is isolated from many medicinal plants from this family including chicory (*Chicorium intybus* L.), and elecampane (*Inula helenium* L.). Up to 45% of the root of dandelion can consist of inulin.[30]

Main therapeutic actions confirmed by research

Antidiabetic

> The bioactive components in dandelion are known to act at target sites of biochemical pathways, especially at sites where glucose metabolism is involved.
>
> —F. E. Wirngo, M. N. Lambert and P. B. Jeppesen[30]

Chlorogenic acid, found in dandelion leaf, roots and flowers, slows down the release of glucose into the bloodstream after a meal. Research demonstrates a direct correlation between the presence of particular 'gut microbiota signatures' (GMS) and inflammatory induced obesity and conditions such as type two diabetes mellitus. Particular types of GMS are linked to something called metabolic endotoxaemia, characterised by specific gram-negative bacteria which have structures called endotoxins on the outside of their cell surfaces.[31] It has been demonstrated that inulin supplementation is capable of modulating both inflammation and metabolic endotoxaemia in women with type two diabetes.[32] This piece of research once again demonstrates the central role of the gut microbiota in our health and wellbeing, and further shows how plant remedies directly influence gut function, the gut microbiota, and therefore our health in general.

Hepatic, cholagogue, digestive stimulant, stomachic, aperient

Dandelion is a classic example of a bitter tonic herb, with all the benefits that this suggests. The beneficial optimisation of the digestive cascade that results from the ingestion of bitters is very well established, and this plants cholagogue and choleretic actions serve not only to optimise bile flow and thus improve the overall health of the liver and gall bladder, but also to aid in the establishment of healthy and robust gut flora in the large intestine.

The interaction between intestinal microbiota and bile acids is not uni-directional. Bile acids can shape the gut microbiota community, and in turn, intestinal microbes are able to alter bile acid pool. In general, gut microbiota actively communicates with bile acids …

—Y. Lee et al.[33]

We would like to make the link between the use of plants for the liver, and the potential benefits to eye complaints; due to the traditional significance of eye (eyeball) problems relating to liver function in some way. The white eye sclera is also one of the first places to show jaundice.

Nutrient

Dandelion root is recorded as having a higher nutritional value than many vegetables. Specifically it has a higher beta-carotene content than carrots. Dandelion greens contain vitamins A, C, B_1, B_2, and B_6, as well as calcium, copper, manganese, silicon, sodium, zinc and iron.[30,34] Likely improvements to gut microbiota from eating wild greens such as dandelion, may also positively impact nutrition, and disease.[35]

Diuretic

Dandelion leaf has an extensive history of use as a diuretic, and is often included in compounds such as spring tonics, aimed at detoxifying the system after the excesses of the winter months. A study in 2009 on human volunteers highlighted this effect.[36]

Taraxacum: Taraxis—**a disorder or disturbance.** *Acas*—**the remedy.** A recent study utilising inulin in combination with vitamin D, isoflavones and calcium, resulted in significant amelioration of symptoms in menopausal women.[37]

Research by Jeon et al.[38] demonstrated potential clinical benefits in the prevention of vascular inflammation, and thus atherosclerosis. This long list of potential sites of action and digestive benefits from the use of dandelion root and leaf, reveal the capacity of this plant to gently stimulate the digestive cascade. It is safe for use for children and the elderly because it is not a strong laxative, nor are its effects addictive-like senna (*Cassia spp.*), for example.

Note: Laxatives. There is a grading system for laxatives; the mildest form is an aperient, then laxative, then purgative and finally the potentially catastrophic cathartic.

There is a wide range of applications for this herb as it will often facilitate the action of other herbs. Gentle stimulation of the digestive cascade may allow correction of processes not correctly 'switched on' since birth and eventual weaning. Stimulation of the digestive cascade allows for regular 'piano practice', correcting peristalsis, improving absorption and elimination and enhancing the environment for the microbiome. The root may be used alone or combined with the leaf.

A gentle detoxification action may be achieved to alleviate pressure on the skin by improving bowel function, by supporting kidney function that will support skin health, and also musculoskeletal tissues like the joints. Dandelion root and leaf may be used in combination with musculoskeletal herbs therefore, as part of a whole-body process for addressing arthritis and rheumatism.[1]

Methods of preparation and use

The uses of dandelion are so many and widespread that it is difficult to pick any specific examples. A dandelion flower infused oil may be used as an external muscle rub for cold and stiff joints (as well as being a useful addition to salad dressings for example).[39] To optimise the nutrient benefit of dande- 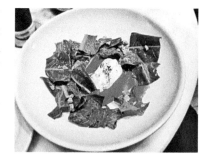 lion, may we suggest adding young fresh dandelion leaves to your spring salads, and using wilted dandelion leaves in simple stir-fries. The Greek pie *spanakopita* can make a delicious meal using wild greens such as nettle, dandelion leaves and wild garlic.

Cautions and care

As you will remember the Asteraceae family have occasionally led to sensitivity reactions in susceptible individuals. This is almost always topical in nature, so picking or brushing against the plant, getting the sap on the skin, especially in the presence of sunlight or water and sunlight seems to prompt a skin rash for a small minority of people (pertinent for florists and gardeners). Occasionally pollen sensitivity has been linked to Asteraceae family members. Despite a powerful capacity as a diuretic, the dandelion plant showed no acute toxicity in LD50 tests.

Textbooks sometimes list bile duct occlusion and obstructive ileus as potential side effects, but there is no data to support this, and it may have arisen from theoretical inference because dandelion is known as stimulating and correcting gall bladder and bile duct function, and these empty into the small intestine.[40] There was one report of a possible poisoning from the 1970s in Germany of a child sucking the flower stems when making a daisy chain with fresh dandelions.

Susun Weed, writing as if she is Dr Dandelion (!) describes dandelion as a hepatic (liver supportive), as a tonic nutritive galactagogue (helps the production and quality of breast milk), as a digestive stimulant, de-obstruent (unblocker of blockages), and also as a hypnotic sedative (the opposite of a stimulant).[41]

In Ayurvedic herbalism dandelion root is used as a way of reducing heat, stagnation and toxicity (Ama) by improving liver and overall digestive function (Agni). It is also used to aid breast milk production, helping suppressed lactation or breast swelling, engorgement and cysts.[42]

Beyond doubt, dandelion is of importance as a reliable organ tonic. For the liver both the root and the leaf have the potential to support liver and gall bladder function, but especially the root, which has blood sugar balancing and bowel toning and digestive enhancing effects. The leaf acts as a kidney organ enhancing herb with its inherent potassium content meaning depletion of potassium and thus strain on the heart is reduced.[1] Dandelion is a cooling bitter herb with a drying nature. Choleric and melancholic constitutions specifically tend to benefit, but this herb has proved to be useful for just about everyone!

Note: **Cleansing the blood—alteratives and depuratives.** A persistent concept within traditional herbal medicine is the idea of 'blood cleansing'—the opening up of modes of elimination by the body or unblocking the 'obstructions of the liver and spleen' as it would have been called in humoural medicinal texts.

Interestingly it is a concept often self-reported by patients themselves with skin complaints—that they feel that they need to 'clean their blood' or open an 'obstruction'. The term **'deobstruent'** can be used with regard to dandelion, as it has the capacity to unblock obstructions to health. This is an empirical observation of health and lacks a proven mechanism. Nevertheless, many herbs were regarded as de-obstruent, alterative or depurative and thus of great use as skin remedies. The skin is thought to take the burden if other organs of elimination are deficient or overburdened themselves. *Urtica dioica* L. and *Galium aparine* L. are two other plants regarded as blood cleansers.

Except in atopic conditions (eczema, asthma, hayfever), which are associated with allergy, most dermatitis and eczema cases are symptomatic of complex conditions often without a clear or apparent cause. Lack of identified cause can make treatment (except palliative treatment) very difficult using conventional medicine. Hence, a range of palliative skin creams is the usual method of treatment.

Using a more traditional herbal medicine view however, it can be useful to consider using a range of 'alteratives', or 'depuratives' that may have a range of tissue affinities, and global effects. Thus dandelion root, with its affinity for the liver and bowel, or cleavers herb with its affinity for the lymphatics and kidney are both useful choices. Other examples might include heartsease (*Viola tricolor* L.) with an affinity for the gut and nervous system, or red clover (*Trifolium pratense* L.) with an affinity for the lymphatic and endocrine system.

Traditionally these de-obstruent herbs may have been combined with skin healing vulneraries and anti-infectives such as *Calendula officinalis* L., or anxiolytics with an anti-inflammatory effect such as *Matricaria chamomilla* L. to address the specifics of each dermatitis case.

Summary of dandelion—three medicines in one

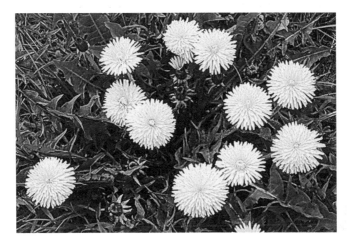

The fresh sap of the flower stem can be used (dabbed on daily then covered under a plaster) to remove warts and benign skin lesions.

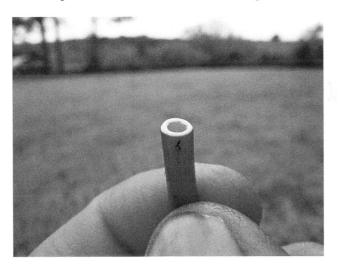

The leaf of the dandelion is an effective diuretic and kidney tonic, gently stimulating the kidney function and removing excess water (oedema) whilst also supporting kidney function, and not depleting potassium levels. The leaf is also a bitter tonic and galactagogue, and can be made into a tincture, or eaten as a salad leaf. Dandelion leaves are also delicious wilted in a cooking pan over a low heat with a very little water, salt and pepper, then served with olive oil and lemon juice. The use of bitter wayside herbs is common in the Mediterranean, and is not always herb-specific, such as 'horta' in Greece, a mixture of wild bitter greens, gently cooked and served with olive oil.

The root of dandelion is most commonly used by herbalists as a gentle liver tonic and depurative. It acts as a gentle aperient—not as an addictive laxative. It aids elimination of normal waste products of metabolism by the liver and kidney, and yet is also mineral-rich; thus dandelion is detoxifying but also nutrient and tonic.

It is gentle enough to use with children and the elderly or infirm. Because of this seemingly paradoxical property, dandelion has been used the world over as a skin remedy. It is often cited as an example of how disparate cultures have reached the same conclusions about the uses of medicinal plants. Dandelion combines well with many other medicinal plants and is commonly used alongside aromatic digestives, other bitters, lymphatics and carminatives, nervines, and tonics. *Dandelion has both stimulating and sedating properties. As such, it is more useful to think of it as a tonic.*

Preparations of dandelion

The leaf can be made easily into a tea, juice or tincture. The root will require a decoction method to extract the beneficial effects, and will also produce an excellent tincture. Stronger tincture preparations are available and manufactured using a process of percolation.

Note: Decoctions, which were formerly popular forms of preparing medicines, have gradually given place to more scientific preparations, and are now seldom used.

The process of decoction is to boil the vegetable substances for from 10 to 15 minutes in water in a covered vessel, and then cool and pour off the liquid.

It is possible to buy dandelion root roasted in small chunks. This is a delicious and nutritious way of taking dandelion with a definite 'tonic' effect. This can be made in a cafetière in a similar way to making coffee. In traditional Chinese medicine some herb roots are roasted or fried to bring out an extra aspect of their healing such as 'tonification' or increasing internal 'heat' and dispelling 'cold' (weakness).

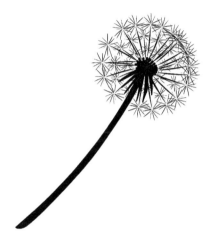

Marshmallow (Althea officinalis *L.*)

Marshmallow, so soft and gentle, and yet so remarkable. The provoking of a pleasurable sensory response is healing in itself. How underrated kindness is. Protector of our exposed surfaces, medicine in root, leaf and flower.

Classification

Marshmallow is a member of the Malvaceae family. If you have ever chewed a tilia leaf, you will not be surprised to find that the Malvaceae are thought to have evolved from Tiliaceae.[1] The Malvaceae family include the cotton plant (*Gossypium hirsutum* L.) and the kapok plant (*Ceiba pentandra* (L.) Gaertn).

A number of beautiful and useful mallows are common to northern Europe including common mallow (*Malva sylvestris* L.) and musk mallow (*Malva moschata* L). We also have the tree mallows often found at coastal regions (*Lavatera* species) and the garden hollyhocks (*Alcea rosea* L./*Althaea rosea*).

Basic botany

Marshmallow (*Althea officinalis* L.) is traditionally and officially the most used medicinally, but if you have common mallow (*Malva sylvestris* L.) growing near you, the flowers in particular make a very soothing and pleasant tisane. Althea—of Greek origin—is derived from the words 'althos', a medicine, and 'althaiein' to heal. A remarkably soft, greyish herb *Althea officinalis* L. is a tall (60–200 centimetres), erect, little-branched herb with velvety leaves (often fan-folded).

- **Leaves** triangular-oval in outline, velvety and toothed into 3–5 lobes.
- **Flowers** on stalks shorter than the upper leaves and are solitary or grouped in arrangements of 1–3. They are a pale pink-lilac colour, 25–40 millimetres diameter. The anthers are purplish red, petals five.
- **Fruit** known as a nutlet and found in a ring formation on the persisting calyx after fertilisation.
- **Root** in commerce it is fibrous in appearance, cream-white when peeled and deeply furrowed longitudinally with some root scars. Roots possess a slight perfumey odour, tasting sweet and quickly becoming mucilaginous.
- **Habitat** found wild on estuarine and marine salt marshes, in ditches and stream sides, at low altitudes.

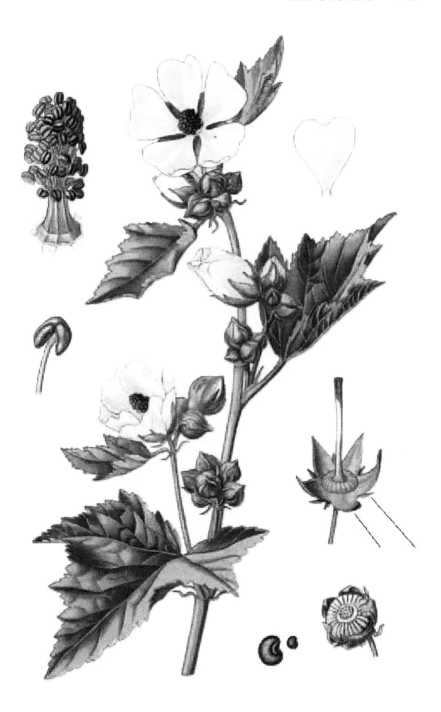

Parts used

- **Roots** (from plants 2–3 years old or more): Harvest in late autumn once the leaves and stems have completely died back, or in early spring when the red growth tips emerge, and before they start to form stems. The root can be split, so that some can be harvested, and some left in the soil to re-grow.
- **Leaves** (fresh or dried): Leaves should be harvested in early mid-summer as the flowers are forming.
- **Flowers**: These are usually harvested along with the leaves and used together. However harvesting common mallow flowers (*Malva sylvestris* L.) and drying them for tea, makes a beautiful lilac herb tea with similar properties to marshmallow leaf.

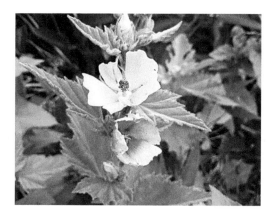

Marshmallow in flower.

Main constituents

- Mucilage (up to and sometimes exceeding 30%) in the roots. About half as much in the leaves, (possibly dependent on the dampness of the habitat).
- A number of polysaccharides have been identified in the mucilage including L-rhamnose, D-galactose, D-galacturonic acid and D-glucuronic acid among others.
- Starches, sugars and pectins (about 35%).
- Mineral salts.
- Asparagine, (a non-essential amino acid, found in roots).

- Phenolic acids (roots).
- Esters of fatty acids (salicylic, caffeic, vanillic and syringic acids) (roots).
- Coumarin (scopoletin) (roots).
- Flavonoids, including kaempferol, quercetin and diosmetin (roots).
- Lecithin and phytosterols (roots).
- Leaf and flower have a small amount of volatile oil (up to 0.02%), and more moderate mucilage content (about 10%).[43]

Main therapeutic actions confirmed by research

The mucilages have proven biological activity beyond vulnerary and anti-inflammatory, including the stimulation of phagocytosis in vitro.[43]

Antibacterial

A recent paper confirmed antibacterial actions for *Althaea officinalis* L. Specifically, this research found that an ethanol extraction of the root was an effective antibacterial agent against *Streptococcus mutans*, a bacteria specifically implicated in the development of dental caries. This would suggest a beneficial role for marshmallow root in mouthwash remedies.[44]

Anti-inflammatory

Sweet, cool and moistening, marshmallow is another one of those gentle yet deceptively effective remedies, eminently safe, soothing and applicable to any hot, dry, irritable condition. In traditional Persian manuscripts, mucilage is one of the most-cited applications of medicinal plants for therapeutic objectives.[45] In northern Pakistan it is still a popular traditional remedy for respiratory illnesses,[46] and recent research has confirmed *Althea officinalis'* effectiveness in the treatment of irritable cough.[47] Research done on the combination remedy 'Cough (EMA) granules' in 2018 highlighted the role of *Althea officinalis* L. in forming a protective layer over the respiratory tract, inhibiting cough, and shielding it from irritants. Cough EMA granules are composed of *Althea officinalis* L., *Sisymbrium irio* L. (Hedge mustard) and *Hedera helix* L., (Ivy). EMA = European Medicines Agency.[48]

Drawing agent

Marshmallow root can also be used as an effective drawing agent. The powder may be mixed with bread or honey and applied either hot or cold to draw out the pus or a foreign object lodged in the skin. If the poultice can be kept in situ overnight or for a few days, it can draw out things the body is having difficulty re-absorbing or dissolving. We have seen this method work for a plumber who had knelt on fine metal filings, and also to draw pus from boils.

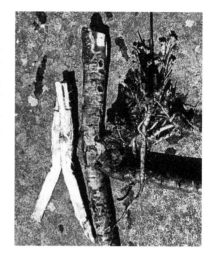

Marshmallow roots.

Miscellaneous

Althea officinalis L. has been the subject of promising research both as an anti-malarial agent,[49] and topically as a potentially effective sunscreen agent.[50]

Methods of preparation and use

Marshmallow absolutely lends itself to the making of a beautiful syrup. Please find here, a good, simple recipe.

Recipe for marshmallow syrup

Ingredients
    50 g dried cut marshmallow root
    500 ml distilled water

Method
    Leave to soak overnight then heat gently to make a decoction.
    Strain carefully and thoroughly through clean dry muslin.
    Now reduce the liquid you have strained, by gently heating to evaporate off sufficient to leave you with 125 ml.

Transfer to a clean saucepan and add 200 g of refined white sugar.
Stir over a gentle heat to dissolve the sugar completely.
Remove from the heat and cool.
Pour into a clean sterile dry bottle (you should have 250 ml of marsh-mallow syrup).

Notes: This quick syrup is ideal for immediate use—say within 12 days (kept in the fridge). To make a syrup with keeping qualities you will need to use refined sugar at a ratio of 2:1 in favour of the sugar and take great care to sterilise everything used throughout the process very thoroughly.

Cautions and care

Marshmallow is considered safe in pregnancy and lactation, no warnings or adverse events have been found.[51] The Drugs and Lactation Database state that:

> *Although no data exist on the safety of marshmallow root during breast-feeding, it is unlikely to be harmful to the breast-fed infant.*
> —Drugs and Lactation Database[52]

It is considered prudent to monitor long-term use where a patient may be taking other medicines. This is due to the possibility that marshmallow could reduce absorbability or gastric emptying. This is however likely to be exaggerated or minor in effect, unlike evidence for the consumption of gel-fibres like fybogel and psyllium husk.[51]

Mucilagenous herbs—an underrated intervention

The word mallow is derived from *moloche* and means softening in the same way as mallow is linked to the word mellow.[25] Its use in ancient times for soothing and healing soreness or ulceration in the stomach was attested by Dioscorides, Dodoens and Ibn Sina. Ibn Sina (Avicenna) added the present-day uses of marshmallow—soothing the urinary tract, the respiratory tract or the skin (topical). Fuchs cites sources earlier than Dioscorides for wounds and quenching the thirst after haemorrhages, and also after dysentery or lung problems such as wheezing and shortness of breath.

Coffin, the lecturer in medical botany from the USA, who spearheaded the revival of herbal medicine in the UK, leading to the formation of the National Institute of Medical Herbalists in 1864, used hollyhock flowers for the throat and stomach, as a tea. He also gave an interesting and classical physio-medical herbal medicine recipe for a conserve of hollyhock flowers to which is added cayenne pepper (*Capsicum annuum* L.), ginger (*Zingiber officinale* Roscoe), poplar bark (*Populus tremuloides* Michx), sugar and cloves (*Syzygium aromaticum* L. Merr & L.M. Perry), for a cough!

Summary of the use of marshmallow in herbal medicine

Marshmallow leaves and roots are a gentle but profound herbal medicine that can be used at any stage of life and with complete safety. The leaves contain a smaller amount of mucilage but therefore work by reflex on the mucous membranes of the respiratory system and urinary system. They are cooling, soothing, healing and anti-inflammatory and can correct catarrhal secretions. The roots have a much greater quantity of mucilage and also have aromatic compounds that make it more suited for use on the membranes it comes directly into contact with (the throat and digestive system). It can be used for short periods of time to alleviate acute discomfort, or over longer periods to act as a constant healing soothing influence.

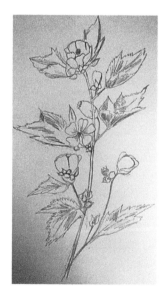

Line drawing of marshmallow.

Cleavers (Galium aparine L.)

Sun loving, sprawling cleavers. Snaking into every crevice. The forgotten system of our body, the lymphatic system, is protected and enhanced by this spring refresher, and therefore, so are we.

Classification

Cleavers is a member of the Rubiaceae family. The Rubiaceae family rather belongs in the tropics where most of the species are found. This illustrious group of plants includes coffee (*Coffea arabica* L.), quinine (*Cinchona spp.*) and the *Gardenias*, which are used in perfumery, and cosmetics dyes. The bedstraw family in Europe consists of a whole array of similar-looking plants known as bedstraws, and includes cleavers (*Galium aparine* L.), but also the dye plant madder (*Rubia tinctorum* L.).

Basic botany

Cleavers is a scrambling green annual which has the ability to stick to your skin and clothing due to downward-pointing prickles on the leaves and the edges of their stems. Variable but often tall, the stems are often brittle and turn dark brown after fruiting. Take a close look with your hand lens!

- **Leaves** occur in whorls on square, or ridged stems (80–180 centimetres long), with 4–12 leaves per whorl. The leaves are 0.5–2 centimetres long with a small point at the tip.
- **Flowers** stalked, white and inconspicuous (1.5–1.7 millimetres), four parted, stamens protruding, with a short corolla tube.
- **Fruit** 3–5 millimetres, green becoming purplish-black. They also stick to anything and everything due to hooked bristles on their rounded surfaces.
- **Habitat** this plant is found almost throughout northern Europe in hedges, ditches, scrubland, disturbed land, and shingle. It is an occasional garden 'weed'.

Parts used

Green herb, leaves and stems are used fresh or dried, but are often preferred fresh and just before or in flower when they are still juicy. Seeds

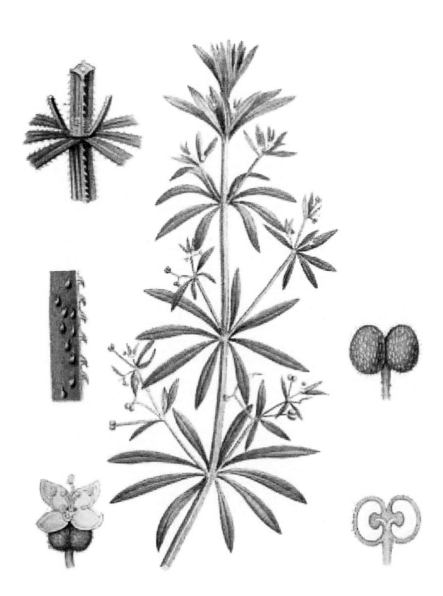

can be harvested (!) and dry roasted to produce a serviceable (if labour-intensive) 'coffee'.

Main constituents

- Iridoids including asperuloside.
- Polyphenolic acids such as caffeic, p-coumaric, gallic and p-hydroxybenzoic acids.
- Anthraquinone derivatives including alizarin and its' derivatives, Xanthopurpurin and its esters, galiosin and simple anthraquinones (in the root, not the herb).
- Alkanes.
- Flavonoids such as luteolin, apigenin and quercetin.
- Tannin.
- Coumarins.

Cleavers contains significant levels of vitamin C (antiscorbutic).

Main therapeutic actions confirmed by research

Diuretic, aperient, tonic, alterative, mild astringent,[53] it is also considered to be anti-inflammatory and slightly hypotensive.[1] It is used largely in herbal medicine for enlarged lymph glands, lymphoedema and for a variety of skin complaints, and urinary problems.

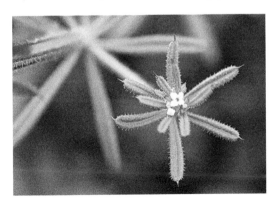

Four sepals; the flowers of cleavers.

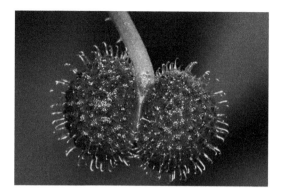

Cleavers fruits are similar inside to coffee fruits.

Anti-cancer

Traditional use of cleavers for 'cancer' may be difficult to interpret in our modern-day understanding of the word,[25] but one study found it had promise as an agent of apoptosis.[54] It has previously been assumed that 'cancer' meant lymph gland enlargement. Certainly cleavers has proved very helpful to our patients with lymphoedema, including women presenting with post-mastectomy lymphoedema.

Anti-inflammatory

Asperuloside can be chemically converted to prostanoid intermediates (prostanoids include prostaglandins and thromboxanes, substances which play important roles in such mechanisms as inflammation). This may prove of benefit in prostatic conditions. It is interesting to consider the huge basin of lymphatics found within the pelvis, and how their function may be helped by the use of herbs such as cleavers.

Immune system modulator

Cleavers is used in the living tradition of Western herbal medicine today with the lymphatic and immune system very much in mind. Recent work by Shinkovenko et al. looked at the herb *Galium verum* L. (Lady's bedstraw), a close cousin of *Galium aparine* L., in terms of its effect on the immune system. In their abstract they concluded:

> *The obtained results enable an assumption of a synergistic effect of PPC and PSC of Galium verum herb fluid extract on the potency of its immunomodulatory activity.*
>
> —I. L. Shinkovenko et al.[55]

(**NB**: PSC = Polysaccharide complex, PPC = polyphenolic complex).

This piece of work touches on the central concept of synergy between phytochemical compounds and reminds us yet again of the dangers of assuming that active constituents act in isolation.

Dermatological healer

Cleavers has a strong association with skin health in traditional herbal medicine. One study using a compound product that included *Galium* extract did not find a meaningful difference between this specific product and placebo.[56] This type of research is disappointing as it does not reflect the way a medical herbalist might utilise *Galium aparine* L. for specific skin complaints in an individualised way. Although cleavers might be used by a herbalist as a supplementary herb in skin conditions such as eczema, it will usually be combined with other skin herbs as appropriate, such as *Viola tricolor* L. (with digestive sluggishness or liver fire), *Trifolium pratense* L. (with flaky dry skin), *Urtica dioica* L. (irritated allergic skin complaints), or *Calendula officinalis* L., *Echinacea angustifolia* DC or *Berberis aquifolium* Pursh, for infected or vulnerable skin.

Antibacterial (MRSA)

Another research paper evaluated the potential effects of *Galium aparine* L. in dealing with methicillin-resistant Staphylococcus aureus strains (MRSA) and found that the methanolic extract of *G. aparine* proved to have high antibacterial activity on MRSA isolates, thus representing promising antimicrobial agents in clinical settings. The research paper stated that plants with higher levels of polyphenols and flavonoids demonstrated greater antibacterial effects, indicating that many other plants rich in these compounds may also prove to be valuable resources in such situations as MRSA.[57]

Galium tea or fresh herb tincture is often used as a lymphatic aid when treating respiratory tract infections, particularly when they are non-responsive, congestive, or have become 'deep' such as in sinusitis or when there is dental involvement. An excellent cleansing herb, cleavers is cooling, soothing and a bit drying. Its slightly salty aspect is reminiscent of our own internal seas. Grieve[58] notes its use dating back to the 14th century as an ointment for scalds and burns, which makes sense, given its energetic properties.

Methods of preparation and use

Cleavers can be dried and used as a tea, and can be consumed in frequent doses, over relatively long periods of time. We have found it to be very helpful for women with lymphedema as a result of radical breast surgery for example, and it has been taken safely over many years. Cleavers lends itself well to being juiced fresh in the spring, or made into a fresh herb tincture. Cleavers can be pounded and used externally as a poultice or bathing herb. It has also found use externally as a wash for sunburn.[58]

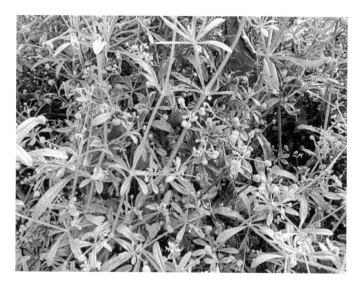

Cleavers (*Galium aparine* L.)

Cautions and care

No adverse reactions have ever been recorded. No drug-herb interactions are expected. No overdoses have been found. No problems in pregnancy or for children. Medical herbalists will be aware of the occasional provocation of skin eruption when using 'depuratives' such as cleavers. These have sometimes been referred to as healing crises.

Exploring the importance of the lymphatic system in herbal medicine

This plant was of great importance to the physicians of Myddfai in Wales, a continuous family practice recorded in 1743, but stretching back to at least the 14th century. The fresh juice was preferred and should be gathered and used quickly, as any left out in foggy or muggy weather would quickly deteriorate and the virtues of the plant would be lost. It was often used as a simple (a single herb, not combined with others), and taken for a magical 9-week duration. It was used to expel and destroy any poisons or disruption of the blood, clearing scrofula, and also illnesses of a more internal nature. Cleavers, rather like figwort (*Scrophularia nodosa* L.), was classically employed as a poultice for any lymphatic swelling (scrofula).

These uses are reflected in modern-day usage and recorded by Bone and Mills,[40] but also in practitioners from the New World such as Felter and Lloyd,[59] Ellingwood and Coffin. Matthew Wood concurs and adds that it is considered 'deer medicine' among native Americans and as such is useful in aiding the nervous system.[60]

The physicians that influenced herbal practice in the late 19th cenruty included the osteopathy and chiropractic movements, who also placed great importance on the lymphatic system. Acknowledgement was made of the anatomical drainage points of the lymphatic system into the vena cava in the upper chest—and so congestion of the lymphatic system could therefore affect the heart and appear to give palpitations for example.

Summary of the uses of cleavers in Western herbal medicine

Cleavers stands in recognition of the importance of the lymphatic system in traditional Western herbal medicine. Cleavers has a gentle but persistent effect in mobilising lymph drainage and as such can assist other herbs in the treatment of all body tissues that are drained by lymph (virtually everything!). In particular cleavers can be used to aid tonsillar and adenoid swellings, or any lymph gland enlargement.

It can also help drain tissues engorged with fluid (oedema) by helping with lymph drainage. It is safe to use whilst breastfeeding and during pregnancy. It can be helpful in cases of mastitis and mastalgia. Cleavers can assist in dealing with acute, chronic or persistent respiratory tract infections and thus support the ear nose and throat, sinuses and lungs, all of which have their own lymphatic vessels. Cleavers may also be of service in grumbling appendix or children's tummy aches whilst they are being investigated, since abdominal discomfort in children can often be lymphatic, and herald an infection.

Cleavers can help with draining engorged and inflamed tissues such as found in acne vulgaris and boils. Other tissues that are highly prone to lymphatic engorgement include breast tissue and testes. *Galium aparine* L. can be extremely useful for swellings, and tenderness in these tissues. Cleavers can also help with the function of the pelvic organs as they also have their own extensive lymphatic vessels and so can aid any condition that appears 'stuck' or 'congested' in origin. This can also be useful when considering the lower skeleton and tissues below the pelvis that may be inflamed as a result of poor venous and lymphatic return.

Cleavers can be serviceable as a mild and gentle diuretic, and may be useful as an adjunct to more powerful urinary antiseptics and anti-inflammatories. By aiding lymphatic drainage, Galium can be a mobilising force in reducing cyst formation and benign cystic skin conditions.

* * *

Our debt to the First Nations people for their herbal knowledge shared:

> To the Cherokee, the use of herbs is only one tool of the many necessary for regaining health. Traditionally it was (and still is) believed that it is crucial to not only heal the body, mind and spirit, but to reintegrate the ill person within the family, the community and with the earth itself.
>
> This is a holistic perspective beyond our culture's limited understanding. None of us can truly be well unless we recognize our connection to the rest of the Great Life.

—David Winston[61]

Bibliography

Millard, E. P., *Applied Anatomy of the Lymphatics*. 1921: Available from: http://www.johnwernhamclassicalosteopathy.com/jwcco-bookshop/

Pengelly, A., *The Constituents of Medicinal Plants: An Introduction to the Chemistry and Therapeutics of Herbal Medicines*. 2004: CABI Publishing.

Pollington, Stephen, *Leechcraft: Early English Charms, Plantlore and Healing*. 2008: Anglo Saxon Press.

Priest, A. W. and Priest L. R., *Herbal Medication: A Clinical and Dispensary Handbook*. 1982: C. W. Daniel.

Revell, Alison, *A Kentish Herbal*. 1984: Kent County Council.

Tierra, Dr. Michael, *American Herbalism: Essays on Herbs and Herbalism by the Members of the American Herbalists Guild*. 1992: The Crossing Press.

References

1. Barker, J., *The Medicinal Flora of Britain and Northwestern Europe*. 2001: Winter Press.

2. Blamey, M. and C. Grey-Wilson, *Wild Flowers of Britain and Northern Europe*. 2003: Cassell.

3. Heinrich, M. et al., *Fundamentals of Pharmacognosy and Phytotherapy*. 2012: Churchill Livingstone.

4. Atanasov, A. G. et al., *Discovery and resupply of pharmacologically active plant-derived natural products: a review*. Biotechnol Adv, 2015. 33(8): pp. 1582–1614.

5. Qadir, M. A., Syeda Kiran Bashir, Asad Munir and Adil Shahzad Shabnam, *Evaluation of phenolic compounds and antioxidant and antimicrobial activities of some common herbs*. International Journal of Analytical Chemistry, 2017.

6. Sakkas, P. C., *Antimicrobial activity of basil, oregano, and thyme essential oils*. J Microbiol Biotechnol. 2017. 28: pp. 429–438.

7. Oliviero, M. et al., *Evaluations of thyme extract effects in human normal bronchial and tracheal epithelial cell lines and in human lung cancer cell line*. Chem Biol Interact, 2016. 256: pp. 125–133.

8. Roby, M. H. H. et al., *Evaluation of antioxidant activity, total phenols and phenolic compounds in thyme (L.), sage (L.), and marjoram (L.) extracts*. Industrial Crops and Products, 2013. 43: pp. 827–831.

9. Altiok, D., E. Altiok and F. Tihminlioglu, *Physical, antibacterial and antioxidant properties of chitosan films incorporated with thyme oil for potential wound healing applications*. J Mater Sci Mater Med, 2010. 21(7): pp. 2227–2236.

10. Kulisic, T., V. Dragovic-Uzelac and M. Milos, *Antioxidant activity of aqueous tea infusions prepared from oregano, thyme and wild thyme. Publisher:* Food Technol Biotechnology, 2005. 44(4): pp. 485–492.

11. Chohan, M. et al., *An investigation of the relationship between the anti-inflammatory activity, polyphenolic content, and antioxidant activities of cooked and in vitro digested culinary herbs.* Oxid Med Cell Longev, 2012. 2012: pp. 627–843.

12. Holmes, P., *The Energetics of western Herbs: Integrating Western and Oriental Herbal traditions.* Vol. 1. 1986: Artemis Press.

13. de Oliviera, J. R., D. D. J. Viegas et al., *Thymus vulgaris L. extract has antimicrobial and anti-inflammatory effects in the absence of cytotoxicity and genotoxicity.* Archives of Oral Biology, 2017. 82.

14. Mills, S., *The Principles and Practice of Modern Phytotherapy*, K. Bone, Editor, Churchill Livingstone.

15. Mennerat, A. et al., *Aromatic plants in nests of the blue tit Cyanistes caeruleus protect chicks from bacteria.* Oecologia, 2009. 161(4): pp. 849–855.

16. Kültür, S., *Medicinal plants used in Kirklareli Province (Turkey).* J Ethnopharmacol, 2007. 111(2): pp. 341–364.

17. Jarić, S. et al., *An ethnobotanical study on the usage of wild medicinal herbs from Kopaonik Mountain (Central Serbia).* J Ethnopharmacol, 2007. 111(1): pp. 160–175.

18. Jarić, S. et al., *Traditional wound-healing plants used in the Balkan region (Southeast Europe).* J Ethnopharmacol, 2018. 211: pp. 311–328.

19. Ahmad, M. et al., *Ethnopharmacological survey on medicinal plants used in herbal drinks among the traditional communities of Pakistan.* J Ethnopharmacol, 2016. 184: pp. 154–186.

20. Benedek, B., B. Kopp and M. F. Melzig, *Achillea millefolium L. s.l.—is the anti-inflammatory activity mediated by protease inhibition?* J Ethnopharmacol, 2007. 113(2): pp. 312–317.

21. Ayoobi, F. et al., *Bio-effectiveness of the main flavonoids of.* Iran J Basic Med Sci, 2017. 20(6): pp. 604–612.

22. Trickey, R., *Women, Hormones and the Menstrual Cycle.* 2011: A&U.

23. Bone, K. and S. Mills, *Principles and Practice of Phytotherapy: Modern Herbal Medicine.* 2nd ed. 2013: Churchill Livingstone.

24. Hoffman, D., *Medical Herbalism: The Science and Practice of Herbal Medicine.* 2003: Healing Arts Press.

25. Tobyn, G., A. Denham and M. Whitelegg, *The Western Herbal Tradition.* 2011: Churchill Livingstone.

26. Von Franz, M.-L., *On Divination and Synchronicity; The Psychology of Meaningful Chance.* 1980: Inner City Books, p. 123.

27. Barker, J., *Notes toward a therapeutic model of phytotherapy in Britain.* British Journal of Phytotherapy, 1991. 2(Spring): pp. 38–46.

28. Elliott, D., *Wild Roots: A Foragers Guide to the Edible and Medicinal Roots, Tubers, Corms and Rhizomes of North America*. 1995: Healing Arts Press.

29. Gamboa-Gómez, C. I. et al., *Plants with potential use on obesity and its complications*. EXCLI J, 2015. 14: pp. 809–831.

30. Wirngo, F. E., M. N. Lambert and P. B. Jeppesen, *The Physiological Effects of Dandelion (Taraxacum Officinale) in Type 2 Diabetes*. Rev Diabet Stud, 2016. 13(2–3): pp. 113–131.

31. Piya, M. K., A. L. Harte and P. G. McTernan, *Metabolic endotoxaemia: is it more than just a gut feeling?* Curr Opin Lipidol, 2013. 24(1): pp. 78–85.

32. Dehghan, P. et al., *Inulin controls inflammation and metabolic endotoxemia in women with type 2 diabetes mellitus: a randomized-controlled clinical trial*. Int J Food Sci Nutr, 2014. 65(1): pp. 117–123.

33. Li, Y. et al., *Bile acids and intestinal microbiota in autoimmune cholestatic liver diseases*. Autoimmun Rev, 2017. 16(9): pp. 885–896.

34. Pizzorno, J. E. and M. T. Murray, *Textbook of Natural Medicine*. 2013, Elsevier.

35. Kassim, M. A., H. Baijnath and B. Odhav, *Effect of traditional leafy vegetables on the growth of lactobacilli and bifidobacteria*. Int J Food Sci Nutr, 2014. 65(8): pp. 977–980.

36. Clare, B. A., R. S. Conroy and K. Spelman, *The diuretic effect in human subjects of an extract of Taraxacum officinale folium over a single day*. J Altern Complement Med, 2009. 15(8): pp. 929–934.

37. Vitale, S. G. et al., *Isoflavones, calcium, vitamin D and inulin improve quality of life, sexual function, body composition and metabolic parameters in menopausal women: result from a prospective, randomized, placebo-controlled, parallel-group study*. Prz Menopauzalny, 2018. 17(1): pp. 32–38.

38. Jeon, D., S. J. Kim and H. S. Kim, *Anti-inflammatory evaluation of the methanolic extract of Taraxacum officinale in LPS-stimulated human umbilical vein endothelial cells*. BMC Complement Altern Med, 2017. 17(1): p. 508.

39. Bruton-Seal, J. and M. Seal, *Hedgerow Medicine Harvest and Make Your Own Herbal Remedies*. 2009: Merlin Unwin Books.

40. Bone, K. and S. Mills, *The Essential Guide to Herbal Safety*. 2005: Elsevier, Churchill Livingstone.

41. Weed, S., *Healing Wise. Wise Woman Herbal*. 1989: Ash Tree Publishing.

42. Frawley, D. D. and D. V. Lad, *The Yoga of Herbs: An Ayurvedic guide to herbal medicine*. 1986: Motilial Banarsidass Publishers.

43. Bradley, P. R. E., *British Herbal Compendium*. Vol. 1. 2006, Bournemouth: British Herbal Medicine Association.

44. Haghgoo, R. et al., *Antibacterial Effects of Different Concentrations of*. J Int Soc Prev Community Dent, 2017. 7(4): pp. 180–185.

45. Heydarirad, G. et al., *Medical Mucilage Used in Traditional Persian Medicine Practice*. Iran J Med Sci, 2016. 41(3 Suppl): p. S41.

46. Kayani, S. et al., *Ethnobotanical uses of medicinal plants for respiratory disorders among the inhabitants of Gallies—Abbottabad, Northern Pakistan.* J Ethnopharmacol, 2014. 156: pp. 47–60.

47. Fink, C., M. Schmidt and K. Kraft, *[Marshmallow Root Extract for the Treatment of Irritative Cough: Two Surveys on Users' View on Effectiveness and Tolerability].* Complement Med Res, 2018. 25(5): pp. 299–305.

48. Khan, M. F. et al., *The evaluation of efficacy and safety of Cough (EMA) granules used for upper respiratory disorders.* Pak. J. Pharm. Sci., 2018. 31: pp. 2617–2622.

49. Sangian, H. et al., *Antiplasmodial activity of ethanolic extracts of some selected medicinal plants from the northwest of Iran.* Parasitol Res, 2013. 112(11): pp. 3697–3701.

50. Curnow, A. and S. J. Owen, *An Evaluation of Root Phytochemicals Derived from Althea officinalis (Marshmallow) and Astragalus membranaceus as Potential Natural Components of UV Protecting Dermatological Formulations.* Oxid Med Cell Longev, 2016. 2016: p. 7053897.

51. Mills, S. and K. Bone, *The Essential Guide to Herbal Safety.* 2005: Churchill Livingstone. Elsevier.

52. MD, B., *Marshmallow.* 2006: Drugs and Lactation Database (LactMed) [Internet]. Bethesda (MD): National Library of Medicine (US).

53. Wren, R. C., E. M. Williamson and F. J. Evans, *Potters New Cyclopaedia of Botanical Drugs and Preparations.* 2nd ed. 1988: Daniel.

54. Atmaca, H. et al., *Effects of Galium aparine extract on the cell viability, cell cycle and cell death in breast cancer cell lines.* J Ethnopharmacol, 2016. 186: pp. 305–310.

55. Shinkovenko, I. L. et al., *The immunomodulatory activity of the extracts and complexes of biologically active compounds of Galium verum L. herb.* Ceska Slov Farm, 2018. 67(1): pp. 25–29.

56. Carello, R. et al., *Long-term treatment with low-dose medicine in chronic childhood eczema: a double-blind two-stage randomized control trial.* Italian Journal of Paediatrics, 6th September 2017.

57. Sharifi-Rad, M. et al., *Anti-methicillin-resistant Staphylococcus aureus (MRSA) activity of Rubiaceae, Fabaceae and Poaceae plants: a search for new sources of useful alternative antibacterials against MRSA infections.* Cell Mol Biol (Noisy-le-grand), 2016. 62(9): pp. 39–45.

58. Grieve, M., *A Modern Herbal.* Reprinted from 1931 ed. 1988: Penguin Handbooks.

59. Felter, H. W. and L. J. U., *Kings American Dispensatory.* Edition 18 revision 3, Vol. 1. ed. 1905: Reprinted in 1983 Eclectic Medical Publications.

60. Wood, M., *The Practice of Traditional Western Herbalism.* 2004: North Atlantic Books.

61. Winston, D., *Nvwoti; Cherokee Medicine and Ethnobotany.* Journal of the American Herbalists Guild, 2001(Fall/Winter): pp. 45–49.

CHAPTER NINE

Swimming upstream: common conditions and therapeutic considerations

Introduction

Following on from Chapter 7, we would now like to look at two more conditions commonly treated by consulting medical herbalists. This will give us a chance to look more closely at both our digestive tracts and our immune systems, two systems which, as we are sure you remember from Chapter 3, work closely together. Again we will contrast the conventional approach to treatment with a Western herbalists approach, and look at where, how and why they differ.

Let's begin with our immune systems, and in particular with infections affecting our respiratory tracts.

Part 1. Respiratory tract infections

What is a respiratory tract infection? How do they come about? Why do they occur? When do they happen? What can we do about them? What do we need to be careful of? Read on ...

Definition—*Respiratory tract infections*: Respiratory tract infections may be defined as any infection which affects the upper or lower respiratory tracts.

Respiratory tract infections sub-categorized as lower respiratory tract infections are more commonly known as chest infections and affect the mucous membranes and tissues of the lungs.

Upper respiratory tract infections affect the mucous membranes of the nose, sinuses and throat, and can involve the ears or eyes (such as otitis media, or conjunctivitis). They include the following:

- Tonsillitis
- Pharyngitis
- Laryngitis
- Sinusitis
- Otitis media (middle ear infection)
- Conjunctivitis
- A head cold

Rhinitis is inflammation in the nasal passages that may occur without infection, such as hayfever or chronic rhinitis.

Lower respiratory tract infections affect the airways (bronchi, and bronchioles) and lung tissues (alveoli and lobes of the lungs). They include:

- Bronchitis
- Bronchiolitis
- Alveolitis
- Lobar pneumonia
- Pneumonia
- Tuberculosis

Chronic persistent inflammation and infection in the lungs usually caused by/resulting in structural changes to the lungs occurs in bronchiectasis, a condition that usually requires life-long management.

The National Institute for Health and Care Clinical Excellence, UK (NICE) define lower respiratory tract infection as:

> *An acute illness (present for 21 days or less), usually with cough as the main symptom, and with at least one other lower respiratory tract symptom (such as fever, sputum production, breathlessness, wheeze or chest discomfort or pain) and no alternative explanation (such as sinusitis or asthma). Pneumonia, acute bronchitis and exacerbation of chronic obstructive airways disease are included in this definition.*

Causes and symptoms; the pathophysiology of respiratory tract infections

Respiratory tract infections are most commonly either bacterial or viral. Most people experience a common or head cold between two and four times a year; children up to eight. Many types of virus can cause the common cold; the most common is rhinovirus, which is thought to account for at least 50% of all colds.

Other viruses that are known to cause common colds include coronavirus (more on this shortly), respiratory syncytial virus, influenza and para-influenza. There are mind-bogglingly over 200 viruses associated with head colds, and there may be more than one type of virus responsible for any given infection. Viruses are not amenable to treatment by antibiotics, but viral infections do respond well to herbal interventions. More of this later …

Flu is shorthand for influenza, very specifically the influenza virus and may become much more serious if left untreated. There are many types of influenza viruses, and they are also changing with new strains emerging all the time. New strains and sub-types of virus can appear to which our immune system has not developed immunity. They can overwhelm our bodies more easily, and spread more rapidly within a population.

The 1918 flu (influenza) pandemic (caused by an H1N1 viral sub-type) infected approximately 500 million people around the world and it is estimated that between 10–20% of those infected died. Unusually it primarily targeted healthy adults rather than the sick or elderly. It is now thought that the virus was not necessarily more dangerous but

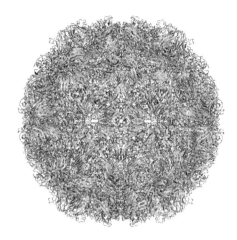

Structure of an influenza virus.

that other factors such as malnourishment, overcrowding in medical camps and hospitals, and poor hygiene interventions, were to blame for the high death toll.

This shocking pandemic has remained strong in race memory, and helps to explain why flu can still engender fear around the world. The following quote is taken from a book written by a herbalist practicing in the UK at that time;

> It is my proud boast that in all my 50 years I have never lost a case of *Pneumonia, Pleurisy or Influenza. This in itself I think has justified my life's work. I leave it on proud record that during the Influenza epidemic of 1918–1919 I dispensed over 15,000 bottles of medicine, that in some houses I had six cases down at once with Influenza or Pneumonia without the loss of a single case.*
>
> —Burns Lingard

This extraordinary statement cuts to the heart of the potential for herbal medicine to treat illness and support the patient, even in seemingly dire situations.

Influenza does have the capacity to spread around the globe, and modern examples include so-called bird-flu (avian flu) and swine-flu (another H1N1 virus) in 2009.

As we write this, the UK is entering week four of a social distancing 'lockdown' imposed by the government as part of a strategy to limit the spread of the virus enticingly named severe acute respiratory syndrome coronavirus 2 (**SARS-CoV-2**), the virus strain currently known as Covid19. Covid 19, which has caused a pandemic, is proving difficult to tackle in terms of a vaccine. There are currently no existing vaccines against human coronavirus, and new technologies are being used, which necessitate thorough safety testing. Cost and distribution will ultimately also factor in. It is thought unlikely that a vaccine will be available to treat the first wave of the pandemic.[1]

This situation is unprecedented in our lifetime, but not unprecedented in terms of the last century (give or take a year). Many people will only suffer mild symptoms, and some will be asymptomatic.

Following the guidelines to stay safe and minimize spread of infection to those in our communities who are vulnerable, is vital.

The potential role of herbal medicine is to ensure that the vulnerable members of our communities are well protected, and that minor infections are contained and, when contracted, prevented from becoming serious. Supporting the human organism, so that the body can better cope with an infection with minimal adverse outcomes, is where the strength of our herbs lies. Each virus is unique, but good, sound and sensible preventative and supportive measures can be employed using tried and tested herbal interventions to minimize the impact of infection, We cannot, and would never claim to, wave a magic wand, or provide a magical cure; that is not what we are about. We do firmly believe however, that there is nothing that cannot be helped.

Influenza or flu, can affect the upper and/or lower respiratory tract—and there are some key differences between influenza and a common cold viral infection.

Symptoms, such as fever, headache, general aches, fatigue, malaise, weakness, sneezing, chest discomfort and cough, can occur with a common cold, but may be much more severe (especially weakness, fatigue and aches) with flu and last for 2–3 weeks rather than 6–10 days.

For people who are more vulnerable (such as asthmatics or those who may be immune-compromised), prolonged viral infections can more easily become chest infections, or secondary bacterial infections. This is where an initial viral infection precedes and possibly allows a bacterial infection to develop over the original viral one. In fact, it is often the complications that can occur during any infection that put people most at risk. So,

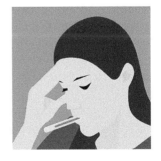

ultimately it comes down to careful management of infections that prevent such complications. More of this later …

Bacteria capable of causing respiratory tract infections include *Streptococcus pneumonia*, *Staphylococcus aureus* and *Haemophilus influenzae*.

Conventional approaches to treatment

Currently a vaccination policy is aimed at vulnerable people including the elderly, and health care workers to try to avoid influenza outbreaks spreading. Unfortunately vaccines have to be updated annually to match probable epidemic strains of the virus. Their effectiveness is also variable from year to year, and can range from 15 to 60% depending on many things, including the strain of the virus and the age of the recipients.

Antiviral drugs can be used for influenza. These work best when administered early, and can shorten the illness by 1–2 days. They may also reduce the likelihood of complications. These antiviral drugs are highly specific and will not be effective against common cold viruses or other virus strains.

Because upper respiratory tract infections tend to be viral in origin, antibiotics are inappropriate and ineffective. Antibiotics used for viral infections may result in prolonged or more severe symptoms. Conventional treatment is most commonly aimed at symptomatic relief. The UK National Health Service—Choices website recommends plenty of rest, drinking plenty of fluids and eating healthily. Conventionally decongestants are used for symptoms such as a blocked nose. Anti-inflammatory drugs and painkillers such as ibuprofen and paracetamol are recommended to deal with high temperature and aches and pains. Some drug preparations combine painkilling and decongestant actions.

There is a wide range of over-the-counter cold remedies available, which are primarily aimed at management of symptoms to relieve the discomfort experienced by someone suffering from a common cold. This often enables people to 'soldier on' with their illness.

Lower respiratory tract infections tend more often to be of bacterial origin, and are usually treated with antibiotics. Like antivirals, antibiotics are quite specific in their effectiveness. This means the correct type of antibiotic must be identified. The length of treatment, whether one or more antibiotic is used, whether glucocorticosteroid

(steroid) treatment is also required, will all depend upon the nature of the individual presenting case. A blood test measuring an inflammation marker known as C reactive protein (CRP) may be used as an indicator of infection, and treatment may be, in part at least, based upon the results of the CRP.

Very interestingly, complementary and alternative medicine treatments are not openly recommended by conventional medical advice, although a recent statement by the UK National Institute of Health and Care Excellence recommends people use honey and home remedies as a first line of defence for a viral infection instead of antibiotics.

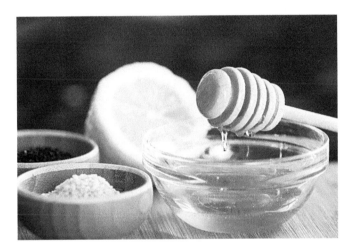

And yet there is very little support from conventional circles for plant-based treatments that were once official medicines available from all UK pharmacies right up to the late 1980s. In particular there has been a total rejection of expectorants that were once commonplace, and known to be reliable—plants such as ipecacuanha and liquorice were often found in conventional cough medicines—revealing the influence of native American (First Nations peoples) herbal medicine and traditional European herbal medicines on UK medical practice.

One outcome of booming health food shop sales has been the use of plant medicines as 'natural versions' of drugs. Frustratingly for the herbal practitioner, people seeking relief will understandably look for a herbal version of say an antibiotic, and the over-the-counter use of echinacea is a prime example of this. This can be seen as applying herbal medicines to a conventional disease model, and can result in disappointing research questions (let alone research outcomes!). You can find plenty of research both proving and disproving the efficacy of *Echinacea species* in the prevention and treatment of the common cold,[2-5] a condition that has incidentally evaded any 'successful' treatment conventional or otherwise.

But for the herbal practitioner we may consider that a viral common cold needs to be managed effectively taking into account a person's unique strengths and weaknesses. This means *echinacea* may be appropriate or not for that person, and will almost certainly benefit from combination with other appropriately targeted herbal medicines—such as herbs to relieve varied and specific symptoms—sore eyes, sore throat, upset tummy, glandular swellings etc. More of this now …

Western herbal medicine approaches to treatment

The human body is constantly exposed to challenges from the outside world which, when we are fit and healthy, we can usually deal with effectively, with minimum impact to our wellbeing. Sometimes, however, things do get through our non-specific defences and can develop into a respiratory tract infection. There are some key concepts that exist in Western herbal medicine:

Causes: Respiratory tract infections are considered to be caused by more than just a virus or bacterium. For example, it may also be possible to identify some sort of deficiency in our capacity to repel a potential invading organism. This may be because we are run-down from overwork, or over worry, lack of sleep or poor dietary choices. Significantly, bereavement is thought to influence the lungs and so chest infections are observed to be more likely following the death of a loved one. Sometimes it is not possible to identify other factors and herbal treatment is nevertheless broadly directed at supporting and managing our innate immune response.

Symptoms: The symptoms of respiratory infections generally correlate with our own body's defence mechanisms moving into action to deal with the situation. For example, raised temperature or fever is a deliberate manoeuvre by the body to make the internal environment hostile to invading pathogens. Excess mucous is produced as a means of flushing away pathogens and cellular debris, as is sneezing. Herbal medicines and other adjuvant advice is targeted at managing these symptoms. Supporting the immune response, preventing mucous from being too thin or too thick, aiding expectoration, reducing inflammation and managing fever without suppressing it are all techniques employed by the herbalist to try to speed up a successful resolution of respiratory infections. Easing symptoms is also appropriate and welcome! It is likely, common and part of being human, to get a respiratory infection at various points in our lives, but it is how we manage the infection that is of interest here.

Despite what we have just said about infections not being solely the result of an infective organism, a herbal strategy will still usually have some sort of antiviral or antibacterial ingredient(s). So many herbal allies can assist us with invading organisms: *Thymus vulgaris* L., *Echinacea purpurea* L., *Salvia officinalis* L., *Commiphora myrrha* (T.Nees) Engl. (syn. *C. molmol*), as examples. *Hypericum perforatum* L. has proven antiviral properties, especially against enveloped viruses.[6]

Recognition of weakness or deficiency will also be a key component. This may involve the use of tissue tonics—such as those supporting the mucous membranes themselves (*Plantago lanceolata/majus* L., *Euphrasia officinalis* L.), the lungs (*Verbascum thapsus* L., *Inula helenium* L.), the sinuses (*Euphrasia officinalis* L., *Baptisia tinctoria* (L.) R.Br), the ears (*Allium sativum* L.), or the throat (*Salvia officinalis* L.), for example.

Careful management of symptoms

Traditions of herbal medicine consider simple respiratory tract infections as an exterior condition—one which affects the body's exposed surfaces—the mucous membranes or the upper respiratory tract and lungs. Treatment strategies are therefore expansive, aiming to push the infective agent out, before it has a chance to become an interior infection. Diaphoretics (herbs that encourage sweating) are a classic example of this. Diaphoresis is seen as beneficial in Western herbal medicine with the employment of such herbs as yarrow herb (*Achillea millefolium* L.), lime flowers (*Tilia x europaea* L.), elderflower (*Sambucus nigra* L. flores) and boneset herb (*Eupatorium perfoliatum* L.). Ideally these herbs are taken as a hot infusion for diaphoresis to be induced.

Preventing excessive fever—fever management may also be required alongside diaphoretics—such as catnip (*Nepeta cataria* L.), meadowsweet (*Filipendula ulmaria* L. Maxim) or lemon balm (*Melissa officinalis* L.).

Note: Dealing with fever. Adults tend not to easily produce a fever whereas children can do so readily.

It is worth remembering that in adults, dealing with a fever by encouraging sweating, can help to fight infection, and ultimately end the fever. This should be done with care not to become excessive, and it should be performed with due regard to convalescence. If you can, seek the guidance of a medical herbalist.

Supporting a fever rather than suppressing it involves giving plenty of fluids such as water, diluted fruit juices and herbal teas that support the immune system and aid fever management such as catnip herb (*Nepeta cataria* L.), yarrow (*Achillea millefolium* L.), elderflowers (*Sambucus nigra* L.), meadowsweet flowering herb, (*Filipendula ulmaria* L.), hyssop herb (*Hyssopus officinalis* L.) and chamomile flowers (*Matricaria chamomilla (L.) Rauchert*). Flavouring these fever management teas with pleasant-tasting but therapeutically valuable herbs such as peppermint, spearmint, or lime blossom can be very helpful as can sweetening with a little honey or apple juice.

Consult your doctor if

- The temperature is higher than 103°F (39.5°C) and does not respond to fever management treatments.
- A child acts confused or loses consciousness.
- A child has rolling eyes or body twitching.
- An infant under six weeks old.
- There is persistent fever accompanied by headache or a stiff neck.

For a small minority of children high fever can cause febrile seizures, seldom associated with any brain damage but frightening nevertheless. They are most likely up to the age of three and seldom after the age of 5.

The first signs of fever are often irritability, grumpiness and a desire to be close to the parent. Cheeks and face may be flushed and warm to touch. The child may feel too hot or too cold, and appetite is often reduced. Sudden onset occurs in babies and toddlers and may occur over a few hours. Extremes and spikes in temperature may occur with relation to the seriousness of the infection. Keep food to a minimum, but keep up fluid intake, especially using the medicinal teas suggested.

With a healthy immune system, most illnesses accompanied by a fever are easily overcome, and can be looked at as a sign of vitality. An excellent resource from an experienced and highly regarded herbalist—Dr Mary Bove ND is her book *An Encyclopedia of Natural Healing for Children and Infants* from which this summary has been taken.[7]

It is interesting to note how we refer to respiratory tract infections here in the West as a 'cold'. Warming the body is a persistent theme in herbal medicine worldwide to increase resistance and vitality. Use of spices, such as ginger, turmeric, cinnamon, black pepper, cardamom, clove, can assist in preventing a cold, or be used during the infection to help reinforce our response.

Anti-inflammatories and pain relief herbs can be used such as those ideal for a sore throat (*Salvia officinalis* L., *Glycyrrhiza glabra* L. and *Commiphora myrrha* (T.Nees) Engl.), or bone aches and pains (*Filipendula ulmaria* (L.) Maxim and *Eupatorium perfoliatum* L.). Encouraging effective expectoration medicinal herbs such as *Pimpinella anisum* L., *Hyssopus officinalis* L., *Thymus vulgaris* L. or *Glycyrrhiza glabra* L. root can be used. Dealing with infections that have gone deep, beyond the exterior (such as sinus and chest infections), may require much more heroic herbal strategies such as *Allium sativum* L., *Hydrastis Canadensis* L., *Baptisia tinctoria* (L.) R.Br, *Thymus vulgaris* L., for instance.

Managing mucous! Mucous has an important role to play in the health and vitality of our mucous membranes. Without it, the membranes are too dry, sore, vulnerable and exposed. Too much or too thick mucous loses its capacity to eject pathogens and debris out of the body, and causes unpleasant symptoms. Herbs used to manage mucous include *Althaea officinalis* L. (root or leaf), *Sambucus nigra* L. flowers, *Plantago lanceolata* L./*P. major* L., *Euphrasia officinalis* L.

Support for the lymphatic system can be really beneficial, especially in cases where swollen lymph glands in the neck are a feature (the patient feels 'glandy'). *Galium aparine* L. and *Echinacea species* would both be indicated here. In addition bitter tonics may be used to increase saliva, patient vitality and restore appetite—this may also improve mucous production. Examples include *Marrubium vulgare* L., as well as many of the herbs already mentioned.

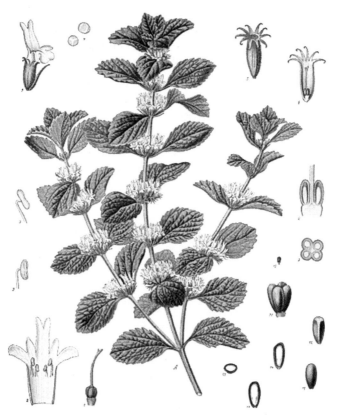

White Horehound (*Marrubium vulgare* L.)

In fact, you may already have noticed how many of the herbs recommended above for respiratory tract infections, are repeated and seem to have multiple effects. This is one of the extraordinary qualities of plant medicines, in that they are complex. They contain multiple compounds and can act at multiple surfaces at once. By combining herbs, it is possible to act in complex beneficial ways to the aid of the person suffering from a respiratory tract infection. Equally every single herb will have multiple benefits to us.

The herbal approach to treatment involves moving to support the body's own defences rather than repress them. This strategy is usually sufficient to effectively deal with conditions such as simple head colds without the danger of them progressing into more serious situations such as chest infections. Adequate rest so the body can direct its energies at effective healing is central to this, alongside treating the situation as early as possible. Feeling poorly could be seen as an attempt by our body to try to make us rest and allow the focus of our resources to be upon the infection.

A simple viral infection left unchecked can potentially become a secondary bacterial infection, bronchitis or even pneumonia, especially in vulnerable people or the elderly or very young. It is therefore important to treat respiratory infections at the first signs of symptoms and stop them from progressing into anything more serious. It may be a person dislikes using conventional treatments for such infections, but avoiding doing anything at all is a mistake. If you wish to avoid using conventional drugs and antibiotics, you are more likely to be successful if you combine rest and herbal medicines.

Problems are more likely to occur in the following situations:

- Someone who is regularly exposed to repeated infections (i.e. teachers, airline workers (recycled air during travel), nurses).
- Someone whose immune system is already compromised (repeated courses of certain drugs such as steroids, stomach acid suppressants and antibiotics), or suffer other conditions such as asthma or emphysema.

A herbal sleep aid may facilitate the patient to rest more successfully at night. Monitor the patient well. Ensure that they are resting, and taking plenty of hot drinks and nourishing foods. If the symptoms do not start to resolve within a few days, seek further advice.

So, when bugs strike, what have you got in your kitchen cupboards? What have you got growing in your gardens? What can the budding herbalist do to help?

Here are a few suggestions to get the ball rolling!

Self-help: the kitchen pharmacy

Sore throats

Something to drink …?

Tea for a sore throat.

- Half a teaspoon of each: peppermint, thyme and sage dried herbs.
- Pour over one mugful of freshly boiled water, and leave to infuse covered for 5 minutes.

- Add a little honey, maple syrup or molasses if desired (to help with the taste and soothing action).
- Drink and/or gargle.

Ideal for sore throats and clearing mucous stuck at the back of the throat.

Something to apply ...?

Compress for a sore throat.

- Make an infusion of thyme herb as described above using 0.5–1 teaspoons of dried thyme leaves (or 1–2 teaspoons of fresh leaves if available).
- Dip a clean cotton scarf in the hot tea (thyme and/or sage), wring it out and wrap it around the throat. Cover with another scarf to hold it in place for around 10–15 minutes. Repeat.

This is one traditional method of treating a sore throat without having to drink lots of liquid. Seek advice in cases of recurrent sore throats.

Blocked nose

Thick or copious mucous can be unpleasant but also slows and stagnates the healing response. Getting things moving, and flowing can be achieved with appropriate herbal treatment.

Mucous mover tea.

- Make a tea blend by mixing equal parts of dried elderflowers, ribwort plantain, eyebright, chamomile and peppermint leaf.
- Use 1 large teaspoon per mug of boiling water.
- Infuse for 4–8 minutes, strain through a tea strainer and drink hot regularly—perhaps as many as 6 cups per day.

Headache

This is one symptom that could be a manifestation of any simple ailment or of an underlying disease. Seek medical advice if the headache persists or become intense or comes with a rash. Simple colds can cause headache usually as a result of the immune response itself and/or nasal or sinus congestion. Easing nasal congestion we have covered above. If additional pain relief is required, you could try adding some meadowsweet herb, or using one of the more 'heroic' recipes from the section on sinusitis (coming up soon).

Bone ache

Using diaphoretics such as boneset, elderflower or yarrow can help the aches and pains of influenza and common colds. Herbs with a natural analgesic effect such as *Filipendula ulmaria* L. (Meadowsweet), which has an array of salicylate compounds that can give ease from aches and pains would also be useful.

Poor sleep

Another diaphoretic herb—linden or lime blossoms (*Tilia x europaea* L.) has a strong reputation in its native Hungary, and across Europe for its mild sedative effects, and therapeutic, relaxation-inducing properties. It makes a gorgeous tasting infusion, and is a welcome pleasant taste among other medicinal bitter-tasting herbs. Many other relaxing and sleep-encouraging herbs may be useful to aid restful sleep at this time— including *Matricaria chamomilla* L., and *Lavandula officinalis* L. or *Passiflora incarnata* L. All can be prepared as an infusion, and taken in small sips, or in a concentrated sweetened mouthful.

Sore eyes

Both chamomile and eyebright can work wonders for sore irritated eyes, having antiviral compounds[8] and being anti-inflammatory, they can be used externally or to supplement internal medication for conjunctivitis. Apply a strong infusion that has been cooled to the closed eye and hold in place for a few minutes. Repeat with a clean cotton swab/pad, as often as necessary.

- Never re-use the cotton swab/pad (it may now carry the infective organism)
- Never place it on the other eye (transmits infection)
- Never dip a used pad back into your beautiful herbal infusion.

The infusion will survive covered in the fridge for 24 hours, then a fresh new batch should be made.

Something for the chesticles!

Anti-infective chest rub

When symptoms threaten to go down to the chest and cause a chest infection, an external chest rub would be a valuable addition to your arsenal. Consider using a good base oil such as almond oil or, even better, marigold or St John's wort flower *infused* oil. You could very gently decoct fresh herbs into this oil, on the lowest heat possible for 2–12 hours: a slow cooker, a stainless steel tin sat inside a pan of hot water would work well for this. Or you could even leave it in a warm airing cupboard! Make sure the heat is nice and gentle; you will lose the therapeutic benefits if you 'cook' the herbs. A quicker method would be to add a few drops of essential oil to the base oil, to give an aromatic, simple therapeutic chest rub. Apply regularly, making sure you cover the chest right to the bases of the lungs, and wear a nice warm woolly jumper over the top.

Suggested herbs for infused oil/decoction

Thyme, sage, aniseed, clove, bay, lavender, fresh garlic, thinly sliced. *Fill the container with the herb material, cover with your plain oil, cover and infuse. Strain before use.*

Suggested essential oils to add to your base oil

Thyme, lavender, eucalyptus, tea tree, pine, frankincense, chamomile, clove. *Approximately I drop essential oil per 10 ml of base oil.*

The must-have all-rounder!

Elderberry syrup

What a fantastic thing to have on stand-by for the treatment of coughs, colds etc. Research has confirmed the long traditional use of elderberries in the prevention and treatment of cold and flu symptoms and, even better, elderberry syrup is delicious!

Clinical trials have supported the traditional use of elderberry for reducing both the duration and severity of fever and for reducing headache, muscle ache, mucus production and nasal congestion associated with colds and flu.[9,10] Flavonoids contained within elderberries have been shown to reduce the flu virus's ability to bind to cell surfaces, therefore reducing their effect on the system.[11,12]

Make plenty during the elderberry season, which is excellent timing when you think about it as it generally precedes the onset of winter

Elderberry and ginger syrup recipe

Ingredients
Ripe elderberries
Sugar
Cinnamon sticks
Root ginger, thinly sliced
Star anise
Cloves

Method
Pick the fruit on a dry day, wash well and drain thoroughly.

Strip the fruit from the stems and put into a pan with spices, adding just enough water to cover.

Simmer for 30 minutes until the berries are very soft.

Strain through a jelly bag or muslin and measure the juice.

Allow equal quantities of sugar to the juice. Heat the juice gently, stirring in the sugar until dissolved.

Boil for 10 minutes and then leave until cold.

The syrup may be frozen in small quantities (such as an ice cube tray) or packed into small, screw-topped, soft drink bottles, which have been sterilised.

and the cough/cold time of year. If you harvested elderflowers in early summer, you will know where the elderberries will be—if you have left enough flowers to become berries!

Elderberry syrups of this kind have been used (at least) since Tudor times as a stand-by against winter colds. The syrup is a cold aperient, relieves all chest troubles, will stop a cold and bring on a sweat. It is normally diluted, allowing 2 tablespoons of syrup to a tumbler of hot water and a squeeze of lemon juice. Drink regularly (every 1–2 hours) with a head cold.

There are no quantities stated in this recipe as things are dependent upon the number of elderberries that you harvest. Spices are added to personal taste, and can be any combination of warming aromatic herbs. Err on the side of stronger tastes rather than weaker. Add other berries such as blackberries or raspberries if you wish. Star anise is particularly recommended for its shikimic acid content, which was used as the basis of the influenza drug Tamiflu.[13]

Diet and lifestyle advice

During the winter months we tend to eat heavier, starchier foods and less fresh fruit, vegetables and salads. This may contribute towards a raised susceptibility to various viruses etc. From the humoural perspective, carbohydrate-rich foods such as breads and pastries are damp and cold. In excess they reduce flow and movement and they increase the effect of the cold damp climate of winter (here in the Northern Hemisphere). They are also lacking in life force as they are farther from their living state than say—a raw carrot! So, consider adding spice, using less refined carbohydrate and finding a way to ingest living food in winter! A spicy winter slaw? A vibrant fresh herb chutney (see also Chapter 5).

Another winter slaw—a quick spicy recipe

- Grate fresh raw cabbage (red, white or green).
- Add half as much raw grated carrot, onion, and finely sliced green, yellow or red peppers.
- Add some raw finely chopped chilli pepper and some garlic. Season well with high-quality sea salt and pepper.

- Add a couple of glugs of cold-pressed oil (hemp seed or olive perhaps), plus either freshly squeezed lemon or lime juice (and zest if they are unwaxed).
- Finally a couple of tablespoons of freshly toasted sesame seeds, or cashew or peanuts.
- Stir well. Leave at room temperature for 1–8 hours before eating—it should feel spicy and zingy!

Then, if there is any left, refrigerate and finish up the next day.

Other strategies

- Rest. Take time off work if necessary. There are two good reasons for this, a) you should give your body a good chance to recover quickly—1 or 2 days off work early on is better than 1 or 2 weeks off if the cold is allowed to get a grip and make you really ill. b) Avoid spreading the cold to others.
- Keep warm, especially if going outdoors. Hats, gloves, scarves etc. are important.
- Drink plenty of fluids (*Not* alcohol). Herbal teas are ideal for this, especially peppermint, yarrow, thyme, chamomile,[14] honey and lemon or elderflower.

  Elderflower, peppermint and yarrow is a classic traditional cold and flu tea. Peppermint acts as a decongestant, yarrow for fever management and elderflower as a nose and throat tonic. Use 1 teaspoon per cup of boiling water and let the tea steep for at least 15 minutes before drinking. Drink the tea freely, 5–6 times a day if possible.

  If you have peppermint in your garden just pick it fresh and make an infusion with hot water. Good old honey and lemon drinks are excellent, especially last thing at night. Add cinnamon and/or ginger for extra effect.
- Rest—mentioned again because it's so important. Don't go to the gym, jog etc. Avoid any housework that is not absolutely necessary.
- Raise your intake of fresh fruit and vegetables. If you own a fruit juicer, use it. It's a great way to take in fresh fruit and vegetables. Kiwi fruit is especially good for its vitamin C content. Some people respond better to high levels of vitamin A so carrot juice is also a good idea. Beetroots are naturally antiviral.

- Avoid eating lots of dairy products whilst you have a cold, and stay away from refined sugars and white carbohydrates—they can be mucous forming.
- Increase your intake of garlic and onions. The volatile oils of both of these related foods contain chemicals with strong antibiotic actions. During World War I the British army used garlic to control infections in wounds. If you eat plenty of garlic and onions during the winter months you are practising preventative medicine by significantly decreasing your chances of contracting a cold. A good traditional recipe for onions is as follows:

Onion milk

Simmer a large onion in milk until tender—about I hour. Eat the softened onion and drink the milk. If you really object to the taste and smell of garlic take garlic capsules.

- Eat a good hot curry with plenty of spices!
- If you have easy access to a sauna, visit it regularly.
- Rest!

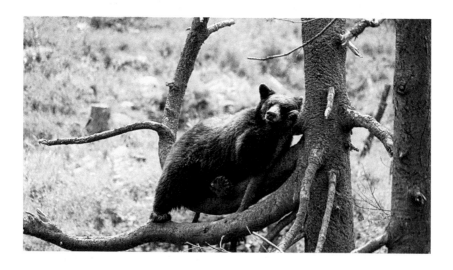

Note: The importance of rest. Note that **rest** plays a crucial role in the above strategy. The BBC News website posted the following article in October 2017!

Patients need rest, not antibiotics, say health officials

By James Gallagher. Health and science reporter, BBC News website 23rd October 2017.

This reports on the latest advice given by Public Health England (PHE), a government department responsible for 'making the public healthier'.

Finally—ladies and gentlemen—we introduce you to (drumroll).

Mustard footbath

- Put 2 teaspoons of ordinary yellow mustard powder into a bucket or basin/washing up bowl (big enough to accommodate your feet comfortably)
- Add hot water, as hot as you can comfortably tolerate.
- Stir
- Soak feet for up to 20 mintes, topping up with hot water as necessary.
- Dry feet well, and put on thick socks.

This is a great thing to do last thing at night before going straight to bed.

The idea here is to stimulate the circulation and therefore vitality and vigour to fight the infection. Our feet are particularly sensitive and can convey a therapeutic agent quickly into the body. Garlic can be taped with medical tape to the feet at night to ease chest and ear infections in children or adults, and footbaths are a worthwhile naturopathic intervention especially if a person does not feel well enough to take medicine by mouth. Finally—as we mentioned before in the section on the circulation, a persistent idea from traditional herbal medicine, is that improving the vigour and 'bounce' in the peripheral circulation will take the strain off the heart and there will be a more harmonious circulatory response of back and forth—central circulation to the periphery.

A special mention for sinusitis

What is happening here when we have sinusitis? You may remember our incredible pairs of sinuses inside the bone of the skull, lined with delicate mucous membranes. Well, firstly we have an 'itis' to contend with here ('itis' simply means 'inflammation of'). Inflammation can occur with, or without infection present. The mucous membranes of our sinuses can become congested and inflamed, and for some people this can be difficult to shift and may lead to chronic problems. This can be brought on by an upper respiratory tract infection, chronic rhinitis or hayfever for example.

Congestion and oedema of the mucosal membranes can allow a bacterial infection to really take hold in these deep and delicate places. An acute bout of sinusitis may be very debilitating in the first instance. Symptoms may include a feeling of pressure behind the nose, a runny or stuffed up nose, green or yellow mucous from the nose, cough, fever and facial pain or headache.

Sinus headaches may be on one side of the face only or bilateral, and feel like a throbbing headache around the area of the sinuses themselves, or up across the crown of the head, which worsens on the movement of the head, on bending forwards and can improve as the day goes on. Changes in temperature (such as going outdoors) can worsen these symptoms. A sinus headache can be mistaken for a migraine, but usually other symptoms associated with sinusitis give the game away. Acute RTI's can self-resolve in the main but inflammation of the sinuses may become entrenched if not dealt with at the time and lead to chronic sinusitis.

Chronic sinusitis can last for at least 3 months, and the facial pain or tenderness can persist, along with such symptoms as post-nasal drip, jaw/tooth soreness, impaired sense of smell and general fatigue. Post-nasal drip occurs because the body is continuing in its valiant efforts to resolve the problem by washing away the irritation with liquid. Unfortunately this isn't resolving the issue, and a constant feeling of mucous at the back of the throat is a big clue pointing towards problems elsewhere which are unresolved. Post-nasal drip can cause a persistent cough, and confuse the diagnosis.

The herbal perspective of sinusitis

The inability to throw off infections and their long-term effects are associated with a certain deficiency—a coldness in the system—a lack of vitality and vigour. Often chronic sinusitis can be traced back to a viral infection that was not adequately treated at the time. The body may not have cleared away all waste products from the original infection, so from a herbal perspective the lymphatic system will need support, and there should be stimulation to circulation.

Treatment strategies would involve:

a) Treating the initial infection. Even if this occurred months (or even years) ago, it should still be treated, and treated robustly. Strong doses of herbal anti-infectives will usually be needed.
b) Support the body's immune and detoxification systems, especially the lymphatic and circulatory system.
c) Return the system to overall health and vigour. Fighting a chronic infection presents a significant challenge to the systems resources and will often have drained vitality from the individual. Tonic herbs are a real blessing here.

So, back to the kitchen cupboard …

If you are unlucky enough to suffer from sinusitis as part of your RTI symptom profile, here are a few things you can do to relieve the situation:

Steam inhalation

Where there is a lot of infection (green mucous, fever, for example) anti-infective herbs can be very helpful. They carry those anti-infective volatile oils to exactly where you need them to be, to help 'fight crime'. Thyme, lavender, rosemary, peppermint and pine leaves may all be used, either together or in combination as a good, strong hot infusion for inhalation purposes. You could also use essential oils if you prefer (including frankincense, tea tree and eucalyptus—use one or two drops only in a bowl of hot, steamy water), although they might not be as gentle, or have as broad-based an action on the mucous membranes as using whole herbs.

Bend your head forwards over the bowl of hot water and cover your head with a towel to make a tent over the bowl and trap the vapours in a steam bath for the head. Inhale slowly. Repeat at least three times a day.

If you have a lot of inflammation of the sinuses (stuffed up, can't breathe), you may want to use a more gentle anti-inflammatory approach and avoid harsh oils. In this case, whole herbs such as chamomile and peppermint can be used as infusions in the steam bath to gently soothe those inflamed, unhappy surfaces. Externally, a balm or lotion may be applied around the nose and cheeks in affected areas, and allowed to penetrate the skin to provide relief. Any combination of the essential oils listed above can be added to a beeswax and oil ointment and applied externally.

Aromatic balms containing such essential oils as clove, pine and eucalyptus can be rubbed externally over sinuses and even up, under the neck and around the lymph glands to encourage opening, drainage and flow to these areas, as well as providing anti-infective compounds. This is a useful adjunct to herbal treatment, but should (as we have previously pointed out) be recognized as being distinct from the use of whole herbs. Essential oils are a highly concentrated form of a specific subset of plant constituents, and are much more intense and targeted than whole plant medicines.

Japanese Shiatsu for a Sinus Headache
Sinus Headache Alleviating Technique

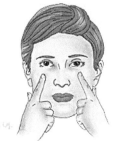 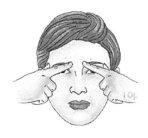

1. Place your index finger on your cheekbones, apply firm pressure & rotate your fingers in a circular motion for 5 to 10 min.

2. Place your index fingers on your forehead right about where your eyebrows begin, apply firm pressure & rotate your fingers in a circular motion for 5 to 10 min.

3. Perform this exercise twise daily.

A lovely herbal tea will also serve to alleviate many of the symptoms of sinusitis. Herbs to include would be: Plantain, sage, thyme, lavender, rosemary, elderflower and chamomile. Drink at least 5 hot cups a day. Take a flask if you go out.

Acute and chronic sinusitis: the herbalist's approach

Medical herbalists might well use many of the herbs mentioned above as part of a home kitchen pharmacy but will also have experience and knowledge of herbs more suited to the art of prescribing. Some of these herbs are restricted by law for use only by practitioners, but they illustrate how circulatory stimulants, and lymphatic support are key parts of a herbalists' strategy. This list is by no means extensive, and practitioners and patients develop their reliable favourites and preferred herbal allies.

Thymus vulgaris L. (thyme)[15]
Commiphora myrrha (T.Nees) Engl. (myrrh)[16]
Hydrastis canadensis L.[17,18] (goldenseal)
Baptisia tinctoria (L.) R.Br. (wild indigo)[10]
Myrica cerifera L. (bayberry)[19]
Phytolacca americana L. (poke root)[20]
Lobelia inflata L. (lobelia: practitioner only)[21]

Big internal doses would be used, often alongside an external preparation, such as this decongestant and antiseptic external sinus rub, given by Simon Mills, MCPP, FNIMH MA. Equal quantities of tinctures of: *Capsicum anuum* L., *Lobelia inflata* L., *Hydrastis Canadensis* L., *Commiphora myrrha* (T.Nees) Engl., *Myrica cerifera* L. Work over affected sinuses for around 10 minutes once or twice a day, Keep away from eyes. Use gloves or wash hands after use.

Garlic powder taken in capsules can be extraordinarily helpful for this condition. Taken in sufficient dose, garlic can be as effective as an antibiotic. Some people need repeated courses of antibiotics to treat sinus infections, so patience may be needed with garlic too.

Ideally take the garlic capsules before each meal, so that your food sits on top of the capsules. This prevents the garlic from repeating on you! 500 mg of powdered garlic (not garlic oil) in capsules can be taken (by a healthy adult) three times daily and more under the guidance of a practitioner, for some people this may disturb the bowel mildly and temporarily but will not do harm. Viruses will also disturb the microbiome and can irritate the lymphatics lining the bowel so digestive disturbances can occur in any case.

Be prepared

A final word about all of this. Be prepared.

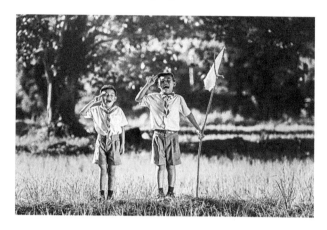

When you are ill you might not want to have to think about any of this. You certainly might not want to mince around making balms, putting teas together and so on. If you know that you are prone to chest infections or have a predisposition for sinusitis, make up as many remedies as you can at the start of the winter season. Chest rubs, balms and so on can all be made in advance. Also, write yourself out a reminder sheet—what to do and where to find it, so you don't have to do too much thinking when you are not feeling your best.

If you are lucky enough to have a lovely minion who will be caring for you, tell them in advance how you would like to be treated and where to find the magic medicines. Show them your care plan, so you can relax and enjoy some good, old-fashioned and much-needed nursing. Either way, plan ahead and make things as easy as possible so you don't have to do anything other than take the medicines and get better.

Red flags

Red flag symptoms are symptoms that may signal a more serious underlying condition and should be looked at more closely or referred to a health care professional/GP. In terms of respiratory tract infections,

seek professional help if the person you are treating exhibits the following symptoms at any time:

- Haemoptysis—blood in the sputum.
- Severe breathlessness. Especially if the person has a history of previ-
  ous hospital admissions for asthma or pulmonary disease.
- Recurrent or poorly resolved chest infections.
- Cough that persists for more than 3 weeks.
- Patients who are immune-compromised. Ie on immunosuppressant
  drugs for any reason. They may need extra support or help.
- Chest pain.
- Development of a rash.
- The elderly. Monitor closely and refer if they do not respond quickly
  to treatment.

Conclusion

Respiratory tract infections are an area where simple home remedies can be remarkably effective and can cut down significantly on
both unnecessary antibiotic use and unnecessary drains on precious
National Health Service resources. The herbal approach differs demon-
strably from that of conventional medicine in that it seeks to support
the body in its endeavours to resolve the problem, rather than to suppress the symptoms so that the person can 'soldier on'. Key to this strategy is allowing the body to rest so that all of its energies can be devoted
to getting better. Using this strategy, chronic issues such as post-nasal
drip, cough etc can be avoided, as can the potential for more serious
complaints such as bronchitis to develop. Be prepared. Rest. Use your
lovely herbs and spices; get going with your care plan. Make herbs into
fabulous medicines whilst the sun shines. Enjoy!

Part 2. Gastro-oesophageal reflux disease

Definition—What is gastro-oesophageal reflux disease (GORD)?
Gastro-oesophageal reflux disease describes a situation where the contents of the stomach reflux backwards into the oesophagus, resulting in
symptoms such as heartburn, bloating and belching, feeling sick. It may
ultimately potentially damage the lining of the oesophagus if it is allowed
to continue unchecked.

NB: In American literature concerning this, you will find that GORD is referred to as GERD, as the oesophagus is spelt with an E (esophagus) in America.

Causes and symptoms: pathophysiology of GORD.

A significant cause of GORD is thought to be hiatus hernia (HH), which is very common, and thought to be present in 30% of people over 50 years of age. The hiatus hernia may or may not result in symptoms for the patient, but the resulting gastrointestinal reflux often does cause an array of unpleasant symptoms, and in some cases may lead to more serious pathologies such as oesophagitis or even oesophageal carcinoma. So what exactly is a hiatus hernia? Let's start with some basic anatomy.

In medicine, the hiatus describes the gap in the diaphragm through which the oesophagus passes to meet the stomach. The muscles of the diaphragm act as a sphincter to prevent stomach contents returning into the oesophagus. This muscular ring, also known as the cardiac sphincter (or oesophageal hiatus) is situated at the hiatus of the diaphragm.

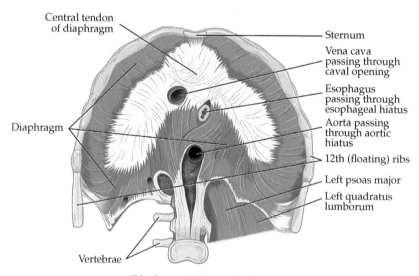

Diaphragm (inferior view)

A hernia is the medical term to describe the movement of an organ beyond its usual anatomical position through an area of muscular weakness in the supporting tissues.

In a hiatus hernia the cardiac sphincter has been stretched to allow the stomach to move upwards beyond its normal anatomical position, so that it is above not below the diaphragm. This will result in stomach contents being able to 'travel backwards' or reflux into the oesophagus.

In conventional medicine this is considered to be the consequence of a sedentary lifestyle common in developed counties. It is often associated with obesity and in particular the deposition of abdominal fat, or many years of straining to void the bowels. Pressure below the diaphragm builds up and puts a strain on the cardiac sphincter. Pregnancy can also put a temporary strain on this sphincter for obvious reasons. Pregnancy hormones compound this problem as they exert a softening and relaxing effect on muscles and ligaments.

Even if a herniation is not evident it is still possible that the function of the sphincter may be weakened resulting in a similar upwards

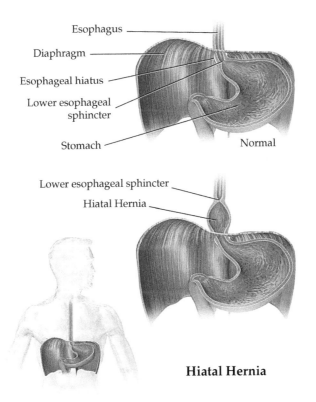

Hiatal Hernia

reflux of stomach contents. Stomach contents are highly acidic, therefore reflux of stomach contents above the level of the cardiac sphincter leads to a cluster of symptoms known collectively as GORD. Most commonly reported is the symptom known as heartburn. This is a sensation, variable in severity, of burning or crushing experienced behind the breastbone (sternum) or below the ribcage (epigastrium). It can feel as if it is rising up, and can also be felt in the throat. Prolonged acidic regurgitation can irritate the lining of the oesophagus causing redness, swelling and pain. This is known as oesophagitis.

Note: These symptoms can be sufficiently severe to mimic a heart attack, and it may only be possible to distinguish between the two by the patient undergoing urgent medical tests in the hospital.

Red flag: All patients who suffer severe, crushing central chest pain should be sent to the hospital emergency department as a matter of urgency.

Other common symptoms include water brash, which is the unpleasant symptom of belching acidic stomach fluid into the mouth. A developing understanding is that even small amounts of regurgitation like this over a prolonged period of time may irritate the vocal cords, or respiratory airways giving rise to symptoms such as cough, hoarseness or even asthma.

Conventional approaches to treatment

Symptoms for GORD can be triggered by bending forwards, or lying down, and therefore conventional advice may include suggestions to raise the head and chest on pillows when trying to sleep. Patients often identify certain food triggers, including obvious suspects such as alcohol, chocolate, coffee and spices. Overeating, smoking and stress are also exacerbating factors. The best approach may well be prevention therefore, and so losing weight, correcting constipation and dietary moderation may all be useful interventions.

Antacid medicines are commonly prescribed to reduce the acidity in the stomach. Currently proton pump inhibitor drugs are very popular (such as omeprazole, lansoprazole etc.). Other drugs such as alginates are considered to be most appropriate for symptoms such as hoarseness, chronic cough, throat clearing and asthma when thought to be caused by GORD.[22]

Drugs to promote the downward movement of peristalsis may also be prescribed to help patients with GORD. Metoclopramide, which promotes peristalsis, acts as a dopamine antagonist and was originally designed as anti-emetic (anti-nausea drugs). Cisapride is another example of a drug to promote peristalsis. It is a serotonin 5-HT3 antagonist (serotonin agonist) and increases gastrointestinal motility. In the most severe cases surgery to tighten the hiatus can be performed using a variety of techniques.

A Western herbal medicine approach to treatment

Herbal medicines have been used in the treatment of reflux for many centuries. Some recent research has focussed on ancient Persian medical texts for example, as a means of sourcing new treatments for this increasingly ubiquitous condition.[23]

Although constipation and straining are seen as potential causative (aetiological) factors in the development of HH and GORD, the phytotherapist sees a more global digestive insufficiency picture as being the focus for treatment. This means that a combination of herbs will be more likely to be used, because multiple points along the digestive tract will be treated at the same time using an array of beneficial plant compounds.

In many European countries (except the UK) it is an area where herbal medicines may still be used as the first choice of treatment. One German pharmaceutical product that is based entirely on herbal medicines for example, is Iberogast (also known in research trials as STW 5) found to be as effective as cisapride, and with an excellent safety profile.[24] It is prepared from nine herbs including bitter candytuft (*Iberis amara* L.), caraway (*Carum carvi* L.), milk thistle (*Silybum marianum* (L.) Gaertn), Lemon balm (*Melissa officinalis* L.) and chamomile (*Matricaria chamomilla* L.). Researchers commented that the broad range of benefit came from a synergy of the herb combination rather than the action of any single herb alone.

You can see how this product contains a mixture of bitters, aromatics and carminatives. Popularly many European cultures still use and

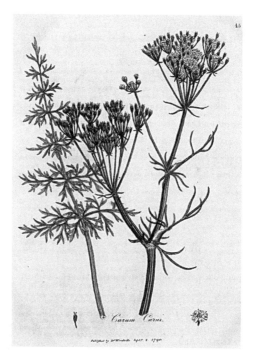

Caraway (*Carum carvi* L.) Common caraway. Medical Botany by Woodville, 1790.

value 'bitters' taken as digestifs, and some of these may be familiar
to you?

Overeating may dampen digestive fire ('understood as the vigour of
digestive function'), but digestive fire may also be dampened through
over-activity of the sympathetic nervous system, or other 'blockages' to the
cascade of normal events in the gut. Thus we can see how working too hard
and/or chronic stress can affect the digestive fire. Western herbalism has
been influenced for many years from all parts of the world, and it is difficult to ignore concepts from other cultures especially the elegant Ayurvedic
concept of GORD being related to liver fire (Pitta disturbance). Thus our
cooling soothing liver herbs will stimulate those parts of the digestive cascade whilst cooling over-activity of the liver and gall bladder. This concept
is echoed in a traditional Chinese formula called Banxia Xiexin Tang (BXT),
used in the treatment of GORD (among other things). A protocol for assessing its efficacy was put forwards in 2018, and the explanation of how the
herbal combination works includes the following statement:

for treating fullness with the accumulation of intermingled cold and heat due to spleen and stomach asthenia. Among the ingredients of BXT, *Radix Scutellariae* Baicalensis and *Rhizoma Copidis* clear heat; *Rhizoma Pinelliae* and *Rhizoma Zingiberis* dispel accumulation and cold; *Radix Ginseng*, *Radix Glycyrrhizae* and *Fructus Jujubae* benefit Qi and cure asthenia. This formula includes both cold and warm drugs and bitter and acrid drugs with descending and expelling effects to invigorate Qi.

—B. Kang et al.[25]

Here you can see how concepts of herbal energetics and how they interact with biological systems are complex, and are echoed the world over.

There is a persistent concept in Western herbal medicine that normal peristalsis can come up against a 'barrier' to the normal one-way direction of flow. This distorts peristalsis and puts pressure on the cardiac sphincter. Rather like the ripples in a pond when they come up against a rock—the ripples bounce back. Bitter and aromatic compounds in herbal medicines, and particularly their complex composition, is thought to broadly stimulate the correct function and with repeated use, break down these 'barriers'.

Just as we saw with the traditional Chinese formulation above, aromatic carminatives are an important adjunct to any bitter remediation. Aromatic carminatives that are popular in Western herbal medicine include:

- Peppermint   (*Mentha x piperita* L.)
- Cinnamon   (*Cinnamonum verum* J. Presyl.)
- Cardamom   (*Elettaria cardamomum* (L.) Maton.)
- Aniseed   (*Pimpinella anisum* L.)
- Fennel   (*Foeniculum vulgare* Mill.)
- Caraway   (*Carum carvi* L.)
- Lavender   (*Lavandula angustifolia* Mill.)
- Rosemary   (*Salvia rosmarinus* L.)
- Coriander   (*Coriandrum sativum* L.)
- Sweet and bitter orange   (*Citrus x aurantium* L.), (C. x aurantium amara L.).

and many more ...

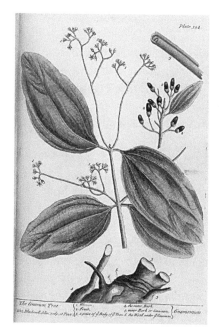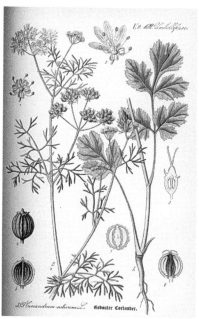

Botanical images of Cinnamon Tree Bark and Coriander herb.

Concurrent herbal anxiolytic use is powerful in its potential to relax the sympathetic nervous system and allow the parasympathetic/enteric nervous system to function unimpeded. Our sympathetic nervous system is engaged when we are active and using our thinking mind and physical body. It can over-ride some activities of the automatic (autonomic) nervous system—the parasympathetic and enteric (digestive) nervous system. Interruptions to normal routine or to the necessary rejuvenation during sleep can be the consequence of over-activity, a lack of rest or interruption to routine and rest.

A functioning cardiac sphincter requires innervation from the parasympathetic nervous system, which can be over-ridden by the all-thinking, all-doing 'active' sympathetic nervous system. This can confuse messages that are directing normal peristalsis, and interrupt this basic function.

Anxiolytics might include:

- Chamomile   (*Matricaria chamomilla* L.)
- Passion flower   (*Passiflora incarnate* L.)
- Skullcap   (*Scutellaria lateriflora/altissima* L.)
- Valerian   (*Valeriana officinalis* L.)

- Lime flower   (*Tilia europaea* L.)
- Lemon balm   (*Melissa officinalis* L.)
- Lavender   (*Lavandula spp* L.)
- Oats   (*Avena sativa* L. (herb))
- St Johns wort   (*Hypericum perforatum* L.)
- Vervein   (*Verbena officinalis* L.)
- Motherwort   (*Leonurus cardiac* L.)

and many more …

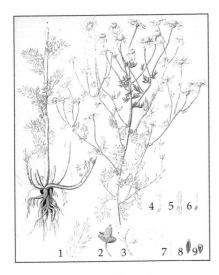 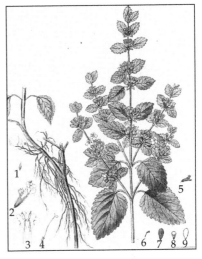

Melissa officinalis   Matricaria chamomilla

It has been suggested by many authors that *insufficient* stomach acid may even act to increase symptoms of GORD because the gastro-intestinal system may go into spasm in response to insufficient gastric acids and enzymes.[26] The herbalist is more interested in restoring function by stimulating corrections to stomach acid, than adding in HCl (hydrochloric acid tablets), or digestive enzymes. Plant bitters and aromatic carminatives can achieve this in most cases.

Correction of the digestive cascade and therefore symptoms of GORD may take the following forms in Western herbalism

A gentle re-weaning approach to diet and eating is a key factor to treatment. See below under self-help strategies for more information on this. Correcting poor sleep, pain and inflammation (particularly if this results in Non-Steroidal Anti-Inflammatory Drugs—NSAID use), or the reasons behind the use of drugs negatively affecting gut function is a key aspect of the herbalists' approach. Improving the quality of sleep will allow cellular regeneration as well as allowing the nervous system of the digestive tissues, and parasympathetics to have unimpeded dominance over the sympathetic nervous system.

Mucilagenous plants can be used to soothe and act as tissue vulneraries and may be included in complex herbal prescriptions. Bitter and aromatic herbs may be used to stimulate digestive and sphincter function. Cooling soothing liver and gall bladder herbs may help reduce symptoms by reducing 'blocks' to peristalsis. Reducing stress and the effects of stress (adreno-corticosteroid hormone production), will help by supporting the enteric nervous system.[27]

Correcting any point of the digestive cascade from mouth to anus, including of course constipation, will also aid peristalsis and the direction of flow within the digestive cascade. Finding alternative symptomatic relief to unpleasant symptoms will often be required, if suppression of vital stomach acidity is to be prevented.

Self-help: the kitchen pharmacy

Firstly, taking greater notice and increased awareness can be valuable in constructing a plan of self-care. Taking time to stop, think, and breathe is an underrated health intervention.

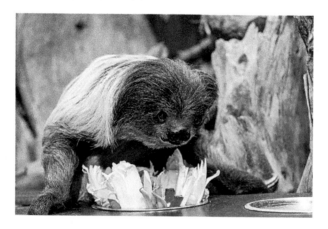

Sloth demonstrating slow eating.

Keeping a diet diary, and an activity diary can be a good start. Being honest with your self about what constitutes healthy eating and writing out a weekly food plan for yourself means you can be realistic. It can also help eliminate unhelpful behaviour. Some things to consider here include concentrating on lightly cooked simple foods eaten in smaller portions. Cooked food is easier to digest and does not require 'warming' by the digestive system. Alternatively grated or lacto-fermented foods will be easier to digest, despite being raw. Chew food thoroughly whilst seated.

Stick as far as possible to regular mealtimes, in a relaxed environment, with adequate time to sit after eating. Avoid late meals, refined carbohydrates, stimulants (alcohol, sugar, caffeine) or other known irritants.

Use of gentle warming spices (cinnamon, fennel, cardamom, cumin, caraway, anise, dill, juniper and turmeric) are recommended especially with cooked vegetables, coconut milk, porridge or yoghurt as appropriate to the individual. Avoiding lots of chilli pepper is usually helpful initially, but later on *Capsicum anuum* L. (Synonym *minimum* Mill.) can be used in small doses to improve digestive vigour. Stimulating gentle warmth in the digestive system will alleviate flatus and prevent 'blockages' further down the digestive tract.

Working out what could be the best healthy snacks and healthy 'fast food' can help you when you are under pressure. Monitoring and improving fluid intake is a good idea, as is not drinking more than just a sip whilst eating or immediately after eating.

Avoiding bread, especially sandwiches and finding non-wheat alternatives helps reduce carbohydrate load. Correct constipation by improving fluid intake, reducing food intake where necessary, and using soluble fibre regularly in the diet. Beans and lentils are a cheap and delicious source of this fibre, as are linseeds (flax), and psyllium husk.

Use a soothing digestive and calming herbal beverage before bed, perhaps a chamomile, marshmallow and mint or chamomile and fennel tea. Change from regular coffee to a dandelion coffee, and regular tea to a non-caffeine variety such as rooibos. If eating out, consider taking an old-fashioned digestive before and/or after your meal. Examples include Angostura bitters in ginger beer, or Campari and soda. Take slippery elm powder as a thick 'drink' dissolved in water before breakfast and before bed as a healing oesophageal agent. Slippery elm can be diluted in plain cold water, warm water, cinnamon, aniseed or mint tea, yoghurt or kefir, or even mashed into half a banana. Cider vinegar diluted in a little warm water (with or without honey) can give relief to many people whose digestion is insufficient. Although counter-intuitive the acids in cider vinegar can help close the cardiac sphincter for some people.

A case history

Elaine (45 years old) began to experience acute stomach acid reflux symptoms that started after she had begun a fitness programme at her local gym 12 months ago. The digestive discomfort was most obvious after meals and as she lay down to try to sleep. It had begun to make her regret trying to take more exercise and get fit. She had been prescribed some drugs by her doctor to reduce the stomach acid, but she was wary of taking them. Elaine often experienced adverse results from taking conventional pharmaceuticals and had learned over time to avoid them. She had been to see a nutritionist who had given her lots of dietary advice, and who had also suggested she see a medical herbalist.

On further questioning, it became clear that Elaine had a long history of severe and chronic constipation, opening her bowels only once per week, and only after taking a laxative she bought from a health food shop. She also had an erratic menstrual cycle, with approximately four menstrual bleeds per year. She nevertheless had adapted to these things, including her periods, that she described as featuring 'terrible' pre-menstrual syndrome (PMS) that often led her to moods and behaviours that threatened to damage her relationships. The physical and the emotional symptoms point to liver congestion or stagnation from a traditional herbal perspective, and resulted in all of the different types of 'blockage' this lady was experiencing.

The dietitian had helped Elaine begin to change her bread-based diet to one rich in other grains such as quinoa, buckwheat and whole grain rice. More beans and lentils, nuts and seeds and green leafy vegetables had also been added to her everyday regimen. She was also trying to switch from drinking multiple coffees to having more water, and herb teas. Accordingly she had noticed her bowel movements were easier and softer although she was still only managing one bowel movement per week, after a laxative.

At the herbal consultation Elaine appeared 'wound up' and admitted to feeling very irritable. She wasn't sleeping well and she had daily acid reflux and heartburn. A plan of herbal therapy to complement the dietary advice was discussed, and she began a herbal prescription in an easy to take liquid tincture format. A combination of marshmallow root (*Althaea officinalis* L.) and chamomile flowers (*Matricaria chamomilla* L.) was used to reduce inflammation and to relax and soothe her digestive system. Lavender flower tincture (*Lavandula angustifolia* Mill.) and valerian root (*Valeriana officinalis* L.) were added to reduce irritability of the liver, gut and nervous system, and burdock root (*Arctium lappa* L.) and dandelion root (*Taraxacum officinale* aggr F. H. Wigg) were included to primarily help ease constipation, whilst energetically cooling the 'Liver'.[28] This prescription contains herbs with bitter properties, aromatic carminatives and is energetically cooling and de-obstruent (unblocking). She was already using peppermint and fennel teas as part of her new dietary regimen.

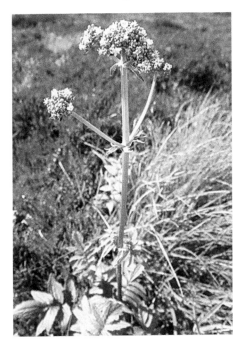

Valerian (*Valeriana officinalis* L.)

After 12 weeks, Elaine reported that she was feeling much better and rarely experienced reflux symptoms. She was now opening her bowels most days, and the stool had become a normal size and was easy to pass. There had been a corresponding improvement to sleep as a result, and this had increased her wellbeing and general happiness. Interestingly,

Elaine had begun to have monthly menstrual cycles, the PMS was much less severe, and only lasted a few hours rather than a few weeks. Elaine returned 4 years later for help with peri-menopausal symptoms. She was still free from gastric reflux symptoms.

Red flags

As mentioned near the beginning of this section, the symptoms of reflux can sometimes mimic those of angina. It is worth repeating here that;

All patients who suffer severe, crushing central chest pain should be sent to the hospital emergency department as a matter of urgency.

Where milder and more chronic symptoms of GORD remain intransigent to treatment, mild angina should be a differential diagnosis. Always seek professional help in these cases.

Conclusion

GORD is an increasingly common complaint, experienced by many people, and can be seen, at least in part, as an almost inevitable corollary to modern-day living. It is also an excellent example of a condition which may be significantly ameliorated or even completely resolved by the patient themselves taking matters into their own hands (helped by gentle and supportive herbs).

Underlying issues such as constipation, imbalanced gut microbiota, poor dietary habits and chronic stress can all be helped by the patient themselves to varying degrees (and the sooner the better). All interactions between patient and herbalist involve working together to resolve issues. We cannot wave magic wands; the patient must do their bit! When this happens, and sufficient time is allowed for new habits to form, the magic can (and does) happen.

References

1. Amanat F. and F. Krammer, *SARS-CoV-2 Vaccines: Status Report*. Immunity. 2020 Apr 14. 52(4): pp. 583–589. doi: 10.1016/j.immuni.2020.03.007. Epub 2020 Apr 6. PMID: 32259480; PMCID: PMC7136867.

2. Shah, S. A. et al., *Evaluation of echinacea for the prevention and treatment of the common cold: a meta-analysis*. Lancet Infect Dis, 2007. 7(7): pp. 473–480.

3. Ross, S. M., *Echinacea purpurea: a proprietary extract of echinacea purpurea is shown to be safe and effective in the prevention of the common cold*. Holist Nurs Pract, 2016. 30(1): pp. 54–57.

4. Karsch-Völk, M. et al., *Echinacea for preventing and treating the common cold*. Cochrane Database Syst Rev, 2014(2): p. CD000530.

5. Schapowal, A., P. Klein and S. L. Johnston, *Echinacea reduces the risk of recurrent respiratory tract infections and complications: a meta-analysis of randomized controlled trials*. Adv Ther, 2015. 32(3): pp. 187–200.

6. Birt, D. F. et al., *Hypericum in infection: Identification of anti-viral and anti-inflammatory constituents*. Pharm Biol, 2009. 47(8): pp. 774–782.

7. Bove, M., *An Encyclopedia of Natural Healing for Children and Infants*. 2nd ed. 2001: McGraw Hill.

8. Koch, C., et al., *Efficacy of anise oil, dwarf-pine oil and chamomile oil against thymidine-kinase-positive and thymidine-kinase-negative herpesviruses*. J Pharm Pharmacol, 2008. 60(11): pp. 1545–1550.

9. Jarić, S. et al., *An ethnobotanical study on the usage of wild medicinal herbs from Kopaonik Mountain (Central Serbia)*. J Ethnopharmacol, 2007. 111(1): pp. 160–175.

10. Roxas, M. and J. Jurenka, *Colds and influenza: a review of diagnosis and conventional, botanical, and nutritional considerations*. Altern Med Rev, 2007. 12(1): pp. 25–48.

11. Chen, C. et al., *Sambucus nigra extracts inhibit infectious bronchitis virus at an early point during replication*. BMC Vet Res, 2014. 10: p. 24.

12. Roschek, B. et al., *Elderberry flavonoids bind to and prevent H1N1 infection in vitro*. Phytochemistry, 2009. 70(10): pp. 1255–1261.

13. Bradley, D. *Star role for bacteria in controlling flu pandemic?* Nature Reviews Drug Discovery, 2005. 4.

14. Miraj, S. and S. Alesaeidi, *A systematic review study of therapeutic effects of Matricaria recuitta chamomile (chamomile)*. Electron Physician, 2016. 8(9): pp. 3024–3031.

15. Hickl, J. et al., *Mediterranean herb extracts inhibit microbial growth of representative oral microorganisms and biofilm formation of Streptococcus mutans*. PLoS One, 2018. 13(12): p. e0207574.

16. Cai, T. et al., *Hibiscus extract, vegetable proteases and Commiphora myrrha are useful to prevent symptomatic UTI episode in patients affected by recurrent uncomplicated urinary tract infections*. Arch Ital Urol Androl, 2018. 90(3): pp. 203–207.

17. Cech, N. B. et al., *Quorum quenching and antimicrobial activity of goldenseal (Hydrastis canadensis) against methicillin-resistant Staphylococcus aureus (MRSA).* Planta Med, 2012. 78(14): pp. 1556–1561.

18. Ettefagh, K. A. et al., *Goldenseal (Hydrastis canadensis L.) extracts synergistically enhance the antibacterial activity of berberine via efflux pump inhibition.* Planta Med, 2011. 77(8): pp. 835–840.

19. Zhang, J. et al., *Biological activities of triterpenoids and phenolic compounds from myrica cerifera bark.* Chem Biodivers, 2016. 13(11): p. 1601–1609.

20. Zhabokritsky, A., S. Mansouri and K. A. Hudak, *Pokeweed antiviral protein alters splicing of HIV-1 RNAs, resulting in reduced virus production.* RNA, 2014. 20(8): pp. 1238–1247.

21. Folquitto, D. G. et al., *Biological activity, phytochemistry and traditional uses of genus Lobelia (Campanulaceae): A systematic review.* Fitoterapia, 2019.

22. Lee, K. Y. and D. J. Mooney, *Alginate: properties and biomedical applications.* Prog Polym Sci, 2012. 37(1): pp. 106–126.

23. Hosseinkhani, A. et al., *An evidence-based review of medicinal herbs for the treatment of gastroesophageal reflux disease (GERD).* Curr Drug Discov Technol, 2018. 15(4): pp. 305–314.

24. Melzer, J. et al., *Meta-analysis: phytotherapy of functional dyspepsia with the herbal drug preparation STW 5 (Iberogast).* Aliment Pharmacol Ther, 2004. 20(11–12): pp. 1279–1287.

25. Kang, B. et al., *Banxia Xiexin tang for gastro-oesophageal reflux disease: A protocol for a systematic review of controlled trials.* Medicine (Baltimore), 2018. 97(17): p. e0393.

26. Wright, M., *Why Stomach Acid is Good For You: Natural Relief From Heartburn, Indigestion, Reflux and GERD.* 2001: M Evans & Co.

27. Gershon, M., *Your Gut Has A Mind Of It's Own: The Second Brain.* 1999: Harper Collins.

28. Predes, F. S. et al., *Antioxidative and in vitro antiproliferative activity of Arctium lappa root extracts.* BMC Complement Altern Med, 2011. 11: p. 25.

CHAPTER TEN

Swimming upstream: common conditions and therapeutic considerations

Introduction

Our third chapter on treating specific conditions brings us up close and personal with our musculoskeletal system, the system that anchors and supports us. Bones are special. Throughout history people from all cultures have worshipped their ancestors via the preservation of their bones. In shamanic practices from around the world, the soul was thought to reside in bones. Resurrection from bones was also thought possible.[1]

When things go wrong at the level of bones, people often face chronic pain and discomfort. We will be considering a number of self-help strategies for short-term treatment plus, of course, the long game, of reducing and possibly reversing the progress of chronic conditions.

Part two of this chapter allows us to explore the process of sleep, so vital for the underpinning of our health generally. Healthy sleep is one of the fundamental pillars of health. Allowing this to happen is therefore key to the treatment of many illnesses. Getting down to the bare bones, let us start with our magnificent musculoskeletal system.

Part 1. Osteo-arthritis

Definition—What is arthritis? What is osteo-arthritis? Arthritis literally means inflammation of the bony surfaces of the body and can take several forms, the commonest being osteo-arthritis (OA). Other diseases of the joints include rheumatoid arthritis (RA) and other forms of auto-immune arthritis such as ankylosing spondylitis and psoriatic arthritis; non-auto-immune arthritis such as gout or infective arthritis (often acute/viral). Osteo-arthritis is a progressive degenerative disorder of the synovial joints. It is the commonest disorder of the joints, affecting women three times more than men.

Causes and symptoms: pathophysiology of osteo-arthritis

Inflammation in or around a joint can be caused either by an injury or strain, or as the result of internal processes. Because OA is a commonly found symptom in people as they age, it is almost seen as 'inevitable' and a normal process of 'wear and tear' on the joints. Many people over the age of 60 will have features of OA on X-ray images, with or without symptoms of OA. This 'acceptance of the inevitable' is one aspect of the conventional medical view of OA that medical herbalists would question.

There seems to be a familial link in certain particularly disabling forms of OA. The development of OA in later life is linked to earlier joint trauma or repetitive stress to the particular joint(s). Statistically women develop OA 2–3 times more frequently than men if they engage in significant amounts of weight-bearing aerobic exercise. Poor alignment of joints may also result in the development of OA. Obesity is thought to increase the likelihood of OA, due to weight-bearing.

Rheumatoid or osteo??

In most textbooks on orthodox medicine you will see a clear differentiation between rheumatoid arthritis and osteo-arthritis in terms of diagnosis. Commonly cited points of comparison include the fact that osteo-arthritis usually affects only one side of the body, whereas RA is bilateral, and that RA is primarily an inflammatory condition, whereas OA does not involve inflammation to anywhere near the same degree. *But facts change.*

More recent research has revealed that symmetrically painful joints are as prevalent in OA as they are in RA.[2] Furthermore, the role of inflammation in both the onset and development of OA is significant.[3] The joints most commonly affected in OA are: hips, knees, ankles and small joints of the fingers, thumbs and hands.

The mechanism of degeneration is poorly understood, but is focussed at the surfaces of the hyaline cartilage, lining the ends of the bones within the synovial joint. In some cases the bone itself degenerates and can become deformed in shape. As the cartilage thins, small spiky bony protrusions can form, called osteophytes (literally meaning bony leaves).

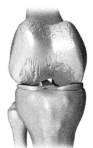

Symptoms

- Ache or stiffness in fingers and/or other joints.
- The ache is worse after rest/sleep, and eases with movement.
- Heat usually helps.
- Puffiness or swelling especially around larger joints can occur.
- An early characteristic sign of OA, especially in women, is the formation of painless deformities at the (distal) joints of the fingertips (Heberden's nodes).

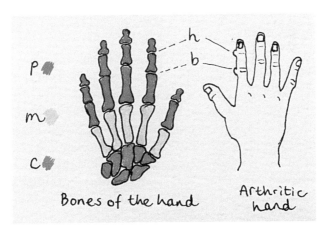

Bones of the hand   Arthritic hand

Bones of the hand can be divided in to: p) Phalanges, m) metacarpels and c) carpels. Heberden's nodes (h) tend to form at the distal (farthest) phalangeal joints, while Bouchard's nodes (b) at the proximal (nearest) phalangeal joints.

- Heberden's nodes can eventually become painful.
- Achy joints, especially the thumb or balls of the feet can occur transiently at peri-menopause. Appropriate treatment will prevent this from becoming OA.
- Deep hip (into the buttock), or knee pain can occur.
- OA can affect the vertebral joints causing pain in the spine.
- Long-term pain can cause weakness and eventual muscle wasting.
- Joint deformity can occur over time.

Conventional approaches to treatment

Many conventional practitioners are happy for their patients with OA to seek treatment with non-conventional practitioners such as medical herbalists, osteopaths and acupuncturists.

The mainstay of conventional treatment often involves pain relief with paracetamol. This is a peculiarity of our medical system because paracetamol has repeatedly failed to produce any significant results in the management or treatment of OA in randomised placebo-controlled trials, and yet it is funded by the NHS in the UK. One clinical review paper assessed 38 clinical trials and found

> There is little evidence to support the efficacy of acetaminophen [paracetamol] treatment in patients with chronic pain conditions.
> —E. A. Grice and J. A. Segre[4]

Conversely, a number of studies have reported significant benefits from well-known herbal medicines. One double-blind study on willow bark extract (*Salix spp.*) demonstrated reduced pain scores for patients with musculoskeletal issues and low back pain.[5-7] Patients taking the willow bark reported improvements even within 1 week of starting the trial. Chrubasik et al. specifically state that salicylate compounds and metabolites found in willow cannot be wholly responsible for the pain relief experienced by patients, and suggest that other compounds present may contribute to the overall analgesic effect. They also mention the significant reduction in side effects experienced by patients, in comparison to those using conventional Non-Steroidal Anti-Inflammatory Drugs (NSAID's).[7] This study demonstrates the benefits of using whole plant medicines for their synergy and low levels of adverse effects.

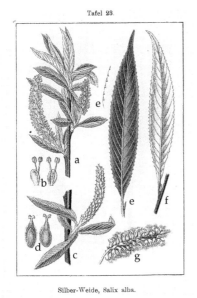

Tafel 28.

Silber-Weide, Salix alba.

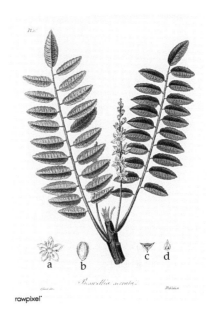

rawpixel

Boswellia serrata.

Willow (*Salix alba* L.) and Frankincense (*Boswellia serrata* Robx.) Trees.

A Cochrane update review demonstrated the efficacy of frankincense (*Boswellia serrata* Robx.) extract in more than one high-quality trial.[8] Further analysis of original gold-standard research also showed patient outcomes continued to be improved/maintained 1 month after herbal treatment had ceased in contrast to the conventional anti-inflammatory used as the control group, where pain scores increased immediately on cessation of NSAID's.[9]

Conventional medicine would now consider relaxation, stretching exercises, and a diet high in antioxidants to all be of help in preventing OA.

Western herbal medicine's approach to treatment

Medical herbalists accept the observation that inflammatory processes found in the joint capsule causing degeneration of the cartilage and eventually bone can be attributed to osteo-arthritis. However, what concerns us is why this is happening. There is a basic requirement for the provision of oxygen and nutrients into the enclosed synovial joint. There is also fundamentally the requirement for waste products of the fluid-filled synovial capsule to exit out of their enclosed position, and be removed from the body.

The cells and tissues of the joint itself are repairing and remodelling themselves all the time, and can potentially develop a faulty 'default' position as a result of any impairment to the processes of generation and breakdown of normal bone and surrounding tissues. A persistent theme within traditional herbal medicine is that OA can be caused by inadequate blood nourishment/supply to the joint capsule resulting in lack of delivered nutrition or resulting in a reduction of effective waste product removal.

Finally, in traditional herbal medicine systems, there is a belief in a strong interrelationship between the kidney and the musculoskeletal system that leads to the selection of certain urinary system herbs as part of a treatment strategy and not just the use of direct herbal anti-inflammatories. Ultimately, there is thought to be a lack of flow at one or many points along the route of elimination to which treatment is directed.

Therefore, any of the following could be possible causes of OA:

- The person's diet could be too high in 'irritant' foodstuffs, creating a problem within the absorbed contents of the blood, or putting an undue burden on the organs of elimination.
- There may be insufficient 'healthy' fluids or excessive amounts of acidic or 'irritant' fluids consumed.
- Circulation to the joint may be impeded directly.
- Injury is not dealt with sufficiently well at the time.
- Poor bowel function could be blocking waste elimination, allowing it to 'build up in the blood' and irritate the fluids in the synovial capsule.
- Poor performance of the liver and/or kidneys could be slowing down the elimination of waste metabolites.
- Extra metabolic waste products are produced through excessive exercise or strain.
- Persistent low vitality (such as persistent infection, chronic insomnia, problematic conventional medication) could be interrupting normal good function at the site of the joints.
- Lowered vitality through exhaustion, depletion or hormone imbalance e.g. menopausal change, results in lowered access to healthy nutrients required for normal cartilaginous repair.

The herbalist seeks to identify possible causes and address these through diet, exercise, internal and external therapies.

Treatment with a medical herbalist therefore could involve one or many of the following protocols (herbs listed are selected as examples):

- Use of herbs with an affinity for the joint (internally or externally) and its nourishment such as, nettle (*Urtica dioica* L.), comfrey (*Symphytum officinale* L.), liquorice (*Glycyrrhiza glabra* L.), and devil's claw root (*Harpagophytum procumbens* (Burch) DC. Ex Meisn) for example.
- Reducing inflammation directly with herbal medicines such as willow bark (*Salix spp.*), turmeric root (*Curcuma longa* L.), frankincense resin (*Boswellia serrata* Robx.), liquorice (*Glycyrrhiza glabra* L.) and meadowsweet (*Filipendula ulmaria* (L.) Maxim.).
- Improving elimination via the kidney perhaps with celery seed (*Apium graveolens* L.), nettle (*Urtica dioica* L.), birch leaf (*Betula pendula* Roth.) or juniper (*Juniperus communis* L.).
- Improving elimination via the liver with nettle (*Urtica dioica* L.), dandelion root/leaf (*Taraxacum officinale* (aggr. F. H. Wigg)), black cohosh (*Actaea racemosa* L. (Synonym Cimicifuga racemosa)), bogbean (Menyanthes trifoliata L.) or burdock (*Arctium lappa* L.).
- Balancing hormones/increasing vitality where appropriate—black cohosh (*Actaea racemosa* L.), liquorice (*Glycyrrhiza glabra* L.), wild yam (*Dioscorea villosa* L.) or devils claw (*Harpagophytum procumbens* (Burch) DC. Ex Meis).
- Improve circulation generally with perhaps chilli pepper (*Capsicum anuum* L.), ginger root (*Zingiber officinale* Roscoe), horse chestnut (*Aesculus hippocastanum* L.) and yarrow (*Achillea millefolium* L.).

Research in 2016 on the Unani Tibb approach to treating osteo-arthritis, found that the use of herbs such as celery seed (*Apium graveolens* L. semen) and European wild ginger (*Asarum europaeum* L.) resulted in a mean percentage in the reduction of pain of 71%. German chamomile (*Matricaria chamomilla* L.) was also used as an external application. It was explained in Unani Tibb terms that:

> *Piper longum and Matricaria chamomilla have anti-inflammatory property. Matricaria chamomilla also has analgesic property. Asarum europeaum, Apium graveolens and Matricaria chamomilla, have diuretic*

property, and hence these drugs eliminate the morbid humours from the body. Asarum europeaum and Matricaria chamomilla have muqawwie asab (nervine tonic) property, and therefore strengthen nerves, increases the muscle tone and power of the muscles, thus preventing peri-articular muscle wasting and make the joints stable.

—A. Tarannum, A. Sultana and K. Ur Rahman[10]

We can see a direct comparison here to the way Western medical herbalists would treat osteo-arthritis. The historical influence of systems of medicine such as Unani Tibb on Western herbal medicine is thus very easy to discern.

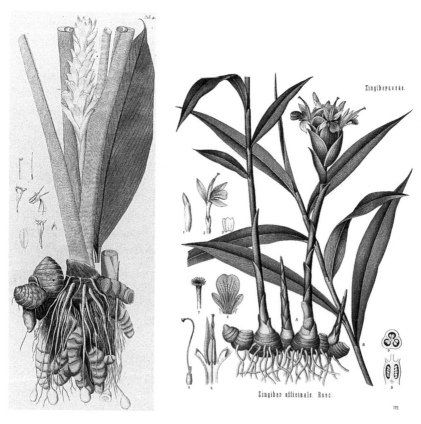

Turmeric (*Curcuma longa* L.)   Ginger (*Zingiber officinale* Roscoe.)

Speaking of chamomile, poultices of healing, anti-inflammatory and circulatory stimulating herbs may be applied externally and can significantly impact on outcomes. Ointments, oils and balms could also be considered.

The herbal approach will usually involve analysis of food and fluid intake with emphasis on:

- Usefulness and practicality of the advice to the patient!
- Avoidance of potentially inflammatory foods—in particular: sugar, refined carbohydrates, wheat or even gluten. There is often a strong correlation between gluten and rheumatoid arthritis (not necessarily OA).
- Avoidance of inflammatory products found in drinks such as fizzy pop, concentrated orange juice, alcohol (quantity and also type may be important), lots of caffeinated, or highly sweetened drinks.
- Increasing helpful fluids such as water, herb tea, dandelion or other root 'coffees' and rooty drinks, probiotic drinks such as kombucha or kefir, or ginger/turmeric ferments.
- Identifying and addressing other potential sources of the inflammatory process such as: 'stress', poor sleep, recurrent infection, recurrent antibiotics, recurrent use of conventional drugs, congestion of tissues locally or globally, constipation, hormone imbalance and so on.

Self-help: the kitchen pharmacy

What can the patient do for themselves? Here are a few suggestions.

- Review and adapt fluid intake. Find alternatives to fizzy drinks/ alcoholic drinks. Drink lots of nettle tea!
- Consider your microbiome! Try making your own lactoferments (lacto refers to lactobacillus not dairy products). See below for a ginger-based fermentation recipe you might like to try.
- Reduce meat in your diet; use more beans, lentils, nuts and seeds.
- Reduce excess cheese, orange juice and refined flour/sugar such as biscuits, pastry, cake and bread.

- Take 10 ml (2 teaspoons) of organic cider vinegar per day. Mix with a little honey and warm water (add a little molasses if you are depleted in nutrients and/or constipated).
- Make your own poultice or balm to apply daily.
- Improve circulation and convalescence to the local area. Take time to gently stretch and massage the affected area. See below for instructions on how to make an anti-inflammatory poultice.
- Don't over-exercise or strain the joint and/or surrounding muscles. Consider stopping repetitive and problematic movement.

Ginger fizz ferment

Ingredients
- I Tablespoon grated organic unpeeled ginger root (healthy wild yeasts). You can add turmeric root to make an excellent combination ...
- I teaspoon raw sugar (stir to dissolve)
- 3 tablespoons filtered water (no chlorine)
  Add ingredients to a clean jar.
  Stir and cover with a clean cloth and rubber band to breathe.
  Leave for 24 hours, at room temperature.
  Repeat daily adding in more ginger, water and sugar and stirring gently.
  Within 3–12 days, it should be bubbling (fermenting).

Once it is fermenting, strain off some of the ginger fizzy liquid, you can add apple juice, fresh fruit pulp or water to it to make a fresh wild fermented drink (filter out the bits of ginger/turmeric). You might drink 30–50 ml per day.

Poultices

The use of poultices should not be underestimated in terms of their healing potential. Poultices work on skin itself or structures and tissues close to the surface. They act to soften surrounding tissues, optimising the transfer of volatile substances across the skin, and increase blood flow. Poultices can exert an osmotic effect, pulling fluid out of cells and into lymphatic tissue. They may help to draw out a pocket of infection. They may be anti-inflammatory, antispasmodic or anti-infective, depending on ingredients. They also provide a simple but highly effective form of self-help for people struggling with conditions such as osteo-arthritis. Coupled with all this they are very cost-effective—an important issue for some patients. Below we have listed a few suggestions for helpful poultice recipes.

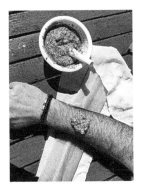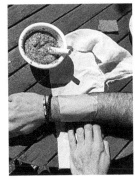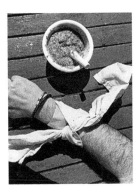

Poultice being applied.

Anti-inflammatory and circulatory stimulating ginger poultice

Ingredients
- A wipe-clean floor or towel protection for your carpet!
- Bandages or large tea towels that can tie around the joint.
- Cling film or greaseproof paper and tape to secure it.
- A food processor or large mortar and pestle and strong arms!
- A fine food grater.
- A large chunk of fresh root ginger.
- Some fresh comfrey leaves (if you do not have these to hand, either omit them and just root ginger or, if you know of a comfrey plant local to you that you can harvest and use safely, please do experiment).

Method
Grate the root ginger finely.
Put the comfrey leaves into a food blender and blend to a pulp.
Add the root ginger and mix well.

Scoop out the pulp and press the pulp all over the affected joint and wrap in cling film, or in greaseproof paper.
Tie in place with a bandage or a clean (but old) tea towel.
Rest with the joint slightly elevated for 20 minutes or even overnight.
Unwrap and remove spent herb material.
Wash skin clean, and pat dry.

A variation of this would involve using ginger powder, which may be mixed with warm water to form a paste, then applied to the joint and held in place with a bandage etc. Some people may experience a burning sensation when the paste is first applied, but this soon passes. This is a slightly easier version of the fresh ginger poultice above and may suit some patients who are less prepared, for various reasons, to take the time required to grate and blend.

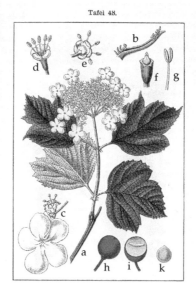

Tafel 48.

Wilder Schneeball, Viburnum opulus.

Cramp Bark (*Viburnum opulus* L.)

Something we have used in acute situations with great success is a hot poultice of the bark of the small tree *Viburnum opulus* L. sometimes known as cramp bark tree.

Cramp bark is ideal for 'spasm' or sudden back pain whilst making an assessment or diagnosis, or after diagnosis, to give relief, allow healing sleep, and to reduce swelling and inflammation and allow healing.

The bark can be harvested from the small branches of the tree by pruning, then scraping off the surface bark into a container.

Antispasmodic cramp bark poultice

- Add bark to cold water and heat on stove fro around 20 minutes
- Add an additional handful of fresh or dried rosemary leaves (if available) in final three minutes of cooking. This is beneficial and also smells gorgeous.
- Strain and compost spent herb material.
- Keep decocted liquid warm and use it to soak toweling or large cotton pads.
- Apply directly to skin over area of spasm or pain.
- Cover with waterproof layer, then apply warm towel or blanket, and finally hot water bottle (if bearable to patient).
- Replace hot poultice liquid as often as feels appropriate, and repeat process for 1–2 hours.
- Repeat for next few days if possible.

Healing/tissue repairing comfrey leaf poultice

Ideal for a joint or muscle injury, especially where internal bruising or minor damage to ligaments or tendons may have occurred. Gather comfrey leaves, fresh or dried. Chop sufficiently to fit into a small saucepan. Use sufficient material to be covered by 500 ml cold water. If available, add 5 cm grated root ginger, or three stems (5 centimetres long) of rosemary, or lavender or sage. Bring the water to a gentle boil, and simmer softly for 5–10 minutes. Strain off the spent herb material through a sieve and compost later when cool. Use the hot liquid now to apply directly to the joint using some towelling, flannel or cotton. Wrap well and keep warm. Repeat as often as desired. Repeat again the following day. Continue as long as necessary.

A non-herbal but nevertheless useful strategy

Epsom salts bath

Use 1–2 mugs of Epsom (magnesium) salts in a full bath of warm water. Immerse yourself, and soak without using other soaps etc for 20 minutes. Get out of the bath, and pat yourself dry without washing off the magnesium-rich bathwater. Climb into warm sleepwear and go to bed as warm as is comfortable. It is possible that the magnesium salts will cause sweating. This is normal and desirable. In the morning shower off, change your sleepwear and, if necessary, your bedding too. Repeat the bath weekly if desired. If getting into a bath is difficult, or only a distal joint is affected, an Epsom salt hand/foot bath can use used; just scale down to using a bowl of warm/hot water and a teacup of magnesium salts. Repeat more frequently, perhaps daily in an acute scenario.

Comfrey infused oil

See Chapter 4, for how to make an infused oil. Dried comfrey leaves work best, as when fresh they have a high water content which can spoil the oil. You might like to add a circulatory stimulating herb at the same time as the comfrey leaf, such as black peppercorns, cloves, or chilli peppers; then strain the oil after cooking slowly for many hours. Rub into the affected area regularly.

Red flags

In some circumstances patients with disorders of their joints will benefit from referral to a conventional doctor for investigation, and/or treatment. Red flags are those symptoms or signs that indicate a referral is to be considered. The following table lists and describes the red flags for disorders of the joints/ligaments and gives some reasoning and expectation of urgency.

1) Intense unexplained persistent shoulder pain lasting for more than 14 days and unrelated to shoulder movement. Although frozen shoulder is the most common cause, excluding a more serious infiltrating

cause from elsewhere is important and would require assessment and imaging.

2) The following common injuries may require imaging and assessment in order to confirm damage and best intervention. Rest/Ice/Compression/Elevation (RICE) should be considered if there is significant inflammation (redness and swelling). Rest is defined as a recognised first-aid measure and may involve complete immobilisation (splints/bandages/slings).

   Traumatic injury to a muscle or a joint with:

   - Sudden onset of pain/swelling in the joint (possible haemarthrosis).
   - Sudden severe pain and swelling around a joint with reluctance to move (possible sprain or fracture).
   - Sudden onset of tender swelling in a muscle (possible haematoma).
   - Locking of the knee joint (Possible tear of meniscal cartilage).

3) Sudden onset low back pain, so severe that walking is impossible; severe sciatica, difficulty urinating or defecating. Seek attention to confirm if vertebrae are intact.

4) Numbness of the buttocks and perineum (saddle anaesthesia). Bilateral numbness or sciatica in the legs, Difficulty in urination/defecation, are all serious symptoms suggesting cauda equina syndrome. Seek medical attention.

5) A single hot, swollen, very tender joint not usually associated with a prior injury. The patient feels generally unwell. Check with patient as may have been caused by a penetrating injury of the joint by a foreign object. Refer to exclude infection.

Conclusion

Osteo-arthritis is a commonly encountered condition, which people often mistakenly consider to be unamenable to improvement and must just be managed. This is often not the case. With sustained use of herbal remedies both internally and externally significant benefits can be achieved. This is not a condition that people should 'just live with'. Much of what can be achieved lies in the hands of the patient. The judicious use of healing poultices provides a great opportunity for fundamental healing to take place and also allows people to interact directly with the plants themselves, forming a healing alliance that will endure.

Part 2. Sleep and insomnia

He was scarcely conscious of her now, for this utterly soft end of a hard day was as soporific as the fabled nepenthe and he could feel himself slipping away, as though his fingertips were relaxing from the edge of the cliff of harsh reality in order that he might drop—drop—through the soft clouds of gathering sleep into the slowly swaying ocean of dreams.

—Isaac Asimov, *The Robots of Dawn*

Nepenthe is an 'anti-sorrow' drug or potion that helps people forget their woes and brings peace, and the ability to forget bad memories. It is often associated with the concept of drifting off to sleep; allowing your worries and cares to slip away into a sea of forgetfulness.

What is sleep?

It is pretty universally accepted that all animals need sleep. How this is managed however, varies depending upon the animal in question and the environmental adaptations that they need to survive. We are animals, and we also need to sleep …

Dolphins and whales can put half of their brains to sleep at a time, so that they can continue swimming whilst sleeping. This is called uni-hemispheric sleep. Birds can also do this, and use it as a survival tactic.

For example, ducks at the perimeter of a flock can detect predators more quickly using this strategy. Birds that spend long periods in the air such as alpine swifts and albatrosses as well as birds on migration employ uni-hemispheric sleep whilst gliding or soaring. Similar brain patterns have been observed in people who experience parasomnias such as sleepwalking. Sleepwalking and other 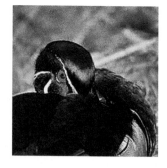 parasomnias like sleep talking, or sleep eating are more common in children, but they do not go away in adulthood for some rare individuals.

Animals like bees regulate sleep by sleeping more deeply rather than sleeping for longer so that they can maximise flying time seasonally. Human neuroscience is slowly discovering what sleep entails, including the functional movement of our memories into longer-term storage centres in the brain, and a physiological cleaning of daily 'toxins'; both of these functions can prevent neurodegenerative diseases. Our thoughts and emotions as well as the physiological functions of our brains use lots of energy, and these areas of the brain require housekeeping and management to keep nerve cells healthy. Chronic sleep deprivation prevents this housekeeping, and is now known to lead to worse health outcomes and shorter life expectancy.

> *From a behavioural stand-point, sleep is a reversible behavioural state of perceptual disengagement from, and unresponsiveness to, the environment.*
> —Dr Simon Kyle, Senior Research Fellow

What happens when we go to sleep?

When we sleep we tend to sleep in sleep cycles comprising of two distinct phases: Rapid Eye Movement (REM) sleep and Non-Rapid Eye Movement (NREM) sleep. NREM sleep is then further divided into four stages, creatively named stages 1 to 4.

The brain has a definite sleep cycle of approximately 90 minutes. These cycles are normally entered through NREM sleep. Those of us lucky enough to call ourselves good sleepers generally experience 4–5 sleep cycles a night.

NREM sleep

We begin the cycle by going into NREM sleep. The four stages of NREM sleep are characterised by changes in brain activity (measured using Electroencephalography [EEG]) and generally reflect the process of going deeper and deeper into sleep as one progresses from stage 1 to stage 4. Stages 3 and 4, known as the slowest wave stages, would be characterised on an electroencephalogram by low frequency, synchronised waves.

People are hardest to wake from slow-wave sleep, indicating greater intensity and depth of sleep. In NREM sleep thought processes are generally absent, or if present, logical rather than bizarre.

REM sleep

REM sleep is named after the rapid, phasic eye movements detected under the eyelids at this time. It is the stage of sleep most often associated with dreaming, and it can result in vivid, colourful and illogical dreams. This may result, in part, from the fact that some specific areas of the brain are as metabolically active during REM sleep as they are whilst we are awake. It is also associated with muscle paralysis, which prevents the sleeper from acting out the dreams that they are experiencing. When this mechanism fails, it is termed REM sleep behaviour disorder (RBD). Typically a normal dream lasts 10–12 seconds. Dream deficit and lack of REM sleep has been linked to serious emotional disorders and psychosis.

> *No live organism can continue for long to exist sanely under conditions of absolute reality; even larks and katydids are supposed, by some, to dream.*
>
> —Shirley Jackson, *The Haunting of Hill House*

It looks like we need to dream.

Sleep cycle composition changes throughout the night. The first third of the night tends to consist of greater amounts of slow-wave or deep sleep (stages 3 and 4). REM sleep is more frequent in the last third of the night, and is linked to a reduction in core body temperature.

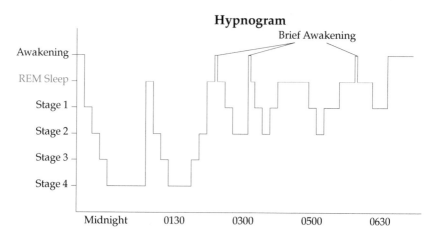

On average, the following figures represent the time spent in the various stages of sleep:

- Wakefulness (5%)
- Stage 1 (2–5%)
- Stage 2 (45–55%)
- Stage 3 (3–8%) [SWS]
- Stage 4 (10–15%) [SWS]
- REM sleep (20–25%)

(**NB.** SWS stands for Slow Wave Sleep)

Hibernation

Hibernation involves a long-term drop in body temperature and metabolism, and the animal enters a coma-like state that takes some time to recover from.

Insert

Bears however, don't experience a significant drop in body temperature during hibernation, and they awake relatively easily. They even move around a bit, and can sometimes leave their den for various reasons. At the other end of the scale, frogs such as the wood frog or the spring peeper actually partially freeze in winter, but a high concentration of glucose in the animal's vital organs prevents them from freezing completely. A partially frozen frog will stop breathing, and its heart will stop beating. It will appear quite dead. But when the frog warms up again, its frozen portions will thaw, and its heart and lungs spring back to life! Finally—did you know that in some parts of the world it was historically traditional for humans to practice a form of hibernation?[11]

Why do we need sleep?

We know that sleep is necessary, otherwise animals would not put themselves into such a vulnerable state for no reason. We have a 24-hour sleep-wake cycle determined by a part of our brain that is influenced by daylight and physical activity—our circadian clock. Even unicellular organisms demonstrate a circadian rhythm. We now know a little about some of the magical things that occur whilst we sleep, but, much like the ocean, the deeper we venture, the more we advance into unchartered waters.

We know that sleep is restorative and serves to promote growth, healing and improve energy reserves. We indulge in tissue repair, hormonal synthesis, muscle growth and much more whilst we are asleep. It has also been observed that we are mentally more agile when we are well-rested, memory recall improves, and we are generally sharper. The processing and storing of memories occurs during sleep.[12]

Brain cells build connections with other parts of the brain as a result of new experience, during sleep. Important neural connections may be strengthened and unimportant ones screened out during sleep. Research has also shown that sleep allows the brain itself to clear out or detoxify on a physiological level. Potentially neurotoxic waste products can be filtered out via a mechanism involving the recently named 'glymphatic system', which allows the exchange of solutes between the cerebrospinal fluid and interstitial fluid. This process is facilitated by glial cells of the brain. Beta-amyloid clearance, among other things, may be enhanced.

Lack of sleep has also been associated with a build-up of inflammatory mediators in the system, which can in turn has been linked to serious chronic health issues. So, in a nutshell, sleep allows a lot of housekeeping to take place in both the central nervous system and the rest of the body.

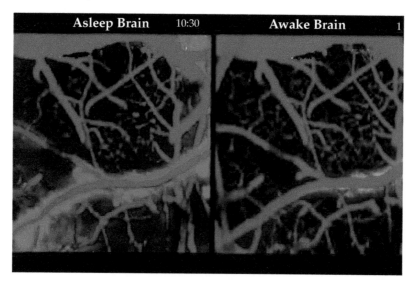

The deep end of the pool

Does anything go on above and beyond housekeeping and general maintenance? Well, here are a few things to consider:

Sleeping on it

A significant number of scientific discoveries have been informed by the act of sleeping on problems, or the solutions of problems presenting themselves in the form of dreams. Dmitri Mendeleev dreamt the layout he devised for the periodic table, Auguste Kekulé discovered the chemical structure of benzene in a dream, and the extraordinary mathematician Srinivasa Ramanujan described how he saw a Hindu goddess in his dreams who showed him mathematical provings.

Further than this there is what many people describe as the pseudoscience area of precognitive dreaming, which seems to be ridiculed and generally experienced in equal measure. In the early 1920s, British aeronautics engineer J. W. Dunne, responsible for designing and building some of the first practical and stable aircraft, wrote a book called *An Experiment with Time*, which recorded his experiences with precognitive dreams. Dunne proposed that our experience of time as linear was an illusion brought about by human consciousness. He argued that past, present and future were continuous in a higher-dimensional reality and only experienced sequentially because of our mental perception of them. To quote Katy Price (lecturer in modern and contemporary literature at Queen Mary University of London):

> *In part, the book functioned as an antidote to the Einstein sensation: Dunne converted the inaccessible, abstruse fourth dimension of relativity theory into something that any reader might explore in their sleep.*
>
> —R. Khanna, J. K. MacDonald and B. G. Levesque[13]

Finally, the hormone melatonin is produced by the pineal gland, located in proximity to the pituitary and hypothalamus. Melatonin is responsible for sleep/wake cycles within us. The pineal gland itself has been linked to

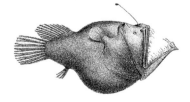

the ancient concept of 'the third eye', and is connected to clarity, concentration, intuition and imagination; it is regarded by many as the gateway to the psychic world.

Just a few thoughts from the deeper end of the pool. Now, read on.

What is insomnia?

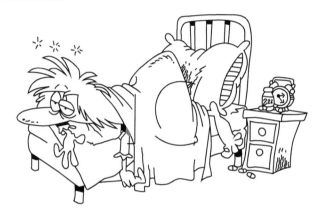

Insomniac woman

We get the word insomnia from the Latin *in* meaning without, and *somnis*, meaning sleep. It is the development of chronic sleep deprivation. Insomnia is characterised by experiencing inadequate quantity and/or quality of sleep night after night for an extended time period. One in ten adults develop chronic insomnia, and sleep disturbance and sleep disorders can also be experienced by children.

Difficulty in falling asleep is the most common complaint. Waking during the night and not being able to get back to sleep is also quite common. Some people complain of early wakening. We are all likely to suffer an occasional sleepless night or two, and can usually deal with this without it impacting on our general health and wellbeing. More than three nights together however will most likely lead to problems. Irritability, daytime sleepiness, relationship issues, poor performance at work and even personality changes can all result from sleep deprivation. Chronic insomnia is most widely defined as:

> ... inadequate quantity or quality of sleep characterized by a subjective report of difficulty with sleep initiation, duration, consolidation,

or quality that occurs despite adequate opportunity for sleep, and that results in some form of daytime impairment and has persisted for at least one month.

—S. Saddichha[14]

How much sleep do we need?

Just like everything else we are all different in terms of sleep requirements. Peoples' desired sleep goals tend to vary between 5 and 10 hours a night, the average being 8 hours. This may also vary depending upon the stage of life that you are in. If the body is doing a lot of growing, developing or healing, requirements may be higher. Young children and adolescents for example, tend to function better with more sleep than the average adult. Neu-

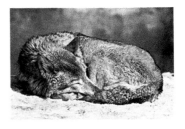

rologists now consider that long periods of sleeping less than 6 hours per night are associated with worse health outcomes for people.

Teenagers have become a specific focus of attention in more recent years, due to their well-known proclivity for 'sleeping in'. Research now is indicating that schools and universities will ultimately achieve better results with students if their operational hours are more suited to the natural sleep patterns of the age group that they are catering for.[15]

If you can wake without needing an alarm clock and if you can make it through the day without flagging or falling asleep whilst reading, you are probably getting enough sleep.

Causes of insomnia

The causes of insomnia are many and varied, and reflect the complexity of the human condition. A bout of insomnia may be triggered by a life event, and then anxiety about not sleeping can develop into chronic insomnia.

The following list of potential causes is large, but not comprehensive:

- Anxiety
- Increased life stress (especially grief)
- Physical pain

- Systemic disorders
- Hypoglycaemia
- Indigestion and heartburn (including eating too late at night)
- Depression
- Certain conventional medications (see below for list)
- Menopause
- Nutritional deficits (especially calcium, magnesium)
- Breathing disorders (such as sleep apnoea, which can wake a person up to 22 times a night)
- Sedentary lifestyles
- Shift work
- Restless leg syndrome
- Electronic devices with artificial light especially smartphones (one in eight people keep mobile phones switched on in the bedroom at night, increasing the risk of disturbed sleep)

Conventional medications linked with insomnia:

- *Antidepressants*: selective serotonin reuptake inhibitors (SSRI's), venlafaxine, bupropion, duloxetine, monoamine oxidase inhibitors.
- *Antiepileptics*: lamotrigine, phenytoin.
- *Antihypertensives*: beta-blockers, calcium-channel blockers.
- *Diuretics*.
- *Hormones*: corticosteroids, thyroid hormones.
- *Non-steroidal anti-inflammatory drugs*.
- *Stimulants*: methylphenidate, modafinil.
- *Sympathomimetics*: salbutamol, salmeterol, theophylline, pseudoephedrine.
- *Oral contraceptives*.

It is worth considering what conventional medications are being used, in case they have a role in causing sleep disorder. Some medications are for example associated with an increased frequency of nightmares. Iatrogenic (drug-induced) causes are more common than might be expected. Electronic media such as smartphones and specifically the growing use of it by adolescents is an area of increasing concern regarding teenagers and sleep patterns. Research conducted in Israel on 470 students aged around 14, concluded that:

Poor sleep patterns in Israeli adolescents are related to excessive electronic media habits and daytime sleep-related problems. These findings raise a public health concern regarding lifestyle and functioning in young individuals.

—B. D Lashkov[16]

It should also be borne in mind that the cause of insomnia might just be something really pragmatic. Maybe too much light is coming in through the curtains. Maybe your partner snores. Maybe you are being woken at the same time every night by a specific noise (a door closing or a dog barking etc). Maybe you are in a draughty room. Is the mattress comfortable? When was it last turned or changed? Does your pillow suit you? Are you warm enough?

Quick case study

Elaine was having trouble sleeping. She lay awake during the night worrying about the many small things in life that bothered her. She could not relax. Herbal remedies were helping a bit but had not managed to alleviate the problem. The insomnia started soon after she moved into her new house. She was happy with the house, liked its location and wanted to stay there. She could not understand what was bothering her. After approximately 2 months, she suddenly decided to move her bed. Her bed had been positioned under the window; it was now on the opposite wall further away from the window. She explained that once she had done this she realised that subconsciously she had been feeling vulnerable as she lived alone. The new arrangement felt 'safer' and she was able to relax and sleep.

This lady's experiences play into both natural survival instincts, and possibly to the sophisticated theory of Feng Shui, which involves the spatial arrangement of furniture in relation to energy flow in a given space. Feng shui tips for a good nights sleep include having a bed with a solid headboard, a good mattress, and no storage underneath, and not having your bed in line with a door. Absence of electronic devices is also encouraged.

Conventional medical treatment of insomnia

The emerging understanding of sleep physiology as the result of technologies such as functional MRI (magnetic resonance imaging) has led to more awareness of the need for good sleep habits. These are now promoted for shift workers including health care workers who regularly work irregular shift patterns. There are some key foundational principles for good sleep suggested for employees at Guy's hospital London that include:

- Ensure you have darkness in the bedroom, and softer lighting leading up to bedtime.
- Try to reduce noise around the time of going to bed.
- Keep your bedroom cool.
- Try to keep to similar times and form a routine.
- Taking a break and having a 15–20 minutes nap during night work will improve your function, and reduce stress.
- Caffeine has positive effects in small doses, especially immediately before a 15-minute nap during a nightshift. At other times, curb your caffeine consumption.
- Wear sunglasses if leaving a nightshift in daylight. Keep lights low as you head off to sleep.
- Reduce electronic light especially from devices such as smartphones. If you have to use them before sleep, change the light levels if the device has night-time lighting options available. Aim to have an electronic light curfew 1 hour before sleep.

In the UK, The National Institute for Health and Care Excellence (NICE) recommend that the underlying reasons for the insomnia should be addressed wherever possible. They do not recommend drug therapy for the long-term management of insomnia. In cases of either severe symptoms or an acute exacerbation of persistent insomnia a short course of a hypnotic drug may be considered, at the lowest dose possible to achieve a result. This should be assessed after 2 weeks. Further prescriptions should not be issued without seeing the person again. They advise caution when prescribing hypnotics for older people.

Hypnotics

Drugs classified as hypnotics work by interacting with gamma-aminobutyric acid (GABA) receptor sites in the body. They enhance the effect of the inhibitory neurotransmitter gamma-aminobutyric acid by increasing the affinity of GABA for its receptor.

Typical hypnotics include:

- Benzodiazepines, such as nitrazepam, flurazepam, loprazolam temazepam
- Non-benzodiazepines, including zopiclone and chloral hydrate[17]

Non-benzodiazepines are very similar to benzodiazepines in their actions but differ in terms of their molecular structure. Potential undesirable effects surrounding the use of hypnotics include: Daytime sedation, poor co-ordination and cognitive impairment, including an increased risk of driving accidents and falls.

Although benzodiazepines encourage sleep, they are thought to reduce the quality of sleep. They are rapid eye movement (REM) sleep–suppressant medications (REM sleep is known to have a role in learning and memory consolidation) and withdrawal often results in episodes of increased REM sleep (REM sleep rebound).

Note: Chronic and long-term sedative/hypnotic use to treat insomnia may cause tolerance to the sedative effect and can contribute to chronic insomnia.[17]

Other conventional medical drugs used for insomnia

Some antidepressant drugs, such as amitriptyline have also been prescribed for insomnia, particularly for people experiencing chronic pain, or for those who have not been helped by anything else. Anti-histamines are also used for occasional insomnia, but the sedative effects may diminish after a few days. Melatonin is a hormone secreted by the pineal gland and responsible for the regulation of the sleep cycle. It may be recommended in tablet form for insomnia in people over the age of 55.

Sleeping pills cannot cure insomnia. They do not go deeply enough into the underlying causes. Also, they may interfere with both REM sleep and the deeper stages of sleep, leading to more problems. Sleep medications are only really recommended for short-term use. Other strategies are recommended by conventional medicine, including cognitive behavioural therapy (CBT), due to its evidence base. CBT aims to help people observe and modify lifestyle patterns that are unhelpful, build more helpful habits and uses cognitive techniques to change thought patterns. CBT is only one of many strategies employed by psychotherapists.

Herbal concepts and treatment strategies

Much like the conventional medical approach, insomnia is generally seen as a surface symptom of something else happening within the life of that person, rather than a condition in its own right. Herbalists recognise the value in changing thought patterns and modifying the environment and behaviour to encourage good sleep-wake habits. The herbal treatment options however may provide a gentler and more flexible approach, as they can encourage the body's own sleep processes.

Have you ever noticed how, if you happen to be awake at 3am, all your problems seem to be insurmountable? Everything appears to be 100 times worse than it actually is, and this anxiety-inducing state is really not helpful in terms of getting back to sleep. Why is this? Well, at around 3am hormones such as cortisol, which help the body cope with stress, are at their lowest. Your ability to cope therefore, with life's difficult challenges is at its lowest ebb. Just knowing this is actually beneficial. You can at least reassure yourself that things are not as bad as they feel. When people have an understanding of why they are feeling the way they do, this can help enormously.

Herbs can gently encourage relaxation. Due to multiple compounds, medicinal plants can encourage relaxation at multiple sites in the body at the same time—for example, the digestive and nervous systems. Although possibly weaker in terms of chemistry, plants work in a restorative way due to their complexity and capacity to act at multiple sites and with synergistic effects. This means that many of the herbs used to help restore sleep patterns, are not forceful and drug-like, and they are also not addictive. They tend to leave the person more likely to sleep well, long after treatment has ceased. Listed in the table below are a few of the more commonly used herbs to encourage relaxation and sleep, and some brief notes concerning them.

Herb	Constituents and actions of the herb	Useful for insomnia with
Matricaria chamomilla L. German chamomile flower	Volatile oils chamazulene, bisabolol, sesquiterpene lactones Antispasmodic, sedative, gentle bitter	Inflammation or spasm in the digestive tract, IBS General underlying digestive issues Children

(*Continued*)

Herb	Constituents and actions of the herb	Useful for insomnia with
Humulus lupulus L. Hop strobiles	Volatile oils, phenolic compounds, bitters. Antispasmodic. Improves bile flow	Nervousness or excitability Restless legs IBS, indigestion
Passiflora incarnata L. Passion flower herb	Indole alkaloids, rutin, luteolin Antispasmodic, anxiolytic, hypotensive	Nervous headaches Panic Palpitations
Scutellaria lateriflora L. Skullcap herb	Flavonoid glycosides, volatile oils, lignans, tannin. Anti-inflammatory, sedative	Nervous system tonic herb. Emotional oversensitivity. Sleeplessness due to exhaustion
Lavandula angustifolia Mill. Lavender herb	Volatile oils, flavonoids, triterpenes Astringent, sedative, antibacterial	Anxiety, depression. Tension headaches. Bloating, digestive complaints

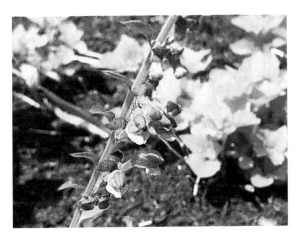

Tall skullcap (*Scuttellaria altissima* L.)

Blending two or more of the above herbs as tea can make for an excellent calming and soothing bedtime drink. Sip slowly, after allowing to draw, covered, for at least 10 minutes. Drink about 30–60 minutes before going to bed. Ideally a regime like this should be continued for several weeks, even months before checking to see if the body can now use its own resources to sleep well.

It is no coincidence that many of these herbs contain volatile oils and/or have an effect on the digestive tract. There seems to be a link here between calming, relaxing herbs and the gut. Think about the gut as being the massive concentration of nervous tissue that it is. No wonder herbs can relax us so effectively via our digestive tracts.

> **Note: The wonderful and reliable *Valeriana officinalis* L.** The dried root of this most interesting herbal medicine has been used for centuries (and more) to aid relaxation, reduce digestive spasm and restore sleep patterns. The name valerian comes from the Latin word *valere*, meaning to be strong or healthy.

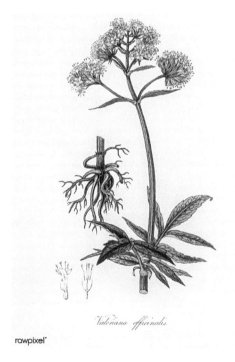

rawpixel

Valerian (*Valeriana officinalis* L.)

Poor cognitive function is often associated with sleep disorders, and yet this incredible plant has even been demonstrated to improve cognitive function, not just sleep alone.[18,19] Like many of the plants mentioned already, valerian contains multiple useful compounds. Estimates run at around 150 to 200 different substances. These include:

- Volatile oils
- Ketones and phenols
- Iridoid esters such as valreotriate, valeric acid
- Alkaloids
- Amino acids such as aminobutyric acid, tyrosine, arginine, glutamine
- Noncyclic, monocyclic and bicyclic hydrocarbons

Like other herbal medicines often used for sleep, there is good evidence for their non-addictive nature and yet their effectiveness in improving falling asleep times and deep sleep cycles.[20] Of course, as insomnia is multi-factorial, herbs for insomnia often work well together rather than in isolation. This may be one reason that research into herbal medicines can have both positive outcomes and yet also be disappointing,[21] as herbs are studied in isolation, not as they would be prescribed by a herbal consultant.

One reliable strategy is to use herbs to help reduce 'stress' during waking hours. Although it may seem counter-intuitive to treat insomnia by taking relaxing herbs during the day, there is plenty of evidence suggesting that over-exertion and mental stress in our waking hours impact negatively on our sleep cycles. As has been shown with valerian, relaxing herbs do not have negative effects on cognitive function, and so can be used safely during the day.

Medical herbalists often combine relaxing herbs with adaptogens for use during the daytime, then a combination of soothing relaxants, nervous system repairing and sleep-encouraging herbs for night-time. This can help accentuate a sleep-wake cycle and help the body find its way back to its own natural circadian rhythm. A strategy like this is best employed over at least 12 weeks. In most cases, this allows the person to eventually cut down and stop their herbal medicines without slipping back. The mechanism of action of these plants is indirect and known to not be addictive.

A gentleman in his early 60s had been suffering from a chronic weeping skin condition for several years. The skin problem would come and go, usually appearing on the palms of his hands, but sometimes on his forearms. It occasionally became infected requiring antibiotics. The severity of the condition was worsening, as were the frequency of attacks and the size of the skin area affected. He was at his wit's end, as it was keeping him awake when he was trying to sleep in the daytime. He had been a night shift worker for many years and although he slept every day, he often experienced only 5 hours of sleep.

A daytime 'tonic' was prescribed, aiming at improving his immune system, and resilience to infection and giving his nervous system a nourishing boost. The herbs included tinctures of:

- Oat flowers (*Avena sativa* L.)
- St John's wort herb (*Hypericum perforatum* L.)
- Chamomile flowers (*Matricaria chamomilla* L.)
- Mahonia root bark (*Berberis aquifolium* Pursh.)
- Echinacea *Echinacea purpurea* L.
- Gotu kola herb (*Centella asiatica* (L.) Urb.)

In preparation for bed, he drank a herbal tea of passionflower (*Passiflora incarnata* L.) and linden blossom (*Tilia cordata* Mill.), and took a small amount of valerian (*Valeriana officinalis* L.) and hops (*Humulus lupulus* L.) tincture. Good sleep habits were discussed, and he was encouraged to take healthier options from home to eat at work.

Interestingly, research supports the long traditional use of hops as an anti-infective skin agent as well as helping sleep patterns.[22] After 6 months he was no longer having skin outbreaks and his sleep had improved sufficiently for him. He returned and used the herbal medicines again when he retired and was able to recover a good sleep pattern after years of night work.

Diet and lifestyle advice

A lot can be achieved by adjusting unhelpful lifestyle habits. The following list is, again, not comprehensive, but the correct combination of strategies can go a long way to ameliorating intransigent insomnia, especially if practised over a period of time.

- Only go to bed when you are sleepy, and prepare for this at a regular time. Reduce noise, dim lighting, stop using your electronic devices.
- Take regular exercise. Exercise in the daytime or early evening, but not before bedtime. Physical exercise can help tire your body, stimulate important hormones, and encourage sleep.
- Avoid heavy meals, caffeine-containing drinks or alcohol late in the evening.
- The amino acid tryptophan helps promote sleep via increasing the levels of both serotonin and melatonin. Foods containing tryptophan include bananas, figs, dates, yoghurt, turkey, milk (the evening milky drink) and tuna.
- The amino acid tyramine can act as a stimulant via increasing the release of norepinephrine. Therefore foods to avoid during the evening include bacon, cheese, chocolate (boo!), spinach, tomatoes and wine.
- Foods such as walnuts, olives, rice, barley, strawberries, cherries, and cow's milk contain natural sources of melatonin.
- Mandarins: In Chinese herbalism, mandarin oranges are believed to calm the spirit and are used to aid memory recall and concentration.
- Don't smoke. Although smokers experience a relaxing effect from cigarettes, nicotine is a neuro-stimulant.
- Minimise your time spent working (especially at computer screens) in the evening.
- Have a hot bath approximately an hour before bed. Soaking in hot water may help relax tense muscles. Use lavender and chamomile in your bathwater. You could make a pint of really strong chamomile and lavender tea and add it to the bathwater, thereby soaking up all those lovely calming volatile oils and other helpful compounds.
- Napping in the day is OK if it is normal for you to do so and does not usually interfere with your night-time sleep. Keep it short, however, less than an hour and don't do it if it's not a normal thing for you to do.

The human body is a cyclical entity. It runs on numerous cycles and feedback loops. This is what it likes. Anyone who experiences the discomfort of constipation associated with a change in day-to-day routines will appreciate the point that is being made here. There are numerous ways in which people encourage relaxation and sleep, but one of the most valuable techniques lies in the tactic of developing a set of habits, or a pre-sleep sleep cycle, that gives your brain very specific signals that you are winding down to rest, and allows it to act accordingly.

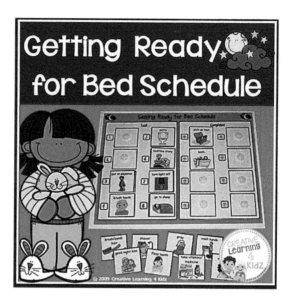

If you are going to adopt some of the strategies listed above, do it as a routine, rather than just trying it for a few nights and giving up. Keeping at it for months so that habits become established is key to success. Specifically going to bed at the same time every evening if possible, and waking/setting your alarm for the same time the following day are really important aspects of this. Even if you wake feeling tired, get up anyway. Establishing the routine is the vital thing.

Domestic medicine/kitchen pharmacy

The above strategies can be supplemented by a few home remedies, for example:

Sleep pillows

One recent story concerning sleep pillows involves a 10-year-old boy who wanted a sleep pillow from his grandmother for Christmas. The lady consulted a herbalist, who supplied lavender newly dried from her herb garden. This was used to fill a sleep pillow made from purple cotton by his grandmother. Sometimes requests for herbal help come from surprising sources!

We all love a good lavender bag, and one discretely tucked under your pillow may help getting off to sleep. Whilst you are at it, hops have also traditionally been used for many centuries in hop pillows. A blend of hops and lavender is an excellent thing!

(See also hot baths under diet and lifestyle.)

Essential oils

If you don't want to go to the bother of making a sleep pillow, or your sewing skills aren't up to much, add a few drops of lavender, or chamomile essential oils to a hanky and leave it in your bedroom. Our sense of smell is located in our emotional centre in our brain. This means that certain smells can trigger certain behaviours, such as relaxation, trust and sleep.

Sprays and mists

Some of the trendier hotels are now supplying sleep sprays to use on your pillow before you go to bed. A good idea, but make sure that there is not too much of the artificial or synthetic about it!

Red flags

Red flag symptoms are symptoms that may signal a more serious underlying condition and should be looked at more closely or referred to a health care professional/GP.

In terms of insomnia, seek professional help if the person you are treating exhibits the following symptoms at any time:

- Significant breathing disturbances during sleep
- Excessive daytime sleepiness in potentially dangerous situations
- Underlying unstable cardiac or pulmonary situations
- Significant sleepwalking
- Violent behaviours or injury to self or others during sleep
- Behavioural changes

Excessive sleepwalking or violent behaviour during sleep can be symptomatic of underlying mood disorders.

Conclusion

How complex seemingly simple things can be. Insomnia truly comes in all shapes and sizes, and is often the product of more than one influencing factor. It is a situation that can be resolved really easily and, in some cases, really pragmatically, or it may be something that can become intransigent, and demand patience and lateral thinking to resolve. It also presents us with a challenge at times, as it may demand a significant change in behavioural patterns on behalf of the patient, as well as having faith in the possibility that things can change. Things can change.

Sleep well.

References

1. Eliade, M., *Shamanism. Archaic Techniques of Ecstasy*. 2004: Princeton University Press.
2. Bergman, M. et al. *FRI0357 Patients with osteoarthritis report symmetrical painful joints in similar numbers and distribution as patients with rheumatoid arthritis*. 2015. 74, 555.
3. Sokolove, J. and C. M. Lepus, *Role of inflammation in the pathogenesis of osteoarthritis: latest findings and interpretations*. Ther Adv Musculoskelet Dis, 2013. 5(2): pp. 77–94.
4. Ennis, Z. N. et al., *Acetaminophen for Chronic pain: a systematic review on efficacy*. Basic Clin Pharmacol Toxicol, 2016. 118(3): pp. 184–189.
5. Vlachojannis, J. E., M. Cameron and S. Chrubasik, *A systematic review on the effectiveness of willow bark for musculoskeletal pain*. Phytother Res, 2009. 23(7): pp. 897–900.
6. Shara, M. and S. J. Stohs, *Efficacy and safety of white willow bark (Salix alba) Extracts*. Phytother Res, 2015. 29(8): pp. 1112–1116.
7. Chrubasik, S. M. et al., *Treatment of Low Back Pain Exacerbations with Willow Bark Extract: A Randomized Double-Blind Study*. The American Journal of Medicine, 2000. 109.
8. Cameron, M. and S. Chrubasik, *Oral herbal therapies for treating osteoarthritis*. Cochrane Database Syst Rev, 2014(5): p. CD002947.
9. Sontakke, S., V. Thawani et al., *Open, randomised, controlled clinical trial of Boswellia errata extract as compared to vaidecoxib in osteoarthritis of the knee*. Indian Journal of Pharmacology, 2007. 39(1): pp. 27–29.
10. Tarannum, A., A. Sultana and K. Ur Rahman, *Clinical efficacy of certain Unani herbs in knee osteoarthritis: A pretest and post-test evaluation study*. Anc Sci Life, 2016. 35(4): pp. 227–231.
11. *Human hibernation*. BMJ, 2000. 320(7244): p. 1245A.
12. Sterpenich, V. et al., *Memory reactivation during rapid eye movement sleep promotes its generalization and integration in cortical stores*. Sleep, 2014. 37(6): pp. 1061–1075, 1075A–1075B.
13. Price, K. J. W. *Dunne and the Popular Promise of Dreams*. Mapping Ignorance, 2014.

14. Saddichha, S., *Diagnosis and treatment of chronic insomnia*. Ann Indian Acad Neurol, 2010. 13(2): pp. 94–102.

15. Wolfson, A. R. et al., *Middle School Start Times: The Importance of a Good Night's Sleep for Young Adolescents*. Behavioral Sleep Medicine, 2007. 5(3): pp. 194–209.

16. Shochat, T., O. Flint-Bretler and O. Tzischinsky, *Sleep patterns, electronic media exposure and daytime sleep-related behaviours among Israeli adolescents*. Acta Paediatr, 2010. 99(9): pp. 1396–1400.

17. Pagel, J. F. and B. L. Parnes, *Medications for the Treatment of Sleep Disorders: An Overview*. Prim Care Companion J Clin Psychiatry, 2001. 3(3): pp. 118–125.

18. Samaei, A. et al., *Effect of valerian on cognitive disorders and electroencephalography in hemodialysis patients: a randomized, cross over, double-blind clinical trial*. BMC Nephrol, 2018. 19(1): p. 379.

19. Hassani, S. et al., *Can Valeriana officinalis root extract prevent early postoperative cognitive dysfunction after CABG surgery? A randomized, double-blind, placebo-controlled trial*. Psychopharmacology (Berl), 2015. 232(5): pp. 843–850.

20. Gyllenhaal, C. et al., *Efficacy and safety of herbal stimulants and sedatives in sleep disorders*. Sleep Med Rev, 2000. 4(3): pp. 229–251.

21. Khadivzadeh, T. et al., *A systematic review and meta-analysis on the effect of herbal medicine to manage sleep dysfunction in peri- and postmenopause*. J Menopausal Med, 2018. 24(2): pp. 92–99.

22. Yamaguchi, N., K. Satoh-Yamaguchi and M. Ono, *In vitro evaluation of antibacterial, anticollagenase, and antioxidant activities of hop components (Humulus lupulus) addressing acne vulgaris*. Phytomedicine, 2009. 16(4): pp. 369–376.

CHAPTER ELEVEN

Swimming upstream: common conditions and therapeutic considerations

Introduction

In this final chapter, dealing with specific treatment protocols for common complaints, we will be looking at the two areas of our magnificent physiology that bring us into the closest contact with the outside world: our skin and our digestive tract. We can view these as being contiguous with each other, and indeed the gut microbiome, and the skin microbiome both star in their respective sections. Taking the relative ratios of the numbers of 'human' cells to 'other' we are after all, only approximately 10% human. Redefining what it means to be human on a genetic level is possibly our next big step in understanding how our bodies function.

Part 1. Skin health (the skinny on skin)

What is skin??

> **Definition—*Skin*:** Skin is composed of three layers: The epidermis, the dermis and the hypodermis. The top or outside layer, the epidermis, is composed of keratin and melanin. Keratin is a fibrous protein which

gives structure to the skin. It is also used by the body to make hair and nails. Melanin refers to a group of pigments in the skin which gives our skin its colour. The epidermis is the layer that we see with the naked eye, and by which we can determine many things about the people around us, including approximate age and general health. We are judging the book by its cover! When we speak of skin this is what we are most commonly talking about. But of course there is more to it than that.

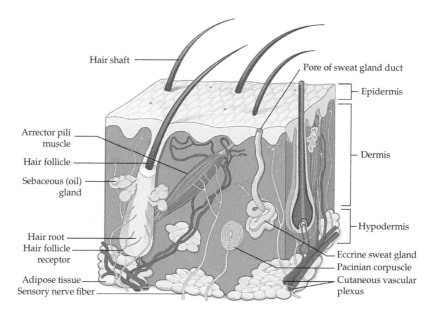

The middle layer, the dermis, has nerve fibres that provide sensory information on pressure, pain and temperature. It also has a network of blood vessels that provide nutrients and help with the elimination of waste products from the skin cells and tissues. Sebaceous glands are also located here, which produce oils to keep the skin supple.

The base layer of our skin, the hypodermis, is largely made up of fat. Subcutaneous (beneath the skin) fat is now regarded as not only a fat store, but as an important endocrine organ in its own right. Two recently discovered hormones produced by this layer of adipose tissue are leptin and ghrelin; they play a major role in how we experience hunger and desire for food.[1]

Functions of skin

- To provide a physical barrier which protects us from toxins, foreign bodies etc.
- To provide an interface with the outside world
- To retain water in the system
- To provide a surface acidic pH as a non-specific defence mechanism against pathogens
- To function as an endocrine gland (sex hormones may also be synthesized by the skin)

We will look at the nature of the interface with the outside world a bit more closely in the section entitled skin microbiome.

Pathophysiology of skin

The area of medicine known as dermatology deals with problems that manifest on the skin. This, in conventional medicine, is often a process of finding a diagnosis for the type of skin condition present, then applying treatment; usually externally.

Eczema is a common condition seen by the practising herbalist. There are two forms of eczema: Atopic, characterised by an increase in blood IgE immunoglobulins, and non-atopic when this is not the case. Around three-quarters of eczema cases are atopic. Raised IgE levels indicate an allergic component to the condition, and it is estimated that around 20% of all children suffer from atopic eczema.[2]

For the medical herbalist, it can be very useful to have a diagnosis for any person presenting with a skin complaint, but it is generally appreciated that the skin, as the most superficial organ of our body, is quite likely to express symptoms as an indicator of more *internal* processes. This is true of the majority of skin complaints that herbalists see, but even such seemingly external issues as melanomas have been found to benefit from common phytochemicals found in a cross-section of herbs, fruits and vegetables.[3]

To provide a list of all of the possible skin conditions recognised by conventional medicine would be outside the scope of this course. However, we will look in more detail at the possible internal imbalances that may give rise to many common skin complaints.

Conventional approaches to treatment

The mainstay of conventional skin management is the application of emollients and skin creams with or without active ingredients such as hydrocortisone. Many of these skin applications are based on petro-chemical byproducts such as vaseline and other petroleum oils. These are used both for short-term relief, and for long-term problems.

It is rare to find oral or internal treatment for skin in conventional der-matology—except in extreme cases of allergy, or serious and acute derma-tological break-outs where oral steroids such as prednisolone may be used. Antibiotics are also used for short-term acute problems, and for the longer-term skin complaints such as acne vulgaris (teenage acne), and other skin problems where infection is present, such as impetigo. Antibiotics in these circumstances may be given orally and/or externally. Antifungal creams and occasionally antiviral creams may be used if appropriate. Antiviral drugs are available for difficult cases of shingles. External applications for scabies and lice can be bought from most chemists.

In serious and long-term dermatitis, oral immune-suppression therapy may be used by consultant dermatologists. Anti-histamine drugs may be used in what appear to be allergic skin conditions.

Conventional medicines and skin reactions

Some skin rashes are well known to be caused by certain drugs especially antibiotics, Non-Steroidal Anti-Inflammatory Drugs (NSAIDs) and tran-quillisers. Medical herbalists often see people with non-specific, chronic dermatitis, especially urticaria-type dermatitis, and would associate these with an 'overload' of conventional medication. Great care needs to be taken with such patients to support their body whilst also giving safe advice about their medication. Often such patients have tolerated an array of conventional medication for many years only to start getting irritating skin itching (pruritis) as they age, and liver metabolism slows.

Western herbal medicine's approach to treatment

Skin from the perspective of the medical herbalist—is produced from within, and is a direct product of the blood (nutrients in, waste products out), and so an assessment of the function of the organs of elimination will be performed. This complex process of skin being nourished and oxygenated, whilst waste products of metabolism are effectively removed by dynamic processes, is seen as being enhanced by the use of herbal alteratives or depuratives. These words are often used in old herbals but refer to a complex metabolic phenomenon, the maintenance of healthy skin.

Depurative

Depurative herbs are considered to have cleansing and detoxifying properties. Historically they would have been referred to as *blood cleansers. Arctium lappa* L. (Burdock) would be a classic example of a depurative.

Alteratives

Alteratives are herbs which are capable of gradually restoring the body to good health by the gentle restoration of healthy function. *Urtica dioica* L. (nettle) would be a good example of an alterative. Nettle is widely regarded as a depurative herb, and Menzies-Trull refers to herbs with this cleansing and detoxifying action as vasotonic alteratives. Monitoring of circulatory function (heat, cold) will allow the practitioner to monitor the distribution of blood within tissues, and how this can be improved with the judicious use of good alterative herbs.[19]

The skin has its own microbiome and is in direct communication with the internal microbiome. Indeed the microorganisms that comprise the microbiota of skin are the same as the ones as found on the mucosa of the digestive tract, although the balance of individual species differs.[4] The herbalist therefore recognises a need to restore health, vigour and function to a disordered microbiome (dysbiosis) inside as well as outside of the body. This means it is important to consider what we put onto our skin, and what cleaning products we use. Will this impact positively or negatively on our microbiome?

Skin microbiome

Our skin is home to an entire ecosystem, which is comprised of many and diverse microbes, including bacteria, viruses and fungi. The distribution of these microorganisms varies depending on location.

Many of these microorganisms have entered into a symbiotic relationship with us. In return for a cosy living habitat, they will protect us from more harmful or pathogenic organisms. It is also thought that they play a role in training our immune systems to recognise their more harmful cousins.[4] It is easy to see how a disruption in the balance between the skin microbiome and the host can result in skin infection or disease.

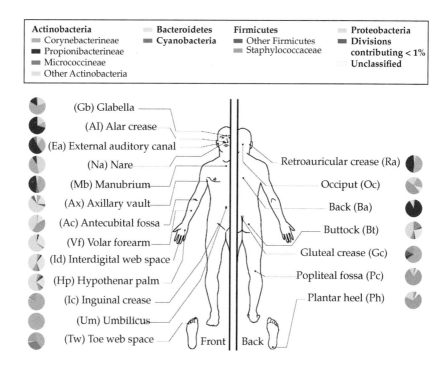

Allergy, by definition, is viewed as a gut microbiome problem affecting our immune response in Western herbal medicine, and so an array of prebiotic herbs/foods and probiotic, or gut-healing herbs/diet will form a major part of any therapeutic strategy.

Skin infections can be treated from within (and without) using herbs with powerful antimicrobial effects; but herbalists will also seek to restore immune function over the longer-term using herbs that are immunomodulatory. The strategy of restoring optimal skin microbiome balance can also play an important role in the resolution of skin disease. Modulation of immune function can also play a vital role in conditions such as atopic eczema where both surface immunity and systemic immunity can be disrupted by 'leaky skin'.[2]

Tinea, candida and other fungal conditions of the skin are seen as opportunistic imbalances of the immune system. In other words—fungal conditions often develop when we are 'run-down' in some way. Boosting the immune system from within is something at which herbal medicine excels. Skin is inter-related to the nervous system (as we have seen in the anatomy and physiology of the skin), and will also respond to the internal environment of a stressed person. Thus using wonderful herbal nervines will often form a major part of any therapeutic strategy.

With an endocrine organ in its own right in the hypodermis, the skin will respond to hormone imbalance within the body. We can see the classic skin reactions to ovarian malfunction such as boils along the jaw-line, excessive hair growth or excess melanisation that can be seen in cases of polycystic ovarian syndrome (PCOS); and there are many other examples, such as types of acne found at adolescence, or at peri-menopause.

Herbal medicine can often provide huge benefits to restore hormone balance whether due to sex hormones or to adrenal hormones—the corticosteroids. Stress hormones can aggravate skin conditions, and herbal alteratives may be ideal here to support and rejuvenate adrenal function. This can accelerate skin repair.

Summary

A quick checklist for the herbalist when seeing someone with a skin problem may well include the following:

- Function of the gut, especially the bowel.
- Function of the urinary system and respiratory system, especially with regard to infection and infection management.
- Nutrition and the microbiome.
- Stress/nervous system—supporting the nervous system and adrenals.
- Age of the person, and potential hormone imbalance that could be related.
- Consideration of conventional drugs—too many? For too long?
- Considerations of what conventional approaches have helped may also give insights into providing a herbal alternative.
- General skincare for everyday—exposure to nasty chemicals or excessive use of soaps/detergents etc. Helping people use natural household products perhaps.

In other words, although herbalists may have their favourite herbs for dealing with specific skin diagnoses, it is often sufficient to apply a broad strategy of internal healing and restoration of function when treating skin complaints. Let's look at some wonderful herbal allies to consider in the key strategies listed above.

1) Gut function!

Looking back at our 15 herbs from the *Material Medica* in this book, herbs that could fall into a digestive category could be:

- Chamomile (*Matricaria chamomilla* L.)
- Fennel (*Foeniculum vulgare* L.)
- Lemon balm (*Melissa officinalis* L.)
- Lavender (*Lavandula angustifolia* Mill.)
- Marshmallow root (*Althaea officinalis* L. radix)
- Dandelion (*Taraxacum offiinale* L. (esp. radix))

Note: Dandelion and burdock. Dandelion and burdock were once the main ingredients of a very popular 'spring cleaning' (alterative/depurative) drink. Fermented drinks of the roots of dandelion and burdock plants were also included in medicinal herb-flavoured meads known as metheglins. The earliest recorded dandelion and burdock drink being made and drunk was 1265. According to legend—taking a walk on a country road one day—Saint Thomas Aquinas prayed to God asking him for inspiration (or maybe a thirst-quenching beverage!!). He made a drink from the first plants that he found (which were dandelion and burdock).

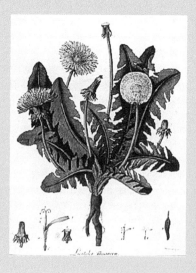

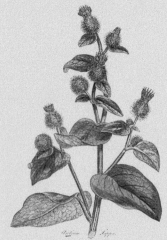

It may not have been as sweet as refined sugars were not available—these were more likely to have been honey or fruits. It is also possible that the dandelion and burdock of the time would contain small amounts of alcohol due to the way in which it was fermented and brewed. Wild ferments are happily enjoying a revival in our time.

Other common depurative/alterative or 'spring-cleaning' herbs used in such drinks were nettle (*Urtica dioica* L.) leaves and yellow dock roots (*Rumex crispus* L.). A revival of root beers was induced by the temperance movement in the 19th century, and by the use of 'tonic' roots from America, such as sarsaparilla (*Smilax ornata* Lem.). Nicholas Culpeper, a critic of the expensive treatments offered by doctors, also commented on the use of cheap, easily available dandelion roots to help people as a medicinal food. He concluded by saying:

> *You see here what virtues this common herb hath, and that is the reason the French and Dutch so often eat them in the spring; and now if you look a little farther, you may plainly see without a pair of spectacles, that foreign physicians are not so selfish as ours are, but more communicative of the virtues of plants to people.*
>
> —Nicholas Culpeper[5]

2) Infection management!

We may need to resort to herbs such as thyme (*Thymus vulgaris* L.) and garlic (*Allium sativa* L.) to help us deal with acute infections, but many herbs can be used to help improve general immunity. One in particular, *Echinacea purpurea* (L.) Moench (purple coneflower) has a real affinity for the skin due to its supportive effects upon the lymphatic system and the microbiome.

3) Microbes!

Our gut microbiome is enhanced and maintained by digestive function and digestive enzyme production. Many herbs are known to improve these important digestive products. You will recall the use of bitter herbs (even simply chamomile, dandelion leaf or meadowsweet from previous chapters), and also the use of aromatic carminatives are viewed as central to the correction of the digestive cascade. Digestive aromatic carminatives we have met already include: *Lavandula angustifolia* Mill., *Melissa officinalis* L. and *Foeniculum vulgare* Mill.

Herbs such as nettle (*Urtica dioica* L.), have anti-allergic effects and provide liver and kidney support—making nettle leaf a fantastic all-rounder for skin health! Plants have their own microbiome that supports our world and soil. Eating wild and raw leaves and fruits with a healthy microbial flora, will encourage our internal and external microbial diversity.

4) Stress!

Nervines are often used in just about every prescription in herbal medicine, because our nervous system reaches just about every part of our body, and our response to stress can often lead to consequences. You will recall key nervines in this book include: *Matricaria chamomilla* L., *Melissa officinalis* L., *Lavandula angustifolia* Mill. and *Tilia europea* L. One more we would like to consider is oat—*Avena sativa* L.

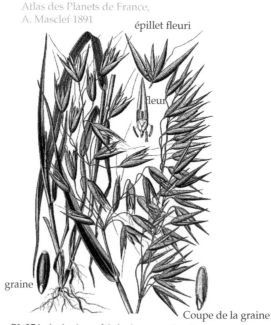

Atlas des Planets de France, A. Masclef 1891

épillet fleuri

fleur

graine

Coupe de la graine

Pl. 374. A. Avoine cultivée. Avena sativa L.
B. Avoine d'Orient. Avena orientalis Schreb.

Although oats are a food, and can be used internally and externally, the plant is considered to be an important stabilising nervine in herbal medicine. Usually—the oat straw or flowers will be used as an internal medicine and this has obvious benefits to those who are sensitive to gluten, as we can access the power of oat without the possibility of gluten being present. We like to imagine the strength and fortitude required by this slender, graceful plant, to stand tall and hold fast in rain, wind and hot sun; a signature for its capacity to increase our own resilience and grace.

5) Hormone balance

A reminder of the amazing amphoteric balancing plant *Vitex agnus-castus* L., and its extraordinary reach of application in almost any hormone imbalance. As the conductor of the hormonal orchestra, chaste tree berries can be of use at many life stages.

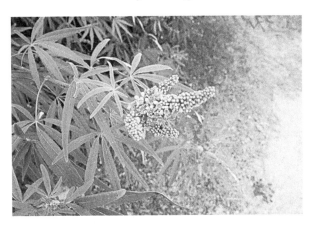

Chaste tree flowers.

We have also looked at adaptogens—one in particular to mention here is liquorice root (*Glycyrrhiza glabra* L.), with its capacity to restore adrenal hormone function and help us adapt to stress, inflammation, and also when trying to reduce corticosteroid drugs and creams. But note that one should avoid 'gross liquorice consumption' which also means gross liquorice *sweets* consumption! Taken orally in large enough quantities glucose acts like a drug and has serious side effects.

6) Lymphatic system support

You will remember our detailed look at the lymphatic drainage supporting herb *Galium aparine* L. (cleavers). Because the skin, like all of our body tissues, is drained by the lymphatic supply, it is no wonder the lymphatic system can become overburdened by inflammation or infection of the skin. Conventional anatomy books do not always focus on the lymphatic system, but supporting the lymphatic system directly with herbs like Galium, is often extremely helpful in any skin condition.

(**NB:** Supporting the liver with medicinal herbs will indirectly aid lymphatic drainage.)

Skin brushing can be useful for general skin health, but should not be used during acute skin problems or where a rash or infection is present. Gentle dry brushing (with a soft bristle brush) of the skin in the direction towards the heart, is thought to encourage the flow of lymph and tone the skin.

Self-help: the kitchen pharmacy

As always, there are definitely things that people can do themselves to help resolve skin disorders and support skin health. They include:

- Avoid—cigarette smoke, excess alcohol and too much ultraviolet light exposure.
- Diet—cut out refined sugars, red meat, soft drinks. Limit tea and coffee. Herb teas make an excellent medicated alternative—especially nettle, heartsease, red clover, chamomile and marigold.
- Lactose intolerance is common in childhood (and sometimes adult) eczema, and so finding dairy alternatives may be worthwhile. It is important to be scrupulous about avoiding dairy for at least 6 weeks to test whether this strategy is going to work.
- Avoiding modern bread and fast-action yeast is also a good strategy for allergic skin problems, due to its adverse effects on the microbiome and therefore our immune system.
- Raise intake of water, fruit, vegetables, nuts, seeds, beans and pulses.
- Add prebiotic foods such as flax seed, slippery elm powder, psyllium husk and chia seeds.
- Raise the intake of foods high in blood cleansing minerals (iron, potassium, sulphur). Radishes (with green tops), spring onions, dandelion leaves, green pepper, watercress, celery, radish, kohlrabi, parsley and carrots will all be beneficial here.

Foods with good quality fats, such as sesame and coconut would be great. Include cold-pressed seed oils like olive oil, and omega oils such as evening primrose, starflower (*Borago officinalis* L. seed) or flax, and hemp seed oils. Fats make up a large portion of our skin, but fats are also essential for immune function and hormone building blocks, so eating good quality fats has an effect on anatomical and hormone structure and therefore potentially on its ability to function well.

Probiotic foods such as lacto-fermented cabbage or beetroot would be ideal to introduce to our diets, and can be introduced to children 1 teaspoon at a time. Raise intake of helpful vitamins and minerals, especially zinc from pumpkin seeds and vitamin C from foods rich in bioflavonoids such as rosehips, watercress, mustard and cress, alfalfa sprouts. Eat more fresh vegetables generally, especially carrots, beets, cabbages and kale. Undertake regular, vigorous exercise where possible to stimulate circulation and relieve stress. Find good de-stressors, do not rely on a glass of wine for example …

External preparations

Good quality external preparations can do much to reduce inflammation, nourish the local area, supply anti-infective agents and generally act as healers and re-balancers of the skin microbiome. A few suggestions include:

Oatmeal baths

Oats can be very soothing and nourishing to inflamed, itchy skin. To make an oatmeal bath:

Oatmeal bath

- Place 2 tablespoons of oatmeal in either a cotton/linen bag with a drawstring , or a clean, old sock.
- Secure the opening (tie a knot in the sock).
- Place the bag in a warm bath of water and gently squeeze to allow the oatmeal to start dissolving into the bathwater. You will find that the bathwater becomes soft and milky.
- Relax in the milky bathwater. You can use the wet bag of oatmeal as a compress or poultice, held against the problem area of skin.

Note: Herbs for external use on skin. It is often safer and more effective to use herbal infusions for weeping eczemas, rather than using a cream (use wet to treat wet). A simple compress, using chamomile for anti-inflammatory purposes or marigold for soothing and healing purposes can often work wonders, especially on conditions such as weeping eczema. Sunburn will also benefit from regular application of a cold marigold compress (or poultice).

Herbal creams for flaking, scaling skin can apply cooling (chickweed), healing (marigold), nourishment (comfrey) and anti-inflammatory (chamomile) effects directly to affected areas. Good quality plant oils (not petroleum oil) provide useful absorbable lipids.

Natural everyday skincare products such as witch hazel and rose water (hydrolats) which are produced as a glorious by-product of the essential oil making process may also be used. Natural deodorants such as skin powders (make your own or try good quality, handmade cosmetics), or hydrolats with small amounts of gentle essential oils such as lavender, lemon or vetiver make effective but gentle deodorants.

We have looked at infused oils earlier in this book. Antiviral herbs such as *Melissa officinalis* L. and *Hypericum perforatum* L. make excellent infused oils for use with cold sores or nerve pain caused by shingles for instance. Adding beeswax to an infused oil creates an ointment. Use oily ointments on thick dry hard skin, such as psoriasis. Try comfrey, lavender or Rose petal oil for this particular ointment.

Herb vinegars, another home pharmacy product we have looked at, have huge versatility. Use a lemon thyme, or rosemary vinegar to clean kitchen and bathroom areas, thus minimising exposure to harsh chemicals. Make a marigold or lavender vinegar to add to bathwater. Just 1 tablespoon in a full bath actually smells lovely, is anti-inflammatory, pH balancing, and leaves skin feeling soft.

Quick tip

Select three or four skin-friendly vegetables. Chop roughly, then drop in a blender with a cup of water and blend for a few minutes. You will end up with a thick, raw, vegetable soup. Drink one glassful a day.

Red flags

Photo-sensitivity. This presents as an urticarial rash after exposure to sunlight. Check prescription medicines.

Regular or easy bruising. Check to rule out more serious issues such as the liver and adrenal disorders.

Moles that change in size or colour, or itch or bleed. (? Melanoma) Refer for further investigations.

Spider naevi. Often harmless, and may occur in pregnancy, but need to be checked out to rule out liver disorders.

Red nodules on the skin which merge together to form a tender, solid plaque, very warm and blanching on pressure. Could be erythema nodosum, inflammation of the layer of fat underlying the skin. May be triggered by inflammatory bowel disease or preceding infection (i.e., sore throat).

Fever, neck stiffness, headache and severe debility with red or purplish spots or a rash that does not blanch on pressure. Meningococcal bacterial/meningitis or sepsis? Always refer.

Any unexplained raised lumps.

Anything that has become infected needs quick robust treatment, and referral if not responsive.

Always refer anything that you are not sure of. Conventional medicine can be good at helping you find a diagnosis—it is then up to you how you wish to treat it!

Conclusions

As with most things, skin disorders tend to be multi-factorial, and therefore respond well to complex interventions. An interesting study in 2016 using data from Taiwan's National Health Insurance Research Database linked the incidence of atopic dermatitis (AD) with the patient's birth month (mechanism remains unknown). People born between October–December apparently run a higher risk of developing AD.[6] Treating skin conditions with a herbal approach can be challenging, but it usually also intensely rewarding, and it is definitely a question of treating primarily from the inside out!

Part 2. Irritable bowel syndrome

Introduction

> **Definition—*What is IBS?*** Irritable bowel syndrome (IBS)! The name
> of this condition actually comes pretty close to describing what is
> going on. The bowel in question is specifically the large intestine or
> colon, and you can perhaps imagine what symptoms people are likely to
> experience when their large intestines are 'feeling grumpy'. The mod-
> ern scientific focus has increasingly come to rest upon disorder in the
> microbiome as a key causative factor—but what causes the disordered
> microbiome?

IBS is an example of what is termed a functional disorder. A functional
disorder is characterised as any condition which impairs the normal
functioning of the body, but for which no disease (pathology) can be
found on either clinical examination or via blood tests or other diagnostic
methods. Previously, the exclusion of any organic disease was sufficient
for considering IBS; however, a diagnosis of IBS, based on the exclusion
of organic pathology alone, is no longer valid according to current definitions. To diagnose a functional bowel disorder like IBS, symptoms need
to persist for more than 6 months—symptoms such as: alternating constipation, diarrhoea, abdominal pain and bowel irregularities.[7] IBS is an
example of a functional gastrointestinal disorder and it affects approximately 15% of people of the industrialised nations worldwide.[8]
    Symptoms of IBS may include:

- Abdominal pain and spasms, often relieved by defecation
- Diarrhoea, constipation or an alternation between the two
- Bloating, trapped wind or swelling of the abdomen
- Rumbling abdominal noises and excessive passage of wind
- The urgency to open bowels
- Incontinence (if a toilet is not nearby)
- Sharp pain or sensitivity inside the rectum
- The sensation of incomplete bowel movement
- Straining
- Mucous with stool
- Dyspepsia

As you can imagine, many of these symptoms may be embarrassing for people, or they are difficult to manage alongside work, other activities or home life. Some people additionally experience related symptoms such as lethargy, nausea, backache and bladder symptoms, and these may be used to support the diagnosis of IBS.

Because many of these symptoms can be found with other conditions and are non-specific, a set of criteria for specifically diagnosing IBS have been defined. These are called the Rome Criteria. On-going updates to the *Rome Criteria* document used for diagnosing IBS, involves an international collaboration of experts from many countries who communicate largely by phone and mail, until the final meeting which takes place in Rome, Italy.

The most recent update on the *Rome Criteria* took place in 2016, and is as follows:

> ### Note: Rome IV Criteria for diagnosing IBS. Recurrent abdominal pain, on average, at least 1 day/week in the last 3 months, associated with two or more of the following criteria:
>
> * Related to defecation
> * Associated with a change in frequency of stool
> * Associated with a change in form (appearance) of stool.
>
> Criteria fulfilled for the last 3 months with symptom onset at least 6 months before diagnosis.

IBS can be further categorised by sub-type. There are three main sub-types:

* IBS-C (predominant constipation)
* IBS-D (predominant diarrhoea)
* IBS-M (mixed bowel habits)

People whose symptoms do not fit into any category are considered to have:

IBS unclassified.

Rome IV has suggested redefining and de-stigmatising functional gastro-intestinal (GI) disorders as disorders of gut–brain interaction, emphasising the interrelationship between the GI tract and the nervous system.[9] Underlying the many symptoms experienced are the following issues:

1. Motility disturbances—the movement of food and waste through the GI tract is compromised.
2. Visceral hypersensitivity—there is a heightened experience of pain in the gastrointestinal tract. Viscera are the organs within the abdomen.
3. Changes in the gut's immune defences, which can result in altered mucosal and immune function. The whole digestive system is lined with mucosa—a mucous membrane.
4. Altered gut microbiota—changes in the community of bacteria in the gut.
5. Altered central nervous system processing—changes in how the brain sends and receives information to and from the gut.

The *Rome Criteria* are most useful as a set of definitions for researchers investigating treatments for IBS. In general practice, guidelines are given to medical personnel that relate to investigations and treatments that are recommended.

One very practical tool used is the Bristol Stool Form Scale—basically a poo chart—this can help people with the unenviable challenge of describing their poo shape and consistency. It can also measure how closely their stool resembles 'normal' or 'type 4' on the chart.

BRISTOL STOOL CHART		
Type 1	Separate hard lumps	Very constipated
Type 2	Lumpy and sausage like	Slightly constipated
Type 3	A sausage shape with cracks in the surface	Normal
Type 4	Like a smooth, soft sausage or snake	Normal
Type 5	Soft blobs with dear-cut edges	Lacking fibre
Type 6	Mushy consistency with ragged edges	Inflammation
Type 7	Liquid consistency with no solid pieces	Inflammation

What are the causes of IBS?

The understanding of how or why IBS develops is still very poorly understood, but a number of predisposing factors have been identified, including previous gut infection or acute gastroenteritis,[10] and antibiotic use.[11] There is acknowledgement of high levels of stress in childhood or self-reported childhood trauma (such as childhood abuse).[12]

Anxiety disorders and depression are common among IBS sufferers and many patients (although not all) will also report worsening of symptoms when they are stressed and/or anxious.

Conventional medical approach to treating IBS in adults

Firstly, it is important to exclude serious causes, and so persistent pain, bloating or change in bowel habit should be investigated. In order to eliminate more serious disease (and cancers), UK doctors are advised to consider doing blood tests such as full blood count, and also inflammation markers such as erythrocyte sedimentation rate (ESR), and C reactive protein (CRP). An antibody test for coeliac disease may also be checked. Faecal calprotectin is a reliable marker for the presence of more serious inflammatory bowel diseases.

Advice to GP's on how to help people manage IBS is evidence-based—or based on the evidence available—and includes the following:

- Have regular meals and take time to eat.
- Avoid missing meals or leaving long gaps between eating.
- Drink at least 8 cups of fluid per day, especially water or other non-caffeinated drinks, for example herbal teas.
- Restrict tea and coffee to 3 cups per day.
- Reduce intake of alcohol and fizzy drinks.
- It may be helpful to limit intake of high-fibre food (such as wholemeal or high-fibre flour and breads, cereals high in bran, and whole grains such as brown rice).
- Reduce intake of 'resistant starch' (starch that resists digestion in the small intestine and reaches the colon intact), which is often found in processed or re-cooked foods.

- Limit fresh fruit to three portions per day (a portion should be approximately 80 g).
- People with diarrhoea should avoid sorbitol, an artificial sweetener found in sugar-free sweets (including chewing gum) and drinks, and in some diabetic and slimming products.
- People with wind and bloating may find it helpful to eat oats (such as oat-based breakfast cereal or porridge) and linseeds (up to 1 tablespoon per day).

The National Institute of Health and Care Excellence UK (NICE) has updated its dietary suggestions to reflect our modern understanding of the benefits of soluble fibre (such as linseed and isphagula husk) as opposed to insoluble fibres such as wheat bran. They have also become more welcoming to the positive effects of probiotics, and encourage patients to continue them for at least 1 month.

Where patients have persistent symptoms, doctors may refer to a specialist in dietary advice and FODMAP exclusion diets. FODMAP is an acronym for Fermentable Oligosaccharides, Disaccharides, Monosaccharides and Polyols. A FODMAP diet is meant to be a diagnostic tool, identifying potential IBS-trigger foods, whilst re-introducing foods that do not trigger symptoms.

Where symptoms are severe or impact is sufficiently problematic—certain drugs can be prescribed:

- Drugs to reduce spasm such as mebeverine, and peppermint oil.
- Laxatives may be appropriate for some people—but not lactulose due to its likelihood to aggravate symptoms. A new laxative for chronic constipation—linaclotide has a role in longer-term cases—but caution should be taken as it can lead to dehydration, a simple thing with potentially serious consequences.
- Sometimes it is suggested to increased fibre intake to treat constipation or use fibre-based treatments such as fybogel or movicol.
- Anti-motility drugs such as loperamide (Imodium) can be recommended for diarrhoea.
- Antidepressants (tricyclic or selective serotonin reuptake inhibitors) may be prescribed but doctors are encouraged to review this regularly with a view to stopping when possible.

- *Psychologic therapies*: Cognitive behavioural therapy, standard psychotherapy and hypnotherapy can be recommended by doctors if drug therapy has not helped within 12 months.

Note the presence of peppermint oil in the recommended treatments for IBS.[13]

Peppermint oil is one of the few 'herbal' remedies that has managed to hang on in the conventional medical pharmacopoeia into the 21st century, a great achievement for a truly wonderful herb. Many scientific papers comment on how herbal medicines could be a great resource for helping sufferers of IBS.[14] Note, however, the use of the isolated essential oil is not at all the same as using the whole range of constituents found in the leaves and therefore is likely to be different to the experience of an infusion of the leaves of *Mentha x piperita* L.

Going back to Rome for a moment—*The Rome IV Criteria* has recognised the importance of an integrated approach to the treatment of IBS and functional GI disorders generally. This approach takes into consideration such things as early life influences, genetics, culture and environment. They say that stress levels, personality, psychological state, coping abilities and amount of social support available to the individual should all be considered, as well as physiological symptoms reported. Gut flora and diet are now recognised as important factors in the development of IBS.

Herbal approach to treating IBS

In the UK, guidelines from NICE have recommended that there should be more research into herbal medicines (Chinese, and other traditions) because 'reviews of herbal medicines suggest a positive effect on the control of IBS symptoms, but the evidence is limited and not sufficient to make recommendations'.

As with all other situations, treating the patient as an individual is key to the treatment of IBS. The *Rome IV Criteria* have come to reflect the broader-based approach to treatment taken by the herbalist when treating IBS. Strategies once only found within complementary medicine are now generally accepted by conventional medicine (such as clear guidance on dietary changes and the use of healing foods).

Herbs remain the mainstay of our treatments as they offer us so much in terms of stress management and enhancement of gut function, both of which are central to positive outcomes. But herbalists will also consider how patients work, rest and exercise, and often act as health-guides to patients who may not have considered the link between lack of exercise, stress and anxiety and their digestive symptoms. Herbalists are also aware of the interconnectedness between other systems in the body—and how the endocrine system, particularly for women, may impact on IBS. We may also recognise ideas from psychotherapeutic professions that 'the body keeps score'[18]—and how life experiences may have lasting impacts for some people. These people can 'manage' their symptoms with drugs, or perhaps instead with a reliable herbal regimen—or both!

With a natural inclination to study healing plants in depth, herbalists view plant based foods as potential medicine (more of this later!). The use of soluble fibre comes precisely from the herbal tradition, and is not limited to isphagula husk and linseed, but may also include healing demulcent plants such as slippery elm bark—*Ulmus fulva* L. (taken as a powder dissolved in water), or mucilage-rich herbs such as marshmallow, chamomile and lime blossom.

Oat milk and slippery elm bedtime drink

Add 1 teaspoon of slippery elm powder to a cup of warm oat (or other milk substitute) milk and stir in well. Add half a teaspoon of blackstrap molasses, stir well. This is ideal as a nourishing drink for the elderly, or underweight, undernourished individuals. Add a few teaspoonfuls of chamomile tea if desired. Making your own oat, seed or nut milk is really easy and contains no artificial ingredients.

The flexibility of the personalised herbal prescription allows us to treat for the differing symptom pictures that IBS presents with. The complex compounds found within every single plant means that great relief can come from the humblest of sources. Even the use of the gentle aperient and anti-inflammatory root of the dandelion (*Taraxacum officinale* aggr F. H. Wigg) has other side-benefits such as aiding micro-biome diversity.[15] Many medicinal herbs will act as prebiotics due to their diverse compounds and the need for plants to maintain their own microbiome.

Any useful research into the herbalists' approach when treating IBS will need to take in to account this patient-centred prescribing. Key considerations when treating IBS within a herbal framework include:

- Nervous system relaxants and tonics.
- Herbs to support the organs of the digestive tract.
- Mucosal anti-infective and anti-inflammatory herbs.
- Digestive antispasmodic herbs.
- Herbs to strengthen and heal damaged mucous membranes (vulneraries).
- Herbs to restore the function of the digestive cascade.
- Herbs and other foods to encourage microbiome diversity.
- Herbal management of related health problems that may negatively impact on a person with IBS, such as recurrent infection, anxiety or hormone imbalance.

One concept which has attracted considerable attention over the years is that of the 'leaky gut syndrome'. In this scenario, damage to the mucous membranes of the gut, and their underlying cell walls, results in poorly digested substances being absorbed into the bloodstream. Auto-immune and allergic mechanisms may be triggered, and gut wall function becomes impaired. This scenario is believed by many to form part of the IBS picture. GAPS, short for Gut And Psychology Syndrome is a school of thought proposing that imbalances in gut microflora result in damage to an unprotected gut wall, ultimately resulting in both physical and emotional ill-health.[16]

The traditional herbal perspective on the development of illness tends to be holistic rather than linear. Therefore, rather than asking the question 'what caused this?' it is more realistic to ask, 'what combination of factors came together at this time to cause this?'

Lets now look at a few of the lovely herbs, and how they can help.

The lovely herbs

Bring on the herbal cavalry!

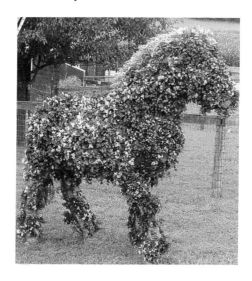

Sedative and nervine tonics herbs

Good old stress and anxiety are strongly represented as underpinning factors in both initiation and exacerbation of the symptom picture. Herbs to choose from here might include (among too many to mention here): Scullcap herb (*Scutellaria lateriflora* L.), valerian root (*Valeriana officinalis* L.) and St John's wort herb (*Hypericum perforatum* L.) which performs better than placebo and has effects on the digestive and nervous system.[14]

Hepatorestorative and choleretic herbs

Liver and gall bladder support will help ease constipation and optimise digestive function. Perhaps choose from: St Mary's thistle (Silybum marianum (L) Gaertn), artichoke (*Cynara cardunculus* L. synonym scolymus)[14] and dandelion root (*Taraxacum officinale* aggr. F. H. Wigg.).

GI tract antiseptic herbs

Where there is a history of serious GI tract infection, which preceded the onset of symptoms, the addition of a few good anti-infective herbs with specific application to the gut may be helpful. Even though the initial episode is historical rather than current, treating for it can often enhance outcome. Consider: Garden thyme (*Thymus vulgare* L.) oregano (*Origanum vulgare* L.), angelica, (*Angelica archangelica* L.), walnut leaf (*Juglans regia* L.) and garlic (*Allium sativum* L.). Gastro-intestinal antiseptics will also help to restore normal bowel flora, and improve the integrity of the gut wall.

> **Note:** With respect to all of the herbs suggested above and below, the use of tinctures, teas, decoctions, etc will of course depend upon the circumstances of the individual. Generally speaking the carminative herbs work well as tinctures and also lend themselves very well to teas in terms of their beautiful flavours. Situations where a degree of inflammation is present will also respond well to a tea, and mucilaginous herbs such as marshmallow are particularly good here as the herb is coming into direct contact with the gut wall. Using both tea and tincture is a good strategy, and offers maximum flexibility.

Mucilage-containing herbs

Slippery elm powder (*Ulmus americana* L. syn. fulva), if there is constipation or diarrhoea. Marshmallow root (*Althaea officinalis* L.) or common mallow (*Malva sylvestris* L.) is kind and gentle to inflamed mucous membranes. Strong chamomile tea is soft and syrupy. Plantain (*Plantago lanceolata or P. major* L.) has a soothing effect on mucous membranes of the gut. Mucilagenous herbs will be helpful in encouraging beneficial gut flora.

Spasmolytic herbs

Relaxation of the gut wall, and the relief of intestinal spasm are usually necessary. Herbs would include any of the aromatic herbs listed below, and also perhaps lavender (*Lavandula angustifolia* Mill.), wild yam (*Dioscorea villosa* L.), catnip (*Nepeta cataria* L.) and valerian root (*Valeriana officinalis* L.).

Carminative prebiotic herbs

Peppermint (*Mentha x piperita* L.), aniseed (*Pimpinella anisum* L.), caraway (*Carum carvi* L.) and fennel (*Foeniculum vulgare* Mill.) are all useful herbs for relieving trapped wind and bloating and settling an upset stomach. Peppermint (*Mentha x piperita* L.) and ginger (*Zingiber officinale* Roscoe) may be beneficial via modification of the perception of visceral organ pain.

Where mucous is part of the symptomatic picture, irritation is most likely to be present. Soothing mucilaginous herbs would be great here, along with gastro-intestinal anti-inflammatories such as meadowsweet (*Filipendula ulmaria* (L) Maxim.) and agrimony (*Agrimonia eupatoria* L.).

Treat constipation gently; with herbs such as yellow dock root (Rumex crispus L.) and dandelion root (*Taraxacum officinale* aggr. F.H Wigg) because they are not strictly speaking laxatives, and are not habit-forming. The seeds and husks of plantain (*Plantago lanceolata or major*) may be used in a similar way to psyllium seeds (*Plantago ovata* Forssk.), ground in a coffee grinder or used whole. Sprinkle on food between once and three times daily. Psyllium seeds can be used dissolved in water (stir and leave for 2–5 minutes, stir again and drink daily before breakfast). They taste clean and fresh, and contribute greatly to bowel health and to the microbiome.[14]

Migraine, and pre-menstrual syndrome are often associated with IBS and it is most important to treat women exhibiting this triad with a hormone-modifying approach and with the guidance of a medical herbalist.

Domestic medicine

So, what can be done about this? We will talk more about diet momentarily, but first, let's look at a few simple home remedies. From the 15 herbs we cover in-depth in this book, the following would be ideal for anyone with IBS symptoms: chamomile, fennel, lemon balm, meadowsweet, marigold, lavender, marshmallow, thyme and dandelion roots.

It is possible to make herbal teas taste great but also be effective—

Minty meditation tea

Combine equal parts of dried or fresh peppermint, spearmint, meadowsweet, and chamomile. Make an infusion by pouring boiling water over 1–2 teaspoons of the herbs, cover to trap the aromatic oils, and leave to infuse for 5–7 minutes. Strain and drink 1–3 cups daily. Ideal if digestive symptoms are 'over-active'.

Marshmallow soother tea

Combine equal parts of marshmallow root, chamomile flowers, fennel seeds and lemon balm. Make an infusion by pouring boiling water over 1–2 teaspoons of dried herbs, cover, and leave to infuse for 5–7 minutes. Strain and drink 1–3 cups daily. Ideal if digestive symptoms are 'sore, raw, or under-active'.

If you are new to herb teas, or are having difficulty persuading children to drink a herbal infusion, you can begin by adding a little herb syrup to sweeten the tea. Over time, most people (children included) will adapt to herb teas without sweetening—but here are two fantastic and useful herb syrups you can make at home to sweeten your IBS tea!

Ribwort syrup

Many people with a garden will have ribwort plantain, or broad-leaved plantain growing in their lawn. Juiced plantain leaves *Plantago lanceolata* L. *or Plantago major* L. can be added to an equal quantity of

Rosebay willowherb syrup

This recipe is taken from Julia and Mathew Bruton-Seals excellent book *Hedgerow Medicine*.[17]

- 20 rosebay willowherb flower-heads
- 500 ml water
- 100 g sugar
- The juice of one lemon

Place flowers and water in a saucepan. Bring to boil and simmer until colour leaves the flowers (5–10 minutes). Then strain.

Return fluid to a pot and add 100 g sugar plus the juice of the lemon.

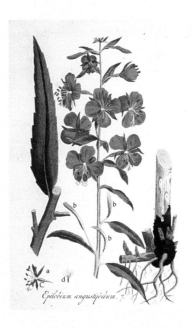

Epilobium angustifolium.

> The liquid will turn bright pink.
> Boil for 5 minutes. Cool. Bottle and label.
> This will keep in the fridge for a few months.
> Dose = I tablespoonful every few hours as needed.

honey and mixed together. Pour into sterilised bottles and store in a refrigerator. Take up to 1 teaspoon of this soothing mix three times daily to help counteract inflammation, or use to sweeten a herbal infusion. Ribwort juice without sugar is also available from herbal suppliers.

Rosebay willowherb leaves are astringent, and in Russia a tea called kapoori is made from them. This tea is also a traditional remedy to take for diarrhoea.

Roasted dandelion root

Perhaps you are a coffee addict? Although coffee has antioxidant properties, it is also very stimulating and even decaffeinated coffee contains acids that can aggravate IBS. A delicious alternative to coffee can be made from roasting dandelion roots and then making into a dark, dense bitter-sweet drink in a cafetière, saucepan or coffee maker—you can even add milk, or a milk substitute, adding perhaps a cardamom pod whilst it brews for extra aromatic antispasmodic effect.

Dig up (lots of) carefully identified dandelion roots before spring and before flowering begins (usually in April in the Northern Hemisphere). Wash them clear of mud using water and a soft brush and slice or cube as small as you can with a knife. Spread out onto a clean tea towel, and dry out in a very low oven or dehydrator until really dry, and then roast the dandelion root for 25–30 minutes on 180°C, 350°F, Gas 4. The roots will become dark brown and will grind in an electric coffee grinder. Use 1–3 teaspoons of the roasted root to make a cup of roasted dandelion root drink—you may prefer to cook it in water in a saucepan for the fullest flavour, or keep it warm whilst it brews in a Cafetière.

Electuary

The aromatic herb powders combined in honey, molasses or tamarind to make the digestive electuary given in Chapter 4 would be great for anyone with wind, bloating or constipation. It is also delicious and nourishing.

Massage oil

Make an infused oil using lavender flowers and a gorgeous cold-pressed oil—sesame, coconut, or sunflower for example. Follow our recipe for an infused oil in Chapter 6. Infused oils can be used to massage the feet before bed, or gentle massage of the abdominal and pelvic area can help relieve spasms and help with constipation. This can be helpful for children as well as adults, and is also useful before or after taking an aeroplane flight—a time when some people can become constipated. Massage in a clockwise direction, following the anatomical direction of the large intestine.

Breathing space

Stress and anxiety can play a major role in the aetiology of this ubiquitous condition. Any techniques that can be incorporated into life to reduce stress and anxiety should be not just considered, but prioritised. Making time to talk through worries and problems, a walk in the country, time to meditate, and spending some time with friends or in peace, quiet and rest can be an invaluable adjunct to treatment. It is often getting people to realise the true importance of these things that is the most difficult task.

Diet

It is not uncommon to meet people suffering from IBS who have significantly restricted their diets to exclude 'problem foods', in an attempt to minimise the symptoms that they are suffering from. For some, this may prove sufficient, and their symptoms may disappear. The food in question really was the only factor causing distress. For many others though, this may only represent a short-term strategy, and over time more and more 'problem foods' are eliminated, until dietary restrictions start to present problems in everyday life.

A restricted diet will also place the health of the micro-biome at risk as variety in the diet serves to optimise a good, broad cross-section of gut flora. *Rome Criteria IV* is a comprehensive document and several new chapters have been added, including one called 'Intestinal Micro-environment and the Functional GI Disorders'. This chapter presents the latest research about the role of the microbiome, food, and nutrition in GI function. This recent inclusion represents a step forward in thinking on a broader level in terms of conventional medical recommendations.

During the initial stages of treatment for IBS it is probably advisable to avoid some of the more pro-inflammatory foods, such as gluten and dairy products, until the gut is stronger. This is when a FODMAP diet may be of use, to identify triggers in the early stages. Cooked foods, especially cooked vegetables are often easier for a compromised digestive system to deal with, so keep raw foods to a minimum in the first instance. Fruit is often easier to digest if cooked. That is after all what baby foods are aiming to do, to gradually prepare the digestive system through a process of weaning. Simple proteins such as cooked eggs, fish or cooked silken tofu, or nut 'butters' (these are finely ground nuts and do not contain butter) may be easier to handle.

It may be a bit ambitious to advise people to launch themselves straight into a fermented food diet, but the gradual introduction of prebiotic herbs and teas will at least begin to gently address the issue. In fact, if dairy products are to be consumed, then fermented dairy products such as yoghurt or kefir are an ideal place to start. People may also find that milk from goats or ewes is easier to tolerate than milk from cows. As symptoms improve there may then be room to steer the diet in a good prebiotic direction. There are plenty of suggestions for this in Chapter 5.

Ultimately, a person would gradually but persistently expand their diet back out to as diverse as it can be, following any sort of exclusion diet. Re-introducing raw foods—especially for the summer months—can be done by starting perhaps with grated raw vegetables left at room temperature (see our slaw recipe from Chapter 5, p. 187), or by adding small spoonfuls of fresh herb chutney (see Chapter 5, p. 186) or lacto-fermented vegetables such as beetroots or cabbage.

Re-connecting with 'wild' foods foraged from healthy wild places near you is also a goal to consider … have you ever tried eating wild garlic, sea beet leaves or nettles!? Once you have correctly identified wild garlic, also known as ramsoms (*Allium ursinum* L.) harvest only a few leaves from each plant, trying to leave other nearby plants healthy and untouched.

Just a few leaves will be ample for making a wild pesto, or they can be sprinkled as a condiment to salads, or cooked into soup or stew.

Ramsons pesto

Place ramson leaves in a blender, (you can add some fresh parsley to reduce the hot garlic taste of the ramsoms a little).

Add enough olive oil to cover them.

Blend until smooth.

Blend now with pine nuts or walnuts and/or some freshly grated parmesan, pecorino or other hard cheese as preferred.

Ramsons sauce

Use I part cider vinegar or white wine vinegar to 3 parts olive oil to cover the ramson leaves before blending. The vinegar will help preserve the ramsons, and the jar will keep in the fridge for many months.

Add a taste of the wild, and a reminder of the gloriousness of the month of May to your pasta or pizza dishes, or pour over vegetable and rice dishes with your lovely ramsoms pesto or ramsoms sauce!

Red flags

The following red flag symptoms are related to gut health generally.
    Seek medical attention for the following:

- Any severe, acute or sudden pain, especially if it prevents a person from being able to walk or sit. May indicate appendicitis.
- Any pain, accompanied by an unexplained swelling or mass, or colic like symptoms and vomiting/constipation, and/or obvious abdominal distension. May indicate hernia or bowel obstruction
- Any yellowing or strange skin colouration. May indicate jaundice or liver damage.
- Prolonged diarrhoea and/or vomiting (24 hours or more) especially in older people or children. May indicate infection.
- Severe, progressive diarrhoea accompanied by nausea or vomiting, bleeding or mucous in stool fever and/or cramps. May indicate inflammatory bowel disease.

Consult your doctor if you notice

- Recent changes in bowel habits. Check to eliminate the possibility of a tumour. Remember tumours can be benign, or more malignant—so it is better to get checked sooner rather than later.
- Coffee grounds vomit (vomit which looks like coffee grounds may be due to blood in the vomit from further down the GI tract).
- Appetite loss, long-lasting, with weight loss or unexplained weight loss.
- Difficulty swallowing.
- Mouth ulcers which do not heal after 2–3 weeks.
- Sudden or unexplained weight gain.
- Any bleeding symptoms-fresh blood, or old darker blood.

Conclusion

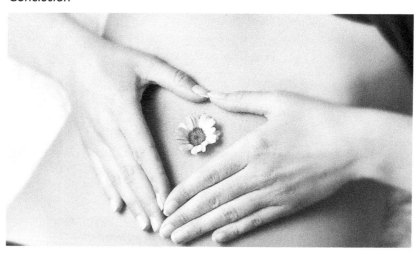

The gastrointestinal tract is at the anatomical core of our being. Our bodies surround and enclose it, allowing us to carry the outside world inside us as we slowly digest, process and absorb it. It's a big and complex task, and it is not difficult to understand how the nature of our interactions with the world on a psychological level can directly affect our dealings with it on the physical one. All of our major homeostatic players are represented here: the nervous system, the immune system, the endocrine system, they all have overwhelmingly significant impacts upon gut health, and likewise, gut health can significantly impact them.

Then we have what is to the scientific community relatively recent *terra nova* to consider: the new and exciting world of the gut microbiome, which in terms of individual microbe cells outnumbers our human cells at least 3:1. The boundaries of self and non-self begin to dissolve. This knowledge then logically permeates out to the microbiome of our immediate environment and the environment from which our food is grown and harvested. It is perhaps why so many people who are interested in plant medicine intuitively feel a deep kinship with the environment and our need to respect and care for it. We emerge from that environment.

IBS has been characterised as a functional disorder as it represents the widespread and subtle shifts in the dynamics of the complexity of our being. In many cases support needs to be as encompassing as possible, and inclusive of the acknowledgement of the impact of stress and anxiety both current and historical. Referral of patients for other strategies such as counselling, cognitive behavioural therapy or hypnotherapy may also be useful to explore more deep-seated emotional issues. Our guts really do have feelings. Sometimes they can express our inner turmoil in a distressingly forthright manner. As with so many things love and understanding (and herbs) will help to win the day.

Bibliography

Buhner, Stephen Harrod, *Sacred and Herbal Healing Beers*. 1998: Brewers Publications.

Corrigan, Desmond, *Indian Medicine for the Immune System: Echinacea*. 1994: Amberwood Publishing.

Greive, M., *A Modern Herbal*. 1st ed. 1931: Penguin.

Griggs, Barbara, *The Home Herbal. A Handful of Simple Remedies*. 1986: Robert Hale Ltd.

Menzies-Trull, C., *Herbal Medicine: Keys to physiomedicalism including pharmacopoeia*, 1st edition, 2003: Physiomedical Herbal Medicine.

Mills, Simon, *Vitex Agnus-Castus: Woman Medicine*. 1992: Amberwood Publishing.

References

1. Adamska-Patruno, E. et al., *The relationship between the leptin/ghrelin ratio and meals with various macronutrient contents in men with different nutritional status: a randomized crossover study*. Nutr J, 2018. 17(1): p. 118.

2. Bell, D. C. and S. J. Brown, *Atopic eczema treatment now and in the future: Targeting the skin barrier and key immune mechanisms in human skin.* World J Dermatol., 2017. 6: pp. 42–51, doi: 10.5314/wjd.v6.i3.42.
3. Pal, H. C. et al., *Phytochemicals for the management of melanoma.* Mini Rev Med Chem, 2016. 16(12): pp. 953–979.
4. Grice, E. A. and J. A. Segre, *The skin microbiome.* Nat Rev Microbiol, 2011. 9(4): pp. 244–253.
5. Culpepper, N., *The British Herbal and Family Physician.* 1816: Halifax.
6. Kuo, C. L. et al., *Birth month and risk of atopic dermatitis: a nationwide population-based study.* Allergy, 2016. 71(11): pp. 1626–1631.
7. Camilleri, M., *Irritable bowel syndrome: how useful is the term and the 'diagnosis'?* Therap Adv Gastroenterol, 2012. 5(6): pp. 381–386.
8. Lovell, R. M. and A. C. Ford, *Global prevalence of and risk factors for irritable bowel syndrome: a meta-analysis.* Clin Gastroenterol Hepatol, 2012. 10(7): pp. 712–721.e4.
9. Team, E., *ROME IV Diagnostic Criteria for IBS.* 2016.
10. Thabane, M., D. T. Kottachchi and J. K. Marshall, *Systematic review and meta-analysis: The incidence and prognosis of post-infectious irritable bowel syndrome.* Aliment Pharmacol Ther, 2007. 26(4): pp. 535–544.
11. Villarreal, A. A. et al., *Use of broad-spectrum antibiotics and the development of irritable bowel syndrome.* WMJ, 2012. 111(1): pp. 17–20.
12. Talley, N. J. et al., *Gastrointestinal tract symptoms and self-reported abuse: a population-based study.* Gastroenterology, 1994. 107(4): pp. 1040–1049.
13. Khanna, R., J. K. MacDonald and B. G. Levesque, *Peppermint oil for the treatment of irritable bowel syndrome: a systematic review and meta-analysis.* J Clin Gastroenterol, 2014. 48(6): pp. 505–512.
14. Rahimi, R. and M. Abdollahi, *Herbal medicines for the management of irritable bowel syndrome: a comprehensive review.* World J Gastroenterol, 2012. 18(7): pp. 589–600.
15. Trojanová, I. et al., *The bifidogenic effect of Taraxacum officinale root.* Fitoterapia, 2004. Volume 75(7–8): pp. 760–763.
16. Lashkov, B. D., *Gaps Guide: Simple Steps to Heal Bowels, Body and Brain.* 2013: Medinform Publishing.
17. Bruton-Seal, J., *Hedgerow Medicine: Harvest and Make your own Herbal Remedies.* 2009: Merlin Unwin Books Ltd.
18. Van Der Kolk, B. A., *The Body Keeps the Score: Brain, Mind, and Body in the Healing of Trauma,* 2014: Viking.

CHAPTER TWELVE

Conclusions: the counter-current revisited

Introduction

Western herbal medicine has its own unique history, context and approach to health and disease. We herbalists who practice from this British—European—American tradition have an eclectic and global heritage. Our roots stretch back to way before the written word, but are deeply infused with ideas and wisdom from the ancient Greco-Roman world, from the Arabic scholars of the early Middle Ages, into the monastic traditions and also the first universities of Europe. Then, uniquely this was all re-enthused with knowledge from the First Nations peoples of the Americas, and a clear divergence from conventional medicine became much more obvious. Many of these herbalists and osteopath-herbalists of the 19th and early 20th centuries evolved their practices as a result of a strongly felt antithesis to conventional medical practices of the time, that were considered to be too barbaric. It is this impulse to reconnect with a healing plant tradition that continues in the herbalists of today, and it is reflected in their slightly different take on anatomy, physiology and pharmacology even now in the 21st century.

Evolution and energetics

The evolution of Western herbal medicine owes a debt of gratitude to many ethnobotanical threads. We mentioned in our introduction the Greco-Roman world, from which we have inherited the basis of the system of humoural medicine. Even today this method of experiencing plants as hot or cold, moist or dry, and of using them accordingly to suit particular constitutions and pathologies still represents a valuable system used by many to optimise a person-centred approach. It is no coincidence that a more energetic approach to health care has been effectively practised the world over for many centuries. There are many reasons why systems such as this have been discredited by conventional medicine, but some of the bigger ones include:

- A basic lack of understanding of the language and terminology used by traditional systems of medicine.
- A total focus on the concept of 'evidence-based medicine' to the point where centuries of empirical evidence have been ignored.
- A devaluation of the data provided by our senses (pharmacognosy).
- An over-emphasis on a reductionist mono-chemical 'magic-bullet' approach.

Modern-day Western herbalists strive to combine the best of all worlds, acknowledging and working with the fantastic advances that the current scientific paradigm has engendered, whilst nurturing and benefitting from a more traditional and sensorial approach to plant-based medicines, which fits well with the nature of them as living entities. The practice of our healing art is informed and strengthened by the diversity of its history. This allows a comprehensive person-centred approach to living and flourishing.

Person-centred medicine

Western herbalists study modern conventional sciences but take a unique approach to the interpretation of health and disease. Herbal medicines are applied to the person, and not as plant-derived versions of drugs. This has resulted in the evolution of a very distinct rationale behind the application of medicinal plants by Western herbalists.[1] A person-centred approach is not just a platitude. It is an acknowledgement that our thoughts, experiences and lived lives contribute to the emergence of our physical body. Our behaviours often represent survival techniques, good or bad and represent our internal stresses manifested. Whilst we can accept the interesting and exciting developments in genetics, for example, we cannot view those developments in isolation: that is to say without taking into account the dynamic interplay that exists between our genetics and our environment. Homeostatic mechanisms in our bodies are designed to nurture and protect our genetic material so that it may function optimally for us. The wider environment in which we live, love and breathe however, impacts on that function in ways that we are still trying to understand. Our co-evolution with the plants that grow in the environment in which we live, provides us with healing gifts that are well suited to our needs as the products of that environment.

Plants and people

Co-evolution of plants and people has been demonstrated in many areas of medicine and pharmacology. Animals share a common ancestry with enzymes and proteins from plants that have led to an evolutionary kinship and allows for a helpful modulation of human enzyme function by medicinal plant use. In addition several important hormonal, and immune-regulatory compounds found in humans have a common ancestor with proteins found originally in rhizobia.

Rhizobia—bacteria that have co-evolved in the root nodules of certain plants and have formed a symbiotic relationship with them; the rhizobia provide the plant with nitrogen, the plant provides the rhizobia with food.

Structural similarities between compounds from key medicinal plants and human steroid hormones, provides another perspective on the hormone-like activity of these plant-derived compounds in humans. Pharmacologists consider today, that our protective cytochromes (intracellular enzyme pathways responsible for processing and making safe the many chemicals that we ingest) have co-evolved so closely with our consumption of plant foods and plant medicines across the millennia, that these human cytochromes have altered genetically to accept them.[2]

It is no wonder that most herbalists would agree they have a deep interest in ecology—an early example of systems theory evolved now into the use of mathematics and physics to study complexity in biology. Many modern practitioners of herbal medicine have found parallels from modern physics with the way herbalists try to manage the complexity of patient and plants.

> You carry Mother Earth within you. She is not outside of you.
>   Mother Earth is not just your environment.
>   In that insight of inter-being, it is possible to have real communication
> with the Earth, which is the highest form of prayer.

—Thich Nhat Hahn

Plant complexity and synergy

Care must be taken, to not ignore synergy in the plant world and how that interacts with our human physiology. It is certainly interesting to discover that certain distinct phytochemicals exert their actions via very specific pre-existing biological pathways in our bodies, and that the results can be measured in vivo. This however is far from the whole story. We increasingly come across statements in research on plant medicines emphasising the importance of synergistic interactions between phytochemical compounds, and how they are responsible for the enhanced benefits found from using whole plant remedies as opposed to individual active constituents. Being mindful of the biochemical dance that flows ever onwards within plants, and how that dance is emphasised once the whole plant is introduced into a living being is crucial to a true understanding of the complexity of plant medicines. To be either unaware of or to ignore this crucial aspect is to fail to establish the true nature of how plants work within us to exert their effects. Research findings are sometimes supportive of the traditional use of a certain herbal medicine, or occasionally they suggest a potentially negative effect from a plant traditionally considered safe. It is often the case that the latter situation results from a failure to consider the dynamic interplay of synergistic interactions that occur in whole plants when they interface with the human body.

Also, research often does not compare like with like. For example, comparisons between the salicylates found originally in spirea (*Filipendula ulmaria* L.) and those manufactured in aspirin (acetyl-salicylic acid) do not match up. Aspirin is a synthetic derivative of salicylic acid, there-fore a) you are not comparing like with like, and b) you are not allowing for pharmacokinetic and pharmacodynamic synergy. It is not scientifi-cally accurate to extrapolate the results of research on isolated com-pounds to explain mechanisms or action of medicinal plants; although of interest, this approach will only ever provide a fragmented picture. Other examples such as phyto-oestrogens and how our understanding of their true function in humans has changed, further demonstrate how plant compounds are so much more than their synthetic counterparts.

Furthermore, we would like to point out that many of these studies are carried out on animal models other than human. The nature of this research is not only abhorrent to most sentient, intelligent people, but is dubious scientifically and not justifiable. Whatever we may learn from research into the individual chemical constituents of plants, it is our interaction with them as wholes that results in an optimal experience of the phenomenon of our healing.

The pan-optimisation of physiological systems achieved by tonic herbs involves a massive amount of complexity. Plant medicine is not about individual active constituents. Nor is it simply about lin-ear relationships, about cause and effect. The multiplicity of support-ive mechanisms of action found in a good *tonic* herb depend upon the presence of the many different families of phytochemicals in the whole plant, and how they interact with, and modify each other and us.

The herbal approach

Using some of the most commonly experienced medical conditions, we have described in a practical way how the medical herbalists' approach is unique. Using case histories we have demonstrated how plants are often given in combination to achieve more than would be possible using single plants (or even single compounds from plants). Our intention has been to demonstrate how complexity in the plant world fits like a glove with the complexity of our human physiology.

We hope you have found our introduction to anatomy and physi-ology has contributed to seeing ourselves as a whole. Interconnected-ness is evident throughout our body. Our complex interactions with plants range from the most straightforward mechanisms, involving them using up our carbon-dioxide and providing us with oxygen, to the most complex, where they interact with a human digestive tract. We normally study anatomy and physiology in the West by way of discrete and well-delineated physiological systems because this is easy and convenient for us. This makes it too easy for us though to fall into the trap of thinking that the body actually works like that. Indeed conventional medicine has organised its hospitals and clinics around this very premise. The reality of course is quite different, and so is the experience of people going through those hospitals and clinics.

Every system in our body works in close collaboration with every other system, and it is hard to think of an illness that does not impact on all systems in one way or another, directly or indirectly. The interrelationships between the immune system, the nervous system and the endocrine system are an excellent example of this web of interrelationships. Herbs are ideally suited to that interconnectedness, containing an array of beneficial compounds with side-benefits. It is also here that we have the real gift of traditionally recognised tonic herbs. Tonic herbs gift us with that unique capacity of many herbal medicines to improve the vitality and integrity of cells, tissues, organs and systems, that is so helpful to people and their experience of wellbeing.

The concept that health is inherently less energy-consuming than disorder, is not a new one. If we are to thrive and not just exist, then we need to be free to function, to be free-flowing to allow optimisation of energy use. Plant medicines seem to encourage free-flow of function that can be seen when complexity models are applied to biological sciences. We are part of the natural world, as are plants. It is no surprise that certain plants may optimise our systems. Working with herbs in this manner, allows us freedom in our approach to treatment and gives us the plasticity of practice to deal effectively with the unpredictable. This has been our experience of herbal practice. Herbal medicine allows us to practice within the framework of universal themes and truths: as the lovely author Sharman Apt Russell describes this—the physics of beauty.[3]

The magic of how we learned about plants

Plants can be (and historically have been) studied by observational, sensorial and contemplative techniques. Our intention has been to demonstrate that modern medical herbalists seek to maintain their deeply acquired familiarity with each plant across all sectors of knowledge. They attempt to hear their patient as a whole unique being *and* find the best 'fit' with various plant allies. This requires a deeper relationship with medicinal plants as whole living beings.

The experience of each plant may differ from place to place, so that plants growing in the area you live, may be as appropriate or even more appropriate than those recognised internationally as having reliable healing properties. There is also recognition that certain plants may be more appropriate for a given climate or season. There is therefore a fundamental need to care for the environment from which those plants came.

Looking at the 15 herbs we have presented here in detail allows us to consider their complexity and their enormous usefulness and crossovers between botanically related and unrelated medicinal plants. We inevitably strayed into pharmacological research in these chapters. We have considered how modern developments in medicine and the biological sciences compares to the traditional use of plants intuited and developed into a system of medicine long before technologies later were able to '*prove*' this. Without pharmacological research herbal medicine is in a vulnerable position regarding its so-called evidence base. Somehow we need to speak to all people and all those with a role in the continuance of herbal practice. Many people do not find an answer to their problems using a conventional medical approach alone. It is our responsibility as practitioners to help plant medicine remain available to such people and to show how the professionally considered use of herbal medicines is not only rational but reliable.

Kitchen pharmacy

We hope you have enjoyed the recipes and sections on domestic medicine and kitchen pharmacy. Herbal medicine operates in a grey area that is not quite just food nor is it 'herbal' drugs. Foods from plants are also seen as having some medicinal benefit nevertheless and can be employed as part of a healing strategy. Herbal medicine throughout history has been partly practised in the home, often by women, and this perhaps is one reason why it remains less-valued by some people today (things falling under the purview of domestic skills being very often undervalued in the Western world). As our environment changes around us, we are not always experiencing the plant compounds or environmental probiotic organisms our ancestors did. Nutrition and dietary advice from herbalists is not based on the latest fad, but has been pretty constant through modern history and certainly in our experience as practitioners over the last 30 years. The value of living vitality in some foods, the return to whole foods along with personalised advice based on all sorts of factors including constitution, is a central theme of herbalism. The only thing that has changed is that more recent research underpinning the vital role of the gut microbiome in our general health has served to verify that unchanging message.

The future of herbal medicine practitioners

As a profession, we need help concerning the development of better research, with methods that apply to our sector and our more complex and dynamic forms of intervention. We also need different legislative rules for both herbal medicines, and the practice of herbal medicine, in recognition of its relative safety and complexity. Human and *humane* research, and patient-centred research needs to be explored to help inform any on-going living system of herbal medicine.

As a society what kind of health service would we thrive in? One that has all that science and technology has to offer, but also does not deny our need for nature as the animals that we are? A health service that can access and connect people with natural foods and natural plant medicine experts when conventional solutions are not available or are too heavy-handed? One of the commonest questions from our patients is why were they not advised to see a medical herbalist by their doctor?

Relying solely on mono-chemicals for our medicine is a mono-culture and a monopoly. We have observed how damaging this is to ecosystems in the natural world. There is still time to welcome back in the wild bramble and use our capacity for complexity to embrace multiple ways of healing.

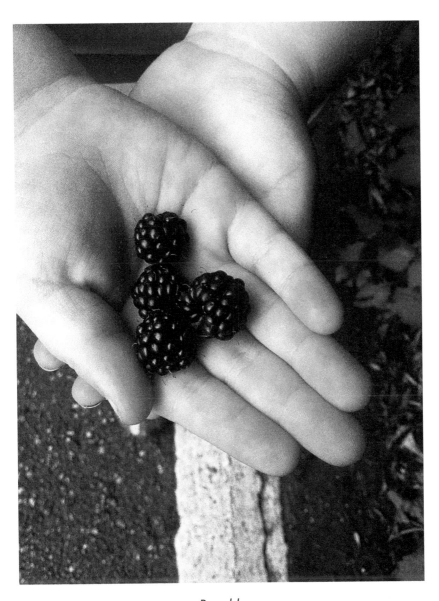

Bramble

References

1. Little, C. V., *Simply because it works better: exploring motives for the use of medical herbalism in contemporary U.K. health care.* Complement Ther Med., 2009. 17(5–6): pp. 300–308.
2. Rahimi, R. and M. Abdollahi, *Herbal medicines for the management of irritable bowel syndrome: a comprehensive review.* World J Gastroenterol, 2012. 18(7): pp. 589–600.
3. Apt Russell, S., *Anatomy of a Rose: Exploring the Secret Life of Flowers.* 2009: Basic Books.

GENERAL INDEX

587

RECIPE INDEX (RECEIPT BOOK)

CASE HISTORY INDEX